Gut Microbiota and their Impact on Disease Pathways and Interventions

Edited by

Sandipan Dasgupta
Department of Pharmaceutical Technology
Maulana Abul Kalam Azad University of Technology W.B.
Haringhata
Nadia-741249, West Bengal, India

&

Moitreyee Chattopadhyay
Department of Pharmaceutical Technology
Maulana Abul Kalam Azad University of Technology W.B.
Haringhata
Nadia-741249, West Bengal, India

Gut Microbiota and their Impact on Disease Pathways and Interventions

Editors: Sandipan Dasgupta, Moitreyee Chattopadhyay

ISBN (Online): 978-981-5324-54-9

ISBN (Print): 978-981-5324-55-6

ISBN (Paperback): 978-981-5324-56-3

First published in 2025.

Bentham Science Publishers Pte. Ltd.
80 Robinson Road #02-00
Singapore 068898
Singapore
Email: subscriptions@benthamscience.net

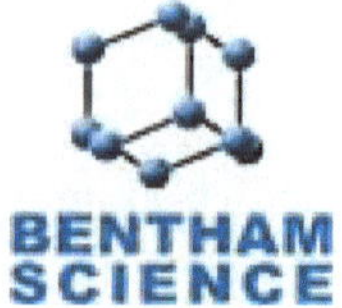

CONTENTS

FOREWORD

Embark on an illuminating exploration into the intricate universe thriving within us: the realm of gut microbiota. This comprehensive book unravels the profound interplay between these microscopic inhabitants and human health, unveiling their pivotal roles in various physiological processes and disease states.

The human gut hosts a vibrant ecosystem, populated by trillions of microorganisms encompassing bacteria, viruses, fungi, and archaea. Collectively, they constitute the gut microbiota—a dynamic community with far-reaching impacts on our well-being. From facilitating digestion and nutrient uptake to modulating our immune responses and influencing mood and cognition, the gut microbiota is a cornerstone in nearly every facet of human health.

Initially, the book establishes a robust groundwork, defining the gut microbiota and examining its multifaceted composition. It explores the varieties of prebiotics that nourish these microbial communities and the metabolites generated by probiotics, illuminating the intricate biochemical processes occurring within our intestines.

Venturing further, the book uncovers the critical role of gut microbiota in conditions such as inflammatory bowel diseases (IBD), obesity, cardiovascular diseases, Type 2 diabetes, and even ocular ailments. Each segment offers an in-depth examination of the respective condition, elucidating the intricate links between gut microbiota dysbiosis and disease development. Additionally, cutting-edge treatment modalities, ranging from microbiota-targeted therapies to innovative interventions were discussed.

A particularly fascinating facet of gut microbiota research is its relevance to neurological disorders, underscoring the profound connection between gut health and brain function. Through the gut-brain axis, the microbiota exerts influence over neurological well-being, potentially unlocking novel therapeutic avenues for conditions like Alzheimer's disease, Parkinson's disease, and depression.

The book also delves into diverse strategies for modulating the gut microbiota, encompassing probiotics, prebiotics, faecal microbiota transplantation, and dietary modifications. These interventions present promising opportunities for fostering a balanced gut microbiome and reducing disease risk.

Exploring the realm of gut microbial metabolites reveals their potential as diagnostic markers and therapeutic targets. From advancing drug development to enabling personalized medicine, these metabolites hold transformative potential for healthcare and disease management.

In the concluding chapters, the future trajectory of gut microbiota research, spotlighting emerging trends, untapped frontiers, and the challenges and prospects on the horizon has been contemplated. The ongoing pursuit to decode the intricacies of the gut microbiota promises to yield fresh insights into human health and disease, catalysing innovative interventions and personalized therapeutic strategies.

I ardently hope that this book serves as an invaluable resource for researchers, healthcare professionals, and anyone captivated by the profound impact of gut microbiota on human health. May it kindle curiosity, stimulate discussions, and guide us towards a deeper appreciation of the microbial cosmos dwelling within us.

Sreenivas Patro Sisinthy
Associate Professor, University of Nottingham, Selangor, Malaysia

PREFACE

The phrase "gut microbiota" has become widely used among scientists and researchers over time. The diverse population of microorganisms directly involved in the body's normal homeostasis and illness states resides in the human gastrointestinal tract. A man's diet and the frequency of infectious diseases determine how much of the microbiota population remains in adulthood after it has grown in the body during infancy.

Before its role in drug absorption was discovered, it was thought that the microbiome was mostly involved in food digestion. Over time, it became clear that the microbiome system is crucial to the body's ability to fight against illness. The particular products of the microbiome are essential to the process of digestion. However, as science advanced and human curiosity grew, it became interesting to see how the microbiota was linked to a number of disorders. After extensive investigation, it was shown that the majority of the diseased state develops as a result of variety in the gut's microbial community.

The idea for writing this book came about as a result of the knowledge regarding the significance of microbiota in human health. The "gut microbiota" plays a role in controlling various systems and is not limited to the alimentary canal. The book's chapters go into greater detail about the role that gut microbes play in the development of conditions like Inflammatory Bowel Disease, Type 2 Diabetes, obesity, cardiovascular problems, neurological disorders, and other conditions. The tactics that would provide an appropriate microbe are also covered here, as the proliferation of the microbiome has become vital in the body.

By reading the book, academics and researchers will gain a grasp of the fundamental physiology and homeostatic changes associated with specific diseases caused by the "gut microbiota," as well as the potential implications of the microbiome and its metabolites for human health.

We sincerely hope that the book will pique readers' curiosity, assist the medical community recognise the significance of the human microbiome in illness prevention and maintaining homeostasis, and provide a natural means of preserving good health for all.

Sandipan Dasgupta
Department of Pharmaceutical Technology
Maulana Abul Kalam Azad University of Technology W.B. Haringhata
Nadia-741249, West Bengal, India

&

Moitreyee Chattopadhyay
Department of Pharmaceutical Technology
Maulana Abul Kalam Azad University of Technology W.B. Haringhata
Nadia-741249, West Bengal, India

List of Contributors

Arijit Mallick	Department of Pharmaceutical Technology, NSHM Knowledge Campus, Kolkata-Group of Institutions, 124, B. L. Saha Road, Tara Park, Behala, Kolkata, West Bengal-700053, India
Atreyee Ganguly	Dr. B. C. Roy College of Pharmacy and Allied Health Sciences, Durgapur, West Bengal, India
Arnab Roy	Department of Biological Sciences (Pharmacology and Toxicology), National Institute of Pharmaceutical Education and Research (NIPER), Hyderabad, Telangana, India
Ansar Laskar	Department of Pharmaceutical Technology, Maulana Abul Kalam Azad University of Technology W.B. Haringhata Nadia-741249, West Bengal, India
Ananya Chanda	Department of Pharmaceutical Technology, Maulana Abul Kalam Azad University of Technology W.B. Haringhata Nadia-741249, West Bengal, India
Anupam	Rameesh Institute of Vocational & Technical Education, Greater Noida, U.P., 201310, India
Bikram Sarkar	Department of Pharmaceutical Technology, Maulana Abul Kalam Azad University of Technology, Haringhata, Nadia, West Bengal, India
Bani Kumar Jana	Department of Pharmaceutical Sciences, Dibrugarh University, Dibrugarh-786004, Assam, India
Bhaskar Mazumder	Department of Pharmaceutical Sciences, Dibrugarh University, Dibrugarh-786004, Assam, India
Deepak Chetia	Department of Pharmaceutical Sciences, Dibrugarh University, Dibrugarh-786004, Assam, India
Falguni Patra	Dr. B. C. Roy College of Pharmacy and Allied Health Sciences, Durgapur, West Bengal, India
Kousik Santra	Department of Pharmacy, Anand College of Education, Paschim Medinipur-721126, West Bengal, India
Kajal Chaudhary	Rameesh Institute of Vocational & Technical Education, Greater Noida, U.P., 201310, India
Mohini Singh	Department of Pharmaceutical Sciences, Dibrugarh University, Dibrugarh-786004, Assam, India
Moitreyee Chattopadhyay	Department of Pharmaceutical Technology, Maulana Abul Kalam Azad University of Technology W.B. Haringhata Nadia-741249, West Bengal, India
Mohamad Taleuzzaman	Department of Pharmaceutical Chemistry, Faculty of Pharmacy, Maulana Azad University, Village Bujhawar, Tehsil Luni, Jodhpur-342008, Rajasthan, India
Manjari Verma	Rameesh Institute of Vocational & Technical Education, Greater Noida, U.P., 201310, India
Prativa Sadhu	Department of Pharmaceutical Sciences, Dibrugarh University, Dibrugarh-786004, Assam, India
Priyakshi Chutia	Department of Pharmacology, School of Pharmacy, The Assam Kaziranga University, Jorhat-785006, Assam, India

Priyakshi Chutia	Department of Pharmacology, School of Pharmacy, The Assam Kaziranga University, Jorhat-785006, Assam, India
Rounak Seal	Department of Pharmaceutical Technology, Maulana Abul Kalam Azad University of Technology, Haringhata, Nadia, West Bengal, India
Rudradeep Hazra	Department of Pharmaceutical Technology, NSHM Knowledge Campus, Kolkata-Group of Institutions, 124, B. L. Saha Road, Tara Park, Behala, Kolkata, West Bengal-700053, India
Rohit Choudhary	Kalka Institute for Research and Advanced Studies, Meerut, U.P., 250103, India
Snehasis Jana	Department of Pharmaceutical Technology, Maulana Abul Kalam Azad University of Technology, Haringhata, Nadia, West Bengal, India
Satarupa Acharjee	Department of Pharmaceutical Technology, NSHM Knowledge Campus, Kolkata Groups of Institutions, 124, B. L. Saha Road, Kolkata 53, India
Sandipan Dasgupta	Department of Pharmaceutical Technology, Maulana Abul Kalam Azad University of Technology, Haringhata, Nadia, West Bengal, India
Soumyadeep Chattopadhyay	Department of Pharmaceutical Technology, NSHM Knowledge Campus, Kolkata-Group of Institutions, 124, B. L. Saha Road, Tara Park, Behala, Kolkata, West Bengal-700053, India
Sakuntala Gayen	Department of Pharmaceutical Technology, NSHM Knowledge Campus, Kolkata-Group of Institutions, 124, B. L. Saha Road, Tara Park, Behala, Kolkata, West Bengal-700053, India
Souvik Roy	Department of Pharmaceutical Technology, NSHM Knowledge Campus, Kolkata-Group of Institutions, 124, B. L. Saha Road, Tara Park, Behala, Kolkata, West Bengal-700053, India
Sabir Hussain	Department of Pharmacology, School of Pharmacy, The Assam Kaziranga University, Jorhat-785006, Assam, India
Sailendra Kumar Mahanta	Department of Pharmacology, School of Pharmacy, The Assam Kaziranga University, Jorhat-785006, Assam, India
Swati Bairagya	Department of Pharmacology/Biotechnology, Delhi Pharmaceutical Sciences and Research University, New Delhi, India
Sanjay Dey	Department of Pharmaceutical Technology, School of Health and Medical Sciences, Adamas University, Barasat-Barrackpore Road, Kolkata – 700126, West Bengal, India
Sk Safiur Rahaman	Department of Pharmaceutical Technology, Maulana Abul Kalam Azad University of Technology W.B. Haringhata Nadia-741249, West Bengal, India
Sabir Hussain	Department of Pharmacology, School of Pharmacy, The Assam Kaziranga University, Jorhat-785006, Assam, India
Sailendra Kumar Mahanta	Department of Pharmacology, School of Pharmacy, The Assam Kaziranga University, Jorhat-785006, Assam, India
Tumpa Sarkar	Department of Pharmaceutical Sciences, Dibrugarh University, Dibrugarh-786004, Assam, India
Tapas Kumar Roy	Department of Ocular Pharmacology and Pharmacy Division, Dr. R.P.Centre, AIIMS, New Delhi, India

CHAPTER 1

Exploring the Microbial Universe: An Overview of Gut Microbiota

Snehasis Jana[1], **Rounak Seal**[1], **Bikram Sarkar**[1], **Satarupa Acharjee**[2], **Kousik Santra**[3] and **Sandipan Dasgupta**[1,*]

[1] *Department of Pharmaceutical Technology, Maulana Abul Kalam Azad University of Technology, Haringhata, Nadia, West Bengal, India*

[2] *Department of Pharmaceutical Technology, NSHM Knowledge Campus, Kolkata Groups of Institutions, 124, B. L. Saha Road, Kolkata 53, India*

[3] *Department of Pharmacy, Anand College of Education, Paschim Medinipur- 721126, West Bengal, India*

Abstract: The gut microbiota, a diverse assemblage of microorganisms inhabiting the gastrointestinal tract, profoundly influences human health and disease. Comprised of bacterial taxa such as Bacteroidetes, Firmicutes, Actinobacteria, and Proteobacteria, this intricate ecosystem engages in symbiotic interactions with the host, exerting regulatory effects on various physiological processes. Prebiotics, indigestible dietary fibers including inulin, oligosaccharides, and resistant starches, selectively nourish beneficial gut bacteria, promoting their proliferation and metabolic activity. Through fermentation, prebiotics yield short-chain fatty acids (SCFAs) such as acetate, propionate, and butyrate, pivotal in supporting intestinal health and function. Probiotics, live microorganisms administered in sufficient quantities, confer health benefits through producing metabolites such as vitamins, enzymes, and SCFAs during fermentation. These bioactive compounds contribute to immune modulation, nutrient absorption, and the preservation of gut epithelial integrity. The profound importance of gut microbiota extends beyond gastrointestinal health, impacting metabolic, immune, and neurological functions. Dysbiosis, characterized by perturbations in microbial composition, has been implicated in a spectrum of disorders, including inflammatory bowel diseases, obesity, and neurodegenerative conditions. Understanding the diversity of gut microbiota and their metabolites is pivotal for devising targeted interventions to modulate microbial communities and optimize health outcomes. Metagenomic investigations have unveiled distinct microbial signatures associated with dietary habits, diseases, and physiological states, underscoring the dynamic nature of the gut microbiome and its potential as a therapeutic avenue.

[*] **Corresponding author Sandipan Dasgupta:** Department of Pharmaceutical Technology, Maulana Abul Kalam Azad University of Technology, Haringhata, Nadia, West Bengal, India; E-mail: sandipan.dasgupta21@gmail.com

Sandipan Dasgupta & Moitreyee Chattopadhyay (Eds.)

Keywords: Dietary metabolites, Gut-brain axis, Gut microbiome, Immune modulation, Probiotics, Prebiotics, Short-Chain Fatty Acids (SCFAs), Vitamin metabolites.

INTRODUCTION

The gut microbiota, which includes bacteria, viruses, fungi, and archaea, is a complex and varied collection of microorganisms that live in the human gut. This microbial ecology affects many body processes, including digestion, immunological response, and even mental health, and is essential to preserving general health and well-being. The complex link between the gut microbiota and human health has been made clear by developments in microbiology and genetics over the last several decades. These developments have highlighted the gut microbiota's potential influence on various ailments, including autoimmune diseases, metabolic disorders, and gastrointestinal disorders. It is becoming increasingly obvious that comprehending this microbial universe is essential to developing novel approaches to the prevention and treatment of a range of medical disorders. The gut flora plays a crucial role in nutrient absorption. These microbes are needed for metabolizing or breaking down necessary components so that the host may absorb them more easily [1].

Beyond its involvement in digestion and nutrient absorption, the gut microbiota also helps to support our body's immunity. The microbial community serves as a barrier to stop dangerous bacteria from colonizing. These beneficial bacteria are added to various vegetable juices, creating what are known as probiotic juices (Fig. **1**). These probiotic juices offer various advantages, as they combine the benefits of a plant-based diet with the presence of beneficial bacteria and high nutritional value.

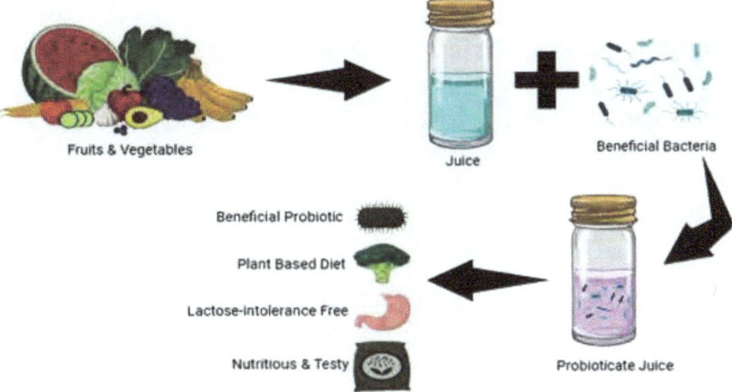

Fig. (1). Stage in probiotic action of fruits and vegetable juice

The gut microbiome's structure is dynamic and influenced by a number of internal and external factors. The microbial community is mostly determined by nutrition, with various dietary habits affecting the variety and abundance of certain bacteria. Poor lifestyle choices, such as stress and inactivity, may change how the gut microbiota functions. Additionally, while antibiotics are often required to cure infections, their usage might upset the delicate balance of the microbial population [2].

What is Gut Microbiota?

A varied population of bacteria called the gut microbiome (MB) inhabits the gastrointestinal tracts of all animals, including humans. This intricate ecosystem is crucial for maintaining health and influencing a variety of physiological activities [3]. The bacteria that live in the human gut are mostly bacteria, with thousands of different species living together. These microbes play an important role in processes including vitamin production, nutrition absorption, and digestion. Additionally, the gut microbiota plays a critical role in maintaining intestinal equilibrium, protecting against dangerous invaders, and strengthening the immune system. Dysbiosis, or an imbalance in the gut's microbial ecology, may lead to many health issues, such as metabolic irregularities, autoimmune diseases, and gastrointestinal disorders [4].

Maintaining a diverse and well-balanced microbial community is important to maintain good complex relationships between general human health and gut microbiota.

COMPOSITION OF GUT MICROBIOTA

A diverse range of bacteria, viruses, fungi, and other microorganisms comprise the gut microbiota, a complex microbial population that resides in the digestive system. The gut microbiota is composed primarily of hundreds of distinct bacterial species and is dynamically influenced by a variety of factors (Detailed impact of different microbes is described in Table **1**).

Individual genetic differences contribute to the early colonization and stability of these bacteria. The quantity and diversity of gut microorganisms are influenced by nutrition, with dietary fiber, probiotics, and prebiotics being important factors. An emerging field of study that holds promise for tailored healthcare methods and possible therapies to support optimum well-being is the recognition of the intricate interactions between the makeup of the gut microbiota and external factors [5].

Table 1. Importance of gut microbiome.

Microbe	Description	Function	Importance	Refs.
Bacteria (Firmicutes, Bacteroidetes, Actinobacteria, Proteobacteria)	Dominant group, with thousands of species.	Vitamin synthesis, pathogen protection, and metabolism.	Overall health, is an intricate link to human well-being.	
Viruses (Bacteriophages)	Target specific bacteria and regulate gut ecosystem.	Potential for novel gut health therapies through understanding interactions with bacteria.	Potential for novel gut health therapies.	[6 - 8]
Fungi (Candida species)	Less abundant than bacteria, contributes to gut community	Complex symbiotic relationship with other microbes.	Deepens understanding of human health.	
Archaea	Adaptable, found in diverse environments		Potential for future gut health therapies.	

Factors Influencing Gut Microbiota Composition Include

Diet

Within the fields of microbiology and nutrition, there is growing interest in the relationship between food and gut health (Fig. **2**).

The connections among immunity, gut health, and dietary fiber are essential as the composition of the gut microbiota influences immune function. A diet high in fiber promotes a diverse microbiota, which is essential for gut health. Short-chain fatty acids (SCFAs), which promote gut integrity and appetite regulation, are produced when gut bacteria digest dietary fiber. These molecules function as energy sources and signaling molecules and influence metabolism, inflammation, and immunological responses. Compounds like polyphenols and antioxidants in fiber-rich diets reduce oxidative stress and inflammation, potentially lowering the risk of metabolic conditions, including type 2 diabetes and obesity [1, 9].

Antibiotics

The complex equilibrium of gut flora is greatly impacted by antibiotics, which are heralded as essential weapons in the fight against bacterial diseases. Human gastrointestinal systems are home to a diverse variety of microorganisms that are essential for everything from immunological protection to digestion. Although antibiotics are very effective at eliminating undesirable bacteria, their careless usage seriously harms the gut's beneficial and harmful microorganisms. This wide-ranging attack may upset the balance, resulting in transient or extreme situations. In the long-term, it changes the composition of microorganisms, known as dysbiosis [10].

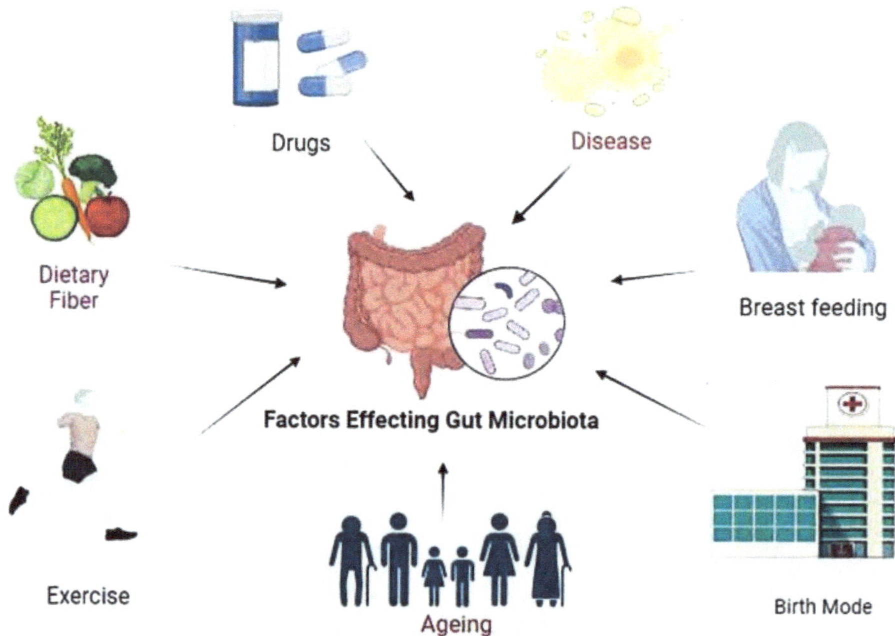

Fig. (2). Gut microbiota-influencing factors.

Antibiotics are essential for treating bacterial infections, but it is important to recognize how they affect the gut microbiota. We may strengthen the resilience of this vital ecosystem and protect our general well-being by maintaining the delicate balance of the gut microbiome.

Genetics

The interaction of the gut and genetis reveals the vast diversity of microbial communities within the human digestive system. Genetic factors encode crucial elements for immune responses, mucin production, and nutrient metabolism, shaping the unique microbial ecosystem. These genetic influences extend to the immune system's interactions with gut microbes, influencing the delicate balance crucial for a healthy microbial community. Understanding how genetic variations affect responses to interventions like diet or probiotics could lead to personalized recommendations for optimizing the gut microbiota. Ultimately, this intricate relationship offers promising avenues for promoting health and addressing various diseases through personalized interventions [11].

Age

The gut microbiota evolves dynamically throughout life, shaping distinct microbial profiles at different stages. This ecosystem plays a vital role in overall well-being and physiological processes. Aging and factors like lifestyle and health status further alter microbial diversity. The gut microbiome ecology is impacted by aging, and this has an effect on the brain and other human organs (Fig. **3**). Understanding this progression is crucial for developing customized therapies that support gut health at all stages of life.

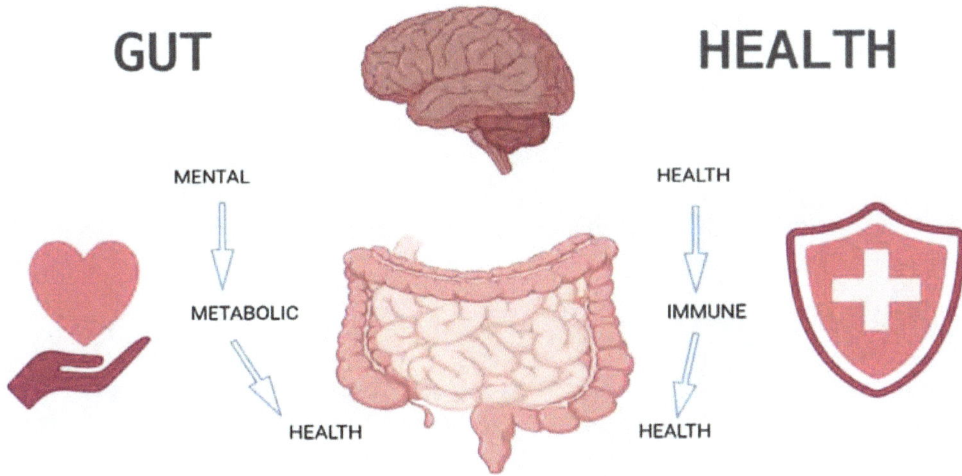

Fig. (3). Relation between GUT and health.

TYPES OF PREBIOTICS AND THE METABOLITES GENERATED BY PROBIOTICS

Prebiotics are indigestible substances that are vital for promoting the growth and health of beneficial microorganisms. Probiotics, which are live microorganisms injected into the body, differ from the bacterial populations that live in the gastrointestinal system.

Prebiotics are substances that serve as a source of nourishment for the existing beneficial microorganisms, encouraging their growth and metabolic activity and supporting the health and function of the gut microbiota. As research in this field progresses, the recognition of prebiotics as essential components for gut health underscores their potential to promote overall well-being by fostering a thriving and diverse microbial community in the gastrointestinal tract. Some common types of prebiotics include:

Inulin

Inulin, a valuable dietary component found in various plants such as chicory root, garlic, and onions, serves as a beneficial soluble fiber with notable impacts on gut health. This carbohydrate, belonging to the group of substances known as fructans, is distinguished by its resistance to digestion in the upper gastrointestinal tract, allowing it to reach the colon intact.

One of the key roles of inulin lies in the proliferation and metabolic engagement of symbiotic bacterial flora within the gastrointestinal tract. Bifidobacteria are recognized for their positive effects on digestive health and their potential contribution to the overall balance of the gut microbiota. Inulin provides more benefits than just the effects of a prebiotic. As a soluble fiber, it forms a gel in the digestive tract, aiding in bowel regulation and promoting digestive health. It also helps maintain stable blood sugar levels and supports weight management by inducing a sense of fullness. Incorporating inulin-rich foods into one's diet, such as chicory root, garlic, and onions, can be a strategic approach to enhance gut health [12].

Fructo-oligosaccharides (FOS)

It represents a group of oligosaccharides similar to inulin, naturally occurring in various fruits and vegetables. As a prebiotic, FOS plays a crucial role in promoting gut health by stimulating the growth of beneficial bacteria. These carbohydrates serve as a fermentable food source for these helpful microorganisms, enhancing their growth and activity in the gut.

Following the fermentation of FOS by these microbial communities, short-chain fatty acids are produced, serving two purposes: supplying a substrate for enterocyte metabolism along the intestinal epithelium and creating an environment that supports the growth of symbiotic microorganisms. Knowing how fructo-oligosaccharides contribute to a varied and healthy microbiome is crucial for researchers and people trying to make the best dietary decisions as interest in gut health grows [13, 14].

Galacto-oligosaccharides

GOS, a type of prebiotic found in human breast milk and certain legumes, plays a vital role in supporting gut health. These oligosaccharides consist of short chains of galactose molecules and function as a food supply for the good bacteria in the gastrointestinal tract.

The presence of GOS in human breast milk underscores its significance in early development and immune system modulation. Bifidobacterium and lactobacilli, two prominent types of beneficial bacteria, thrive on GOS. These microorganisms ferment GOS to generate short-chain fatty acids., contributing to the overall well-being of the digestive system. GOS, found naturally in legumes like chickpeas, lentils, and beans, is crucial for a balanced diet, alongside breast milk. These legumes offer a dietary source of GOS, promoting a diverse gut microbiome. Research highlights the importance of a varied gut microbiota for overall health, extending beyond digestion. Including GOS-rich foods or supplements can help cultivate beneficial gut flora, supporting a healthy microbial community.

Lactulose

This is commonly recognized for its laxative properties and serves a dual role as a prebiotic, contributing to the promotion of beneficial bacteria within the gut. Initially developed to alleviate constipation, lactulose works by drawing water into the colon, softening stools, and facilitating bowel movements. However, its impact extends beyond the digestive process. As a prebiotic, lactulose provides a food source for the gut's beneficial bacteria, including lactobacilli and bifidobacteria. These microorganisms thrive on the fermentation of lactulose, producing short-chain fatty acids (SCFAs) in the process. SCFAs are essential for preserving gut health by creating an acidic one that encourages the development of good bacteria while preventing the spread of dangerous diseases.

The bifunctional nature of lactulose, both as a laxative and a prebiotic, underscores its potential in promoting a healthy, balanced gut microbiome. This dual functionality positions lactulose as a compound with therapeutic potential beyond its conventional use for relieving constipation.

Resistant Starch

Resistant starch, a unique form of starch, plays a distinctive role in the digestive process, impacting our health in ways beyond typical starch consumption. Unlike regular starches, resistant starch is difficult to digest. Inside the small intestine's boundaries, it refrains from succumbing to digestion; rather, it traverses undisturbed to the colon, where it assumes the role of a substrate for microbial fermentation. Found in certain foods like green bananas, raw potatoes, and legumes, resistant starch contributes to the complex relationship between diet and gut health. Because this starch resists digestion in the small intestine, it reaches the colon relatively unchanged. Once there, it becomes a source of nourishment for the diverse community of microorganisms that make up the gut microbiota. There are some examples like resistant starch, found in foods like green bananas, raw potatoes, and legumes, which represents a unique dietary component that the substance exhibits resistance to enzymatic breakdown within the confines of the small intestine, persisting until it traverses its path towards the colon, where it undergoes microbial fermentation, highlights its role in supporting gut health and influencing various physiological processes.

METABOLITES GENERATED BY PROBIOTICS

Probiotics are good bacteria that digest prebiotics in the gut to create a variety of metabolites. The host's general health benefits from these metabolites. Some key metabolites include short-chain fatty acids, vitamins, and bioactive compounds, playing crucial roles in immune function, digestion, and overall well-being. Some key metabolites include:

Short-Chain Fatty Acids (SCFAs)

These vital substances are produced in the gastrointestinal system by the fermentation of prebiotics and dietary fibers. Acetate, propionate, and butyrate are the major SCFAs, and they are all crucial for gut health. Some short-chain fatty acids, produced through the fermentation of dietary fibers and prebiotics, play multifaceted roles in gut health. These SCFAs play a crucial role in the complex interactions between gut microbiota and general health, supplying energy to colonocytes, controlling the immune system, and bolstering a robust gut barrier. Gaining knowledge of and using the advantages of SCFAs might lead to the creation of focused therapies that support and preserve gut health.

Lactic Acid

Lactic acid, a vital component of gut health, is produced by lactic acid bacteria, of which certain probiotic strains are particularly important. This organic acid is essential for establishing an acidic environment in the gastrointestinal system, which improves gut health in general. Probiotic supplements often include lactic acid bacteria, which are common components of the gut microbiota and include Lactobacillus and Bifidobacterium species. Lactic acid may be produced as a byproduct of the fermentation of carbohydrates by these microorganisms. This fermentation process helps maintain the ideal pH balance in the stomach in addition to facilitating the breakdown of complex carbs for energy [15]. Lactic acid-producing probiotics that are not incorporated into the diet or supplements can optimize gut microbiota by enhancing symbiotic interactions. Understanding these nuances is crucial for overall wellness. Harnessing lactic acid's benefits could improve digestive health and prevent gastrointestinal disorders.

Biogenic Amines

Biogenic amines, a group of naturally occurring compounds, have gained attention in the realm of gut health, particularly in the context of probiotic bacteria and fermented foods. Probiotics, beneficial bacteria known for their positive impact on the gut microbiota, have been found to produce biogenic amines, including histamine and tyramine.

Histamine and tyramine are biogenic amines that serve important roles in the body, such as neurotransmission and immune response modulation [16]. However, when present in excessive amounts, they can have varying effects on health. High levels of histamine, for instance, have been associated with allergic reactions and inflammatory responses. These include foods like aged cheeses, sauerkraut, and fermented meats.

B Vitamins

It plays a crucial role in supporting various physiological functions within the body, and certain probiotic strains have been identified as contributors to their synthesis. Probiotic bacteria, including certain strains of Lactobacillus and Bifidobacterium, have been shown to produce riboflavin in the intestines. This synthesis represents a potential additional source of this vital vitamin, complementing dietary intake [17].

IMPORTANCE OF GUT MICROBIOTA

The gut microbiome plays a very crucial role in maintaining a norm, healthy lifestyle. They have different roles in lipid metabolism, insulin sensitivity, gut-brain communication, the production of vitamins, and the production of the immune system (Fig. **4**). Thu, these microbiota are also found to be very effective in the treatment of different disorders, which are briefly described in Table **2**.

The Importance of Gut Microbial Colonization During Infancy for Immune System Development

The gut microbiota plays a pivotal role in shaping the immune system, especially during infancy when immune maturation is most critical. Early microbial colonization influences immune responses, enhances immune tolerance, and provides protection against diseases. From birth, the gut is populated by microorganisms that interact with immune cells to support the development of T and B cells and stimulate the production of immunoglobulin A (IgA), strengthening gut immunity. This microbial exposure helps train the immune system to differentiate between harmful and harmless antigens, reducing the risk of allergies and autoimmune conditions. The process of early microbial colonization is influenced by several factors. The mode of delivery plays a significant role, as infants born vaginally acquire beneficial maternal microbiota that aids in immune system development. On the other hand, infants born *via* cesarean section may experience delayed colonization and lower microbial diversity, potentially affecting immune regulation. Feeding practices also contribute to microbial colonization. Breastfeeding provides essential probiotics and prebiotic materials that promote healthy gut microbiota, reducing the risk of infections and inflammatory diseases. On the other hand, formula feeding leads to a different microbial profile, which may impact immune responses. A balanced gut microbiota protects against immune-related diseases by regulating immune responses and maintaining the gut barrier. Infants with a diverse microbiome are less likely to develop conditions like allergies, asthma, and autoimmune diseases. Disruptions in early microbial colonization can lead to chronic inflammation and immune imbalances. Establishing a healthy gut microbiota during infancy is crucial for optimal immune function and long-term health. Ensuring proper microbial colonization through natural birth, breastfeeding, and minimal antibiotic exposure supports immune resilience and disease prevention [35].

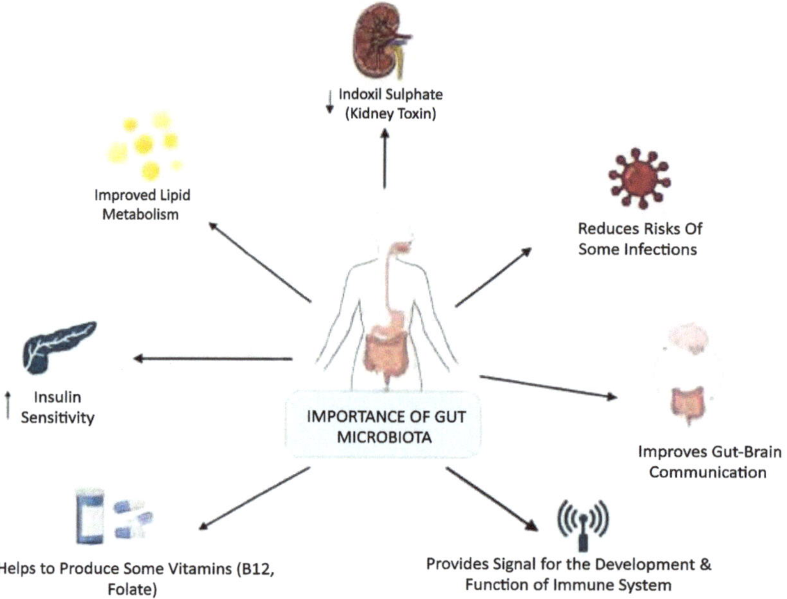

Fig. (4). The significance of gut microbiota.

Table 2. Role of MB in different disorders.

Disease	Role of Gut Microbiota	Treatment
Type 1 diabetes	Factors like diet, genome, and digestive microbiota are linked to T1D development. The stomach microbiota promotes resistance to the disease, and T1D patients' intestinal mucosa is more susceptible to bacterial mucin debasement, causing the body to produce antibodies. Cardwell's group found that Caesarean section children are more likely to develop T1D [18].	Like probiotics, prebiotics, or fecal microbiota transplantation, these strategies aim to restore microbial balance, enhance immune regulation, and potentially delay or prevent the onset of T1D [19].
Type 2 diabetes	The gut microbiota plays a significant role in T2DM development, with patients having an alternate stomach microbiota with a lower proportion of bacteria and Bifidobacteria. This balance aids in energy elimination from food and can produce endotoxins and other diseases. F. Prausnitziias could be a valuable microbial objective for managing glucose homeostasis in T2DM patients [20, 21].	Targeting gut microbiota through probiotics, prebiotics, or dietary changes can improve metabolic health, reduce disease complications, and offer new therapeutic interventions [22].
System of the Heart	A study using targeted metabolomics identified pathways linking dietary lipid intake, atherosclerosis, hypertension, and the gut microbiota. Three phospholipid metabolites in the diet, phosphatidylcholine, betaine, and trimethylamine N-oxide (TMAO), were identified as independent indicators of clinical vascular events. The gut microbiota generates the precursor to TMAO, increasing the rate of cardiovascular events in patients with higher levels [23].	Modulating gut microbiota through diet, probiotics, or fecal transplantation shows promise in CVD management by reducing lipid deposition and hypertension [24].
The stomach-brain axis	The stomach microbiota influences the brain and spinal cord through immune system adjustments, digestion, and metabolites. It also influences the central nervous system by producing neuroactive particles and fats. The vagus nerve transmits hormone levels and neuronal activity to the brain, creating a link between the brain and the stomach-related system. Weight also influences the stomach microbiota [25, 26].	The gut microbiota is crucial in the stomach-brain axis, affecting mood, cognition, and behaviour. Imbalances can lead to anxiety, depression, and neurodegenerative diseases. Treatment strategies like probiotics, prebiotics, and dietary interventions can improve mental health outcomes by modulating the stomach-brain axis [27].

(Table 2) cont.....

Disease	Role of Gut Microbiota	Treatment
Diseases of the nervous system	Digestive microbiota can convert sugars into short-chain starches unsaturated fats (SCFAs), causing neuropsychiatric problems. SCFAs inhibit gastrointestinal motility and promote glucose digestion. Propionate can cause chemical imbalances in rodents, leading to chemical imbalance range disorder (ASD). Changes in microbiota can also cause mood, depression, and tension issues. Stomach microbiota is believed to be significant in disease pathogenesis [28].	Treatment strategies include probiotics, prebiotics, dietary changes, and fecal microbiota transplantation to restore balance and improve neurological function, potentially alleviating neurological symptoms [29].
Parkinson's disease	Parkinson's disease is a neurodegenerative condition affecting the central nervous system, patients have more Enterobacteriaceae species in their stool, leading to increased α-synuclein production and unusual collapsing. Excessive Enterobacteriaceae levels cause cytokine production and inflammation, controlling the progression of Lewy bodies and dopaminergic neuron death. Probiotics containing lactobacilli and bifidobacteria have been shown to reverse the PD-like state [30].	Modulating gut microbiota through probiotics, prebiotics, or fecal microbiota transplantation shows promise in ameliorating PD symptoms by reducing inflammation and improving gut-brain communication, offering a new treatment avenue for Parkinson's disease [31].
Alzheimer's disease	Alzheimer's disease is a neurodegenerative condition causing hyperphosphorylated tau neurofibrillary tangles and beta-amyloid plaques in the brain, leading to memory, language, and behavior issues. Alzheimer's patients have a diverse stomach microbiota, with more Bacteroidetes and less Firmicutes and Actinobacteria. Bacterial metabolites cause inflammation, increasing the blood-cerebral barrier and digestive permeability, leading to beta-amyloid production. N-methylamino-L-alanine, a neurotoxin produced by intestinal bacteria, can lead to neurodegeneration and cognitive impairment [32, 33].	Modulating gut microbiota through probiotics, prebiotics, or dietary interventions shows promise in AD management, potentially mitigating neurodegenerative processes and improving cognitive function. Understanding this relationship offers new therapeutic interventions targeting the gut-brain axis [34].

Early-Life Gut Microbiome: The Significance of Mother and Child Inputs in Its Development

The formation of the gut microbiota in the early years of life is impacted by both maternal and baby factors, and it is essential for overall health. The mother has a significant influence on the microbial community that forms during the early microbial colonization in babies, which lays the groundwork for the immune system and general health. At birth, bacteria quickly invade the baby's intestines. This process is significantly influenced by the manner of delivery: children delivered vaginally are exposed to the intestinal and vaginal microbiota of their mothers, while infants born by cesarean section are exposed to other microbiota. Another important component is breastfeeding, which promotes the development of a healthy gut microbiota by supplying prebiotics and good bacteria. In contrast, immune system imbalance and long-term health issues may result from disturbances in early microbial colonization caused by things like antibiotic usage or not nursing. Both maternal and newborn factors have a substantial impact on how the gut microbiota develops throughout infancy. The development of the child's immune system and long-term health are supported by ensuring adequate microbial colonization *via* natural delivery, nursing, and a healthy mother environment [36].

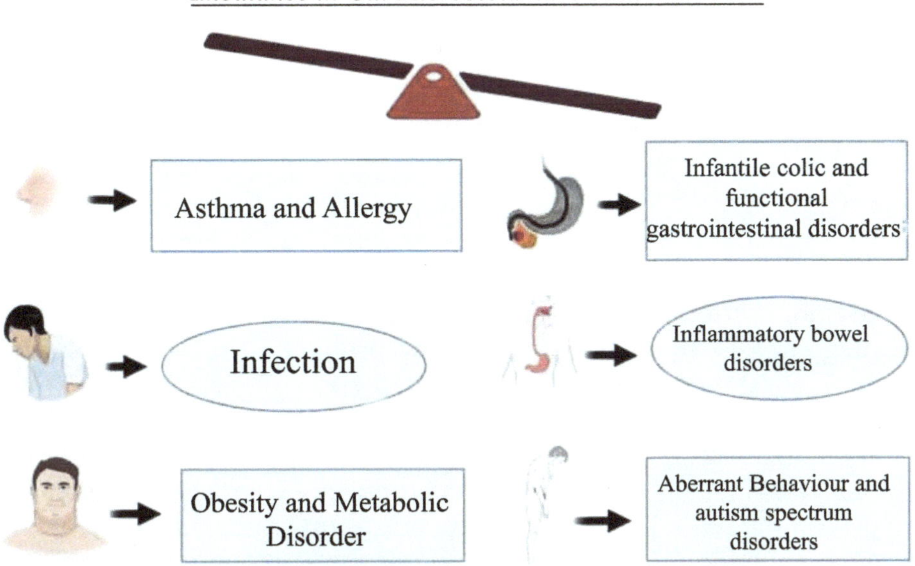

Fig. (5). Imbalance in the microbiota of the gut.

The Gut Microbiota's Function in Nutrition and Health

The microbial populations that inhabit various parts of the human gut influence many aspects of health. The gut microbiome provides vitality to the body in a healthy condition. They also maintain a balance with the host's immune system and digestive system. However, adverse effects may include gastrointestinal disorders, causing irritation and contamination, and perhaps diabetes and obesity. The chemical composition of the microbial community may be significantly impacted by food over the long and short term, which could lead to new options for diet-based health management. Maintaining physiological homeostasis and building a robust immune system are two distinct functions of the microbiota in a typical, healthy human life (Fig. **6**).

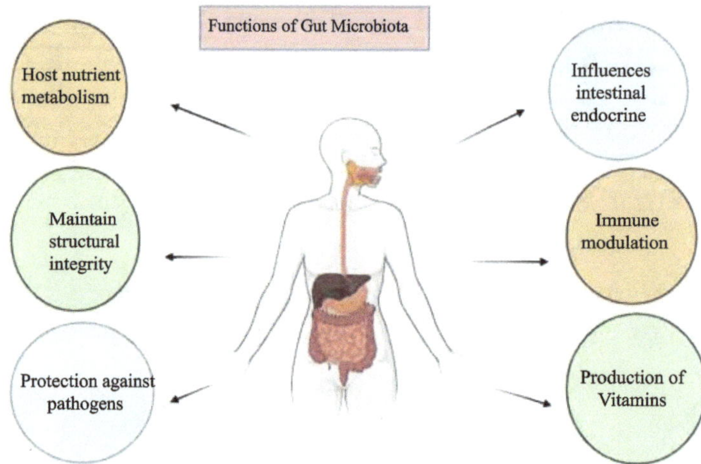

Fig. (6). Gut microbiota function.

The group of bacteria in our digestive tract, known as the gut microbiota, is essential to both nutrition and general health. It facilitates the breakdown of fiber and complex carbohydrates, resulting in the production of healthy short-chain fatty acids (SCFAs) that promote gut health and give off energy. Additionally, the microbiota produces vital vitamins that are necessary for many body processes, such as vitamin K, folate, and B12. Also, the gut flora influences glucose control, energy storage, and metabolism, all of which impact weight and the risk of illness. It interacts with the brain *via* the gut-brain axis to influence mood, mental health, and cognitive function. Disturbances in the microbiota have been connected to neurological illnesses such as anxiety and depression. By inhibiting the growth of dangerous pathogens and lowering inflammation, the gut microbiota aids in immune system regulation. Inflammatory bowel illnesses, metabolic disorders (such as diabetes and obesity), and autoimmune diseases are all associated with dysbiosis or an imbalance in the microbiota [37].

TYPES OF GUT MICROBIOTA AND ITS METABOLITES

The gut microbiota (MB) is the diverse community of microorganisms (viruses, bacteria, fungi, and other microbes) present within the gastrointestinal tract. These microorganisms participate in the metabolism of different dietary components. These metabolites have significant impacts on human health [38]. The list of vital gut microbiomes and their metabolites are given below:

Bacteroidetes

These bacteria, belonging to a specific phylum, are commonly found in the human gut microbiota. They play a significant role in maintaining gut health and overall well-being [39]. In the digestive process, they break down complex carbohydrates and extract energy from food [40]. Additionally, these bacteria also contribute to the synthesis of essential vitamins like folate and biotin. These compounds are used to maintain normal metabolic function within the human body and can also modulate the immune system [41]. They promote the balance of microbial communities and prevent the colonization of harmful pathogens. If there is any alteration of the abundance of Bacteroides, it causes different types of health-related issues and causes obesity, inflammatory bowel disease, and metabolic disorders. The metabolites produced by these bacteria include short-chain fatty acids (SCFAs) such as acetate, propionate, and butyrate. (Table **3**). These SCFAs are important for energy metabolism and maintaining gut health [42, 43].

Firmicutes

Firmicutes are a dominant phylum in the human gut, comprising a significant portion of the total gut microbiome. These gram-positive bacteria play a multifaceted role in our health, influencing digestion, immunity, and even metabolism. *Lactobacillus* and *Bifidobacterium* are examples of firmicutes well-known for their probiotic properties, aiding in nutrient absorption and immune function [44, 45]. Others, like members of the Clostridium genus, specialized in breaking down carbohydrates that humans can't digest, producing short-chain fatty acids in the process. A higher population in the firmicutes-to-bacterias ratio has been associated with a severe disorder like obesity and inflammatory bowel disease [44]. Metabolites produced by Firmicutes are short-chain fatty acids (SCFAs) (Table **3**).

Actinobacteria

Actinobacteria is gram-positive, having the characteristics of both fungi and bacteria, which contain high amounts of cytosine and guanine in their DNA.

Actinobacteria are involved in the production of compounds, such as bacteriocins (Table **3**), which have antimicrobial properties. They also contribute to the fermentation process in the gut [46].

Proteobacteria

Proteobacteria are one type of gram-negative bacteria. These are a complex and diverse group of bacteria found in abundance within the human gut microbiome.

Among them, some species play an essential role in maintaining human health, while some species can also be harmful pathogens and cause urinary tract infections, food poisoning, and stomach infections. That means in the complex ecosystem of our gut, they act like a captivating double-edged sword. They can modulate the inflammatory response and immune function, and their overgrowth in the gut can lead to severe disorders. It is essential to understand the factors that contribute to their virulence to prevent disease. Proteobacteria, one of the most abundant phyla, is present in about 35-40% of the total gut microbiome population [47]. The gut environment encompasses a diverse array of species with differing metabolic capabilities and ecological niches. Salmonella enteric, Helicobacter pylori, E.coli, and some beneficial genera like Synechococcus and Desulfovibrio are common members of this proteobacteria family [48]. Proteobacteria play a significant role in carbohydrate breakdown and energy and protein production. Some proteobacteria can produce lipopolysaccharides (LPS), which can have pro-inflammatory effects when released into the bloodstream (Table **3**) [49]. However, not all proteobacteria are associated with negative health effects.

Table 3. Gut microbiota and metabolites.

Name of the Gut Microbiota	Name of their Major Metabolites
Bacteroidetes	Short-chain fatty acids (acetate, propionate, and butyrate)
Firmicutes	Short-chain fatty acids
Actinobacteria	Bacteriocins
Proteobacteria	Lipopolysaccharides
Fungi	Mycotoxins
Archaea	Gaseous metabolites (methane)

Fungi

When it comes to the gut microbiome, there is very little abundance and a much smaller number in comparison with bacteria. Although less understood, fungi also play a major role in this complex ecosystem, contributing to maintaining healthy conditions and modulating immune system function. Some common genera present in the human gut include candida, Saccharomyces, and Malassezia. Fungi in the gut can produce various metabolites, including secondary metabolites like mycotoxins (Table **3**) [50].

Archaea

Archaea, often overshadowed by bacteria, represent another vital element of the human gut microbiome, although they exist in significantly smaller proportions (approximately 1.2%). Despite the ongoing emergence of research on this captivating group, their potential contributions to our health remain intriguing.

Methanogens are majorly present among all of the gut archaea, especially the genus named Methanobrevibacter, known for the production of methane gas as a byproduct of their metabolism (Table **3**), this is a part of the complex microbial interactions in the gut. There is a very less abundant archaea group like nitrososphaera, which has a vital role in the nitrogen cycling inside the human gut. Archaea in the gut primarily produce methane during the metabolism of certain substrates [51].

Viruses (Bacteriophages)

Bacteriophages, viruses that infect bacteria, can influence the abundance and diversity of bacterial populations in the gut, which have an indirect role in the production of different metabolites.

METABOLITES PRODUCED BY THE GUT MICROBIOTA

Gut MB and its Carbohydrate Metabolites

The diet substances that reach the large intestine are mainly complex polysaccharides, and they have a bond that remains indigestible by the enzyme that is present inside the upper GI tract. Various types of complex glycan monosaccharides disciplines are also unable to absorb completely from the upper GI due to the incomplete digestion process due to the unavailability of the respective digestive enzyme for their metabolism and they are available for metabolism by the colonic microbiome [52].

In the large intestine, the gut microbiota degrades complex polysaccharides and synthesizes SCFAs, which serve as an energy source for the host; for example, acetate, Propionate, butyrate. This small chain fatty acid can regulate energy homeostasis by controlling glucagon-like peptide (GLP-1) and grilling (the two main intestinal hormones that maintain energy homeostasis). There is also another pathway that regulates the stored energy and reduces fat and glycogen by increasing energy expenditure that is called the AMPk pathway. This small-cell fatty acid can activate the AMPk pathway and indirectly control the energy expenditure process [53, 54].

The microbiome also influences the function of fat-inducing adipocyte factor (FIAF), thus affecting fat storage within the host. FIAF can block another pathway, the lipoprotein lipase pathway, which normally promotes triglyceride (TG) storage in adipose tissue [55]. SCFAs can interact with different receptors. Among SCFAs, propionate binds with GPR41, and GPR43, acetate binds with GPR43, and Butyrate can bind with GPR41. The GPR43 and GPR41 receptors activate leptin expression and stimulate adipogenesis aiding in energy utilization, respectively [56, 57, 59]. Propionate also plays a role in gluconeogenesis and reduces glucose production, leading to reduced adiposity and thus maintaining energy homeostasis [58, 59].

SCFA decreases the process of cell proliferation and suppresses apoptosis. If there is any reduction in the level of SCFA concentration, that may sometimes cause malignant tumors in the distal colon and lead to colorectal cancer [60, 61] (Fig. 7).

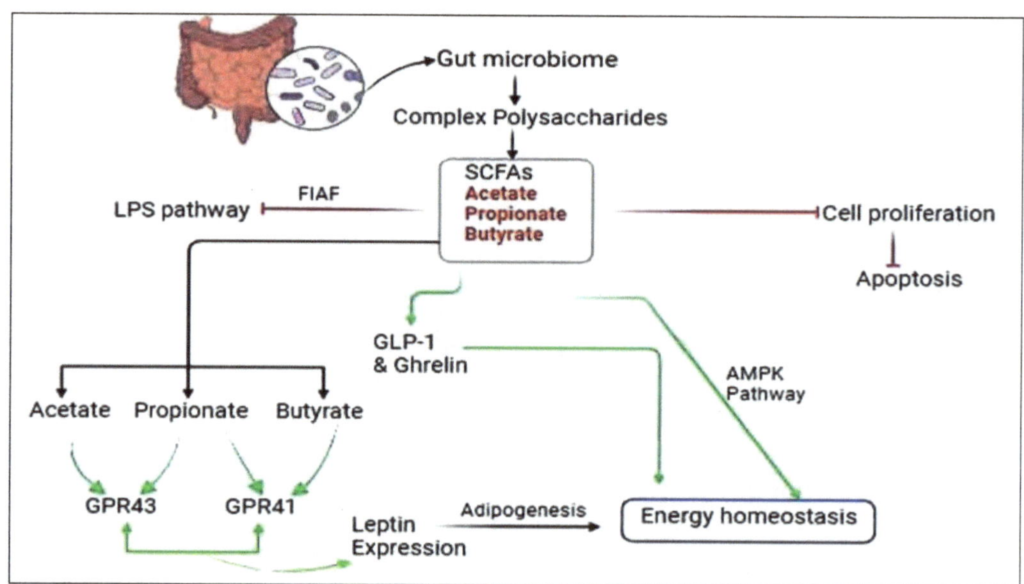

Fig. (7). Carbohydrate metabolites of gut microbiome and their different physiological responses.

Gut Microbiome and Lipid Metabolism

The Microbiota can regulate the metabolism of lipids in the liver and serum. In adipose tissue, the lipoprotein lipase inhibitor is suppressed by the gut microbiome thus, it has a favorable action on lipid metabolism and fatty acid reabsorption. The gut microbiome also alters lipid absorption by manipulating different genes like Sterol response element binding protein 1 (SREBP1), fatty acid synthase, *etc.* [62, 63]. Pancreatic lipase plays a great role in the digestion of lipids, which is regulated by the expression of colipase. Bacteroides can influence the expression of this particular gene and increase lipid hydrolysis [64] (Fig. **8**).

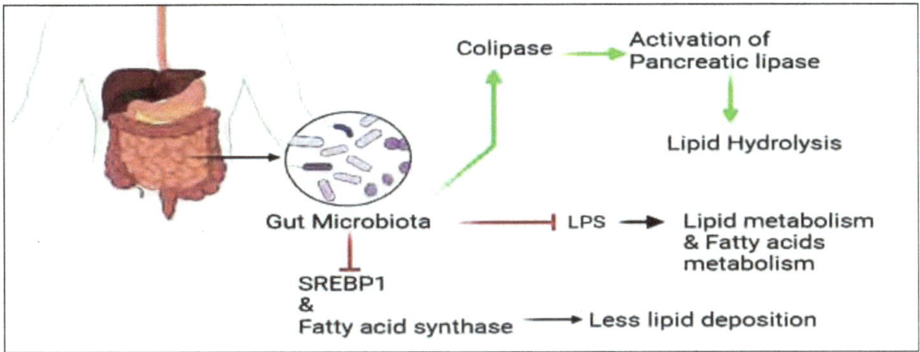

Fig. (8). Lipid metabolites of gut microbiome and their different physiological responses.

Gut Microbiome and Bile Acid Metabolism

Bacteroides species synthesized Conjugated linoleic acid (CLA) is obtained from the unsaturated fatty acids. It is therapeutically active against diabetes, atherogenesis, carcinogenesis, and hyperlipidemia. It also has some immune modulatory properties [65]. The gut microbiome deconugates and dehydrates bile acid to form secondary bile acids. This bile acid is the major metabolite of cholesterol compounds produced by the gut microbiome [66].

The secondary bile acid metabolites bind with the TGR5 receptor and regulate glucose and energy homeostasis, reduce the expression of inflammatory mediators, and stimulate the action of GLP-1 inside the host body [67, 68] (Fig. **9**).

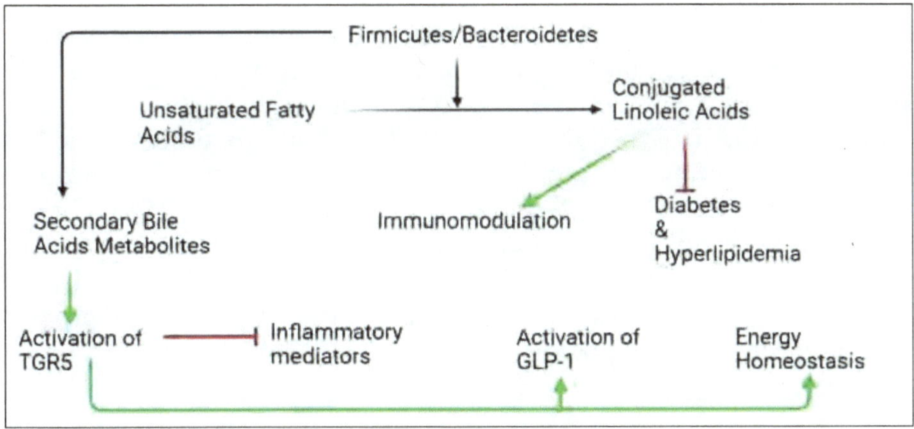

Fig. (9). Bile acids metabolites of the gut microbiome and their different physiological responses.

Gut Microbiome's Vitamin Metabolites

The gut microbiota participates in the synthesis of vitamins such as vitamin K, B vitamins (folate, nicotinic acid, cobalamin), and biotin. These vitamin metabolites also help maintain plasma prothrombin levels [69, 70].

Gut Microbiome and Gas Metabolites

In the anaerobic system in the digestive tract, different types of gases can be produced by microbial fermentation. That is why prebiotics and probiotics can reduce the formation of gas inside the intestinal tract, for example, hydrogen, carbon dioxide, and methane, but the most abundant is hydrogen gas [69]. The two major types of bacteria that produce these gases as metabolites are Clostridium and Bacteroides. Hydrogen-utilizing microorganisms, such as methanogens and hydrogenotrophic acetogens, are essential for intestinal fermentation [71, 72]. The second most abundant gas is carbon dioxide, which is recycled by methanogenesis and acetogenesis and helps maintain homeostasis [71, 73]. Changes in the amount of these gases within the gastrointestinal tract may be associated with diseases like inflammatory bowel syndrome. The recycling process of these gases is also important; otherwise, it may cause pneumatosis cystoides intestinalis [74].

Gut Microbiome in the Metabolism of Amino Acids

The gut microbiome plays a vital role in amino acid recycling and metabolism. The gut microbiome uses these amino acids as building blocks and sometimes produces metabolites like NO, H_2S, and NH_3 through fermentation [75]. They can contribute to maintaining the body's amino acid pool by synthesizing some amino acids. Furthermore, they convert amino acids into various intracellular signaling molecules by facilitating the transport of amino acids from the body into the intestinal lumen. The gut microbiome has the capability of catalyzing most of the amino acids. The metabolites are aspartate, glutamine, glycine, leucine, valine, and isoleucine [75, 76]. The other fermented products are SCFAs, and branched-chain fatty acids (BCFAs). After amino acids metabolism, they produce some gases like hydrogen, methane, hydrogen sulfide, carbon dioxide, aromatic compounds like phenol, organic acids like lactate and succinate, neurotransmitters like GABA, Serotonin, histamine, DOPA, tryptamine, *etc.* They also modulate the expression of various genes, which, in turn, participate in the production of different amino acid-metabolizing enzymes [77].

CONCLUSION

In summary, the gut microbiota is a dynamic, complex ecosystem with broad effects on human health. Composed of a wide range of bacterial taxa, including Firmicutes, Actinobacteria, Proteobacteria, and Bacteroidetes, this microbiome interacts symbiotically with its host. The gut microbiota regulates the immune system, affects metabolic and neurological processes, and preserves intestinal health through processes like the fermentation of prebiotics into short-chain fatty acids (SCFAs). Prebiotics and probiotics provide viable ways to support the development and activity of beneficial microorganisms, improving general health and reducing dysbiosis-related ailments such as obesity, neurodegenerative diseases, and inflammatory bowel diseases. The gut microbiota is diverse and dynamic, and metagenomic research has shed light on its dynamic nature and its potential as a therapeutic target. Continued exploration of microbial diversity and metabolite production will be essential for developing targeted interventions aimed at optimizing health outcomes and managing diseases.

CONSENT FOR PUBLICATION

All authors have consented to publish the book chapter "Exploring The Microbial Universe Within: An Overview of Gut Microbiota" in this book.

ACKNOWLEDGEMENTS

We are grateful to the Department of Pharmaceutical Technology, Maulana Abul Kalam Azad University of Technology, Haringhata, Nadia, 741249, West Bengal, India, for providing all support and facilities.

REFERENCES

[1] Gupta, A., Gupta, R. and Singh, R.L., Microbes and environment. Principles and applications of environmental biotechnology for a sustainable future, 2017; pp. 43-84.

[2] Karl JP, Hatch AM, Arcidiacono SM, *et al.* Effects of psychological, environmental and physical stressors on the gut microbiota. Front Microbiol 2018; 9: 2013. [http://dx.doi.org/10.3389/fmicb.2018.02013] [PMID: 30258412]

[3] Barko PC, McMichael MA, Swanson KS, Williams DA. The gastrointestinal microbiome: A review. J Vet Intern Med 2018; 32(1): 9-25. [http://dx.doi.org/10.1111/jvim.14875] [PMID: 29171095]

[4] Parizadeh M, Arrieta MC. The global human gut microbiome: genes, lifestyles, and diet. Trends Mol Med 2023; 29(10): 789-801. [http://dx.doi.org/10.1016/j.molmed.2023.07.002] [PMID: 37516570]

[5] Minor L. Discovering precision health: predict, prevent, and cure to advance health and well-being. John Wiley & Sons 2020. [http://dx.doi.org/10.1002/9781119672715]

[6] Emencheta SC, Olovo CV, Eze OC, *et al.* The Role of Bacteriophages in the Gut Microbiota: Implications for Human Health. Pharmaceutics 2023; 15(10): 2416.

[http://dx.doi.org/10.3390/pharmaceutics15102416] [PMID: 37896176]

[7] Possemiers S, Grootaert C, Vermeiren J, *et al.* The intestinal environment in health and disease - recent insights on the potential of intestinal bacteria to influence human health. Curr Pharm Des 2009; 15(18): 2051-65.
[http://dx.doi.org/10.2174/138161209788489159] [PMID: 19519443]

[8] Eckburg PB, Lepp PW, Relman DA. Archaea and their potential role in human disease. Infect Immun 2003; 71(2): 591-6.
[http://dx.doi.org/10.1128/IAI.71.2.591-596.2003] [PMID: 12540534]

[9] Gowd V, Karim N, Shishir MRI, Xie L, Chen W. Dietary polyphenols to combat the metabolic diseases *via* altering gut microbiota. Trends Food Sci Technol 2019; 93: 81-93.
[http://dx.doi.org/10.1016/j.tifs.2019.09.005]

[10] Makokha, W.S., Characterization of Escherichia coli strains and Salmonella enterica serovars isolated in gallus gallus and their antimicrobial susceptibility (Doctoral dissertation, Kenyatta University), 2010.

[11] Ventura M, Turroni F, Canchaya C, Vaughan EE, O'Toole PW, van Sinderen D. Microbial diversity in the human intestine and novel insights from metagenomics. Front Biosci 2009; Volume(14): 3214-21.
[http://dx.doi.org/10.2741/3445] [PMID: 19273267]

[12] Dogra S, Chung C, Wang D, Sakwinska O, Colombo Mottaz S, Sprenger N. Nurturing the early life gut microbiome and immune maturation for long term health. Microorganisms 2021; 9(10): 2110.
[http://dx.doi.org/10.3390/microorganisms9102110] [PMID: 34683431]

[13] Peled S, Livney YD. The role of dietary proteins and carbohydrates in gut microbiome composition and activity: A review. Food Hydrocoll 2021; 120: 106911.
[http://dx.doi.org/10.1016/j.foodhyd.2021.106911]

[14] Yoo S, Jung SC, Kwak K, Kim JS. The Role of Prebiotics in Modulating Gut Microbiota: Implications for Human Health. Int J Mol Sci 2024; 25(9): 4834.
[http://dx.doi.org/10.3390/ijms25094834] [PMID: 38732060]

[15] Rabiu BA, Gibson GR. Carbohydrates: a limit on bacterial diversity within the colon. Biol Rev Camb Philos Soc 2002; 77(3): 443-53.
[http://dx.doi.org/10.1017/S1464793102005961] [PMID: 12227522]

[16] Erdag D, Merhan O, Yildiz B. Biochemical and pharmacological properties of biogenic amines. Biog Amines 2018; 8: 1-14.

[17] Gulzar N, Saleem IM, Rafiq S, Nadeem M. Therapeutic potential of probiotics and prebiotics. Oral Health by Using Probiotic Products. Intech Open 2019.
[http://dx.doi.org/10.5772/intechopen.86762]

[18] Ryan PM, Delzenne NM. Gut microbiota and metabolism. The gut-brain axis. Academic Press 2016; pp. 391-401.
[http://dx.doi.org/10.1016/B978-0-12-802304-4.00018-9]

[19] Fujimura, K.E., Slusher, N.A., Cabana, M.D. and Lynch, S.V., Role of the gut microbiota in defining human health. Expert review of anti-infective therapy, 2010; 8(4), pp. 435-454.
[http://dx.doi.org/10.1586/eri.10.14]

[20] Andoh A. Physiological role of gut microbiota for maintaining human health. Digestion 2016; 93(3): 176-81.
[http://dx.doi.org/10.1159/000444066] [PMID: 26859303]

[21] McCallum G, Tropini C. The gut microbiota and its biogeography. Nat Rev Microbiol 2024; 22(2): 105-18.
[http://dx.doi.org/10.1038/s41579-023-00969-0] [PMID: 37740073]

[22] McCallum, G. and Tropini, C., The gut microbiota and its biogeography. Nature Reviews

Microbiology, 2024; 22(2), pp. 105-118.
[http://dx.doi.org/10.2152/jmi.63.27]

[23] Robles Alonso V, Guarner F. Linking the gut microbiota to human health. Br J Nutr 2013; 109(S2) (Suppl. 2): S21-6.
[http://dx.doi.org/10.1017/S0007114512005235] [PMID: 23360877]

[24] Li D, Wang P, Wang P, Hu X, Chen F. The gut microbiota: A treasure for human health. Biotechnol Adv 2016; 34(7): 1210-24.
[http://dx.doi.org/10.1016/j.biotechadv.2016.08.003] [PMID: 27592384]

[25] Selma MV, Espín JC, Tomás-Barberán FA. Interaction between phenolics and gut microbiota: role in human health. J Agric Food Chem 2009; 57(15): 6485-501.
[http://dx.doi.org/10.1021/jf902107d] [PMID: 19580283]

[26] Jandhyala SM, Talukdar R, Subramanyam C, Vuyyuru H, Sasikala M, Nageshwar Reddy D. Role of the normal gut microbiota. World J Gastroenterol 2015; 21(29): 8787-803.
[http://dx.doi.org/10.3748/wjg.v21.i29.8787] [PMID: 26269668]

[27] Ramakrishna BS. Role of the gut microbiota in human nutrition and metabolism. J Gastroenterol Hepatol 2013; 28(S4) (Suppl. 4): 9-17.
[http://dx.doi.org/10.1111/jgh.12294] [PMID: 24251697]

[28] Thursby E, Juge N. Introduction to the human gut microbiota. Biochem J 2017; 474(11): 1823-36.
[http://dx.doi.org/10.1042/BCJ20160510] [PMID: 28512250]

[29] Wang B, Yao M, Lv L, Ling Z, Li L. The human microbiota in health and disease. Engineering (Beijing) 2017; 3(1): 71-82.
[http://dx.doi.org/10.1016/J.ENG.2017.01.008]

[30] Conlon M, Bird A. The impact of diet and lifestyle on gut microbiota and human health. Nutrients 2014; 7(1): 17-44.
[http://dx.doi.org/10.3390/nu7010017] [PMID: 25545101]

[31] Suvorov A. Gut microbiota, probiotics, and human health. Biosci Microbiota Food Health 2013; 32(3): 81-91.
[http://dx.doi.org/10.12938/bmfh.32.81] [PMID: 24936366]

[32] Sekirov I, Russell SL, Antunes LCM, Finlay BB. Gut microbiota in health and disease. Physiol Rev 2010; 90(3): 859-904.
[http://dx.doi.org/10.1152/physrev.00045.2009] [PMID: 20664075]

[33] Chen Y, Zhou J, Wang L. Role and mechanism of gut microbiota in human disease. Front Cell Infect Microbiol 2021; 11: 625913.
[http://dx.doi.org/10.3389/fcimb.2021.625913] [PMID: 33816335]

[34] Harmsen, H.J. and De Goffau, M.C. The human gut microbiota. Microbiota of the human body: Implications in health and disease, 2016; pp. 95-108.
[http://dx.doi.org/10.1007/978-3-319-31248-4_7]

[35] Janssen AWF, Kersten S. The role of the gut microbiota in metabolic health. FASEB J 2015; 29(8): 3111-23.
[http://dx.doi.org/10.1096/fj.14-269514] [PMID: 25921831]

[36] Khan, I., Yasir, M., I Azhar, E., Kumosani, T., K Barbour, E., Bibi, F. and A Kamal, M., Implication of gut microbiota in human health. CNS & Neurological Disorders-Drug Targets (Formerly Current Drug Targets-CNS & Neurological Disorders), 2014; 13(8), pp. 1325-1333.

[37] von Martels JZH, Sadaghian Sadabad M, Bourgonje AR, *et al.* The role of gut microbiota in health and disease: *In vitro* modeling of host-microbe interactions at the aerobe-anaerobe interphase of the human gut. Anaerobe 2017; 44: 3-12.
[http://dx.doi.org/10.1016/j.anaerobe.2017.01.001] [PMID: 28062270]

[38] Morrison DJ, Preston T. Formation of short chain fatty acids by the gut microbiota and their impact on human metabolism. Gut Microbes 2016; 7(3): 189-200. [http://dx.doi.org/10.1080/19490976.2015.1134082] [PMID: 26963409]

[39] Rinninella E, Raoul P, Cintoni M, *et al.* What is the healthy gut microbiota composition? A changing ecosystem across age, environment, diet, and diseases. Microorganisms 2019; 7(1): 14. [http://dx.doi.org/10.3390/microorganisms7010014] [PMID: 30634578]

[40] Flint HJ, Scott KP, Duncan SH, Louis P, Forano E. Microbial degradation of complex carbohydrates in the gut. Gut Microbes 2012; 3(4): 289-306. [http://dx.doi.org/10.4161/gmic.19897] [PMID: 22572875]

[41] Hill MJ. Intestinal flora and endogenous vitamin synthesis. Eur J Cancer Prev 1997; 6(2) (Suppl. 1): S43-5. [http://dx.doi.org/10.1097/00008469-199703001-00009] [PMID: 9167138]

[42] Silva YP, Bernardi A, Frozza RL. The role of short-chain fatty acids from gut microbiota in gut-brain communication. Front Endocrinol (Lausanne) 2020; 11: 25. [http://dx.doi.org/10.3389/fendo.2020.00025] [PMID: 32082260]

[43] Du Y, He C, An Y, *et al.* The role of short chain fatty acids in inflammation and body health. Int J Mol Sci 2024; 25(13): 7379. [http://dx.doi.org/10.3390/ijms25137379] [PMID: 39000498]

[44] Stojanov S, Berlec A, Štrukelj B. The influence of probiotics on the firmicutes/bacteroidetes ratio in the treatment of obesity and inflammatory bowel disease. Microorganisms 2020; 8(11): 1715. [http://dx.doi.org/10.3390/microorganisms8111715] [PMID: 33139627]

[45] Krajmalnik-Brown R, Ilhan ZE, Kang DW, DiBaise JK. Effects of gut microbes on nutrient absorption and energy regulation. Nutr Clin Pract 2012; 27(2): 201-14. [http://dx.doi.org/10.1177/0884533611436116] [PMID: 22367888]

[46] Salwan R, Sharma V. Molecular and biotechnological aspects of secondary metabolites in actinobacteria. Microbiol Res 2020; 231: 126374. [http://dx.doi.org/10.1016/j.micres.2019.126374] [PMID: 31756597]

[47] Mendes R, Garbeva P, Raaijmakers JM. The rhizosphere microbiome: significance of plant beneficial, plant pathogenic, and human pathogenic microorganisms. FEMS Microbiol Rev 2013; 37(5): 634-63. [http://dx.doi.org/10.1111/1574-6976.12028] [PMID: 23790204]

[48] Salillas S, Sancho J. Flavodoxins as novel therapeutic targets against Helicobacter pylori and other gastric pathogens. Int J Mol Sci 2020; 21(5): 1881. [http://dx.doi.org/10.3390/ijms21051881] [PMID: 32164177]

[49] Jeong MY, Jang HM, Kim DH. High-fat diet causes psychiatric disorders in mice by increasing Proteobacteria population. Neurosci Lett 2019; 698: 51-7. [http://dx.doi.org/10.1016/j.neulet.2019.01.006] [PMID: 30615977]

[50] Nesic K, Ivanovic S, Nesic V. Fusarial toxins: secondary metabolites of Fusarium fungi. Rev Environ Contam Toxicol 2014; 228: 101-20. [PMID: 24162094]

[51] Hoegenauer C, Hammer HF, Mahnert A, Moissl-Eichinger C. Methanogenic archaea in the human gastrointestinal tract. Nat Rev Gastroenterol Hepatol 2022; 19(12): 805-13. [http://dx.doi.org/10.1038/s41575-022-00673-z] [PMID: 36050385]

[52] Macfarlane GT, Macfarlane S. Bacteria, colonic fermentation, and gastrointestinal health. J AOAC Int 2012; 95(1): 50-60. [http://dx.doi.org/10.5740/jaoacint.SGE_Macfarlane] [PMID: 22468341]

[53] Fluitman KS, De Clercq NC, Keijser BJF, Visser M, Nieuwdorp M, IJzerman RG. The intestinal microbiota, energy balance, and malnutrition: emphasis on the role of short-chain fatty acids. Expert

Rev Endocrinol Metab 2017; 12(3): 215-26.
[http://dx.doi.org/10.1080/17446651.2017.1318060] [PMID: 30063458]

[54] Tolhurst G, Heffron H, Lam YS, *et al.* Short-chain fatty acids stimulate glucagon-like peptide-1 secretion *via* the G-protein-coupled receptor FFAR2. Diabetes 2012; 61(2): 364-71.
[http://dx.doi.org/10.2337/db11-1019] [PMID: 22190648]

[55] Conterno L, Fava F, Viola R, Tuohy KM. Obesity and the gut microbiota: does up-regulating colonic fermentation protect against obesity and metabolic disease? Genes Nutr 2011; 6(3): 241-60.
[http://dx.doi.org/10.1007/s12263-011-0230-1] [PMID: 21559992]

[56] Lin HV, Frassetto A, Kowalik EJ Jr, *et al.* Butyrate and propionate protect against diet-induced obesity and regulate gut hormones *via* free fatty acid receptor 3-independent mechanisms. PLoS One 2012; 7(4): e35240.
[http://dx.doi.org/10.1371/journal.pone.0035240] [PMID: 22506074]

[57] Gomes AC, Hoffmann C, Mota JF. The human gut microbiota: Metabolism and perspective in obesity. Gut Microbes 2018; 9(4): 1-18.
[http://dx.doi.org/10.1080/19490976.2018.1465157] [PMID: 29667480]

[58] Brown AJ, Goldsworthy SM, Barnes AA, *et al.* The Orphan G protein-coupled receptors GPR41 and GPR43 are activated by propionate and other short chain carboxylic acids. J Biol Chem 2003; 278(13): 11312-9.
[http://dx.doi.org/10.1074/jbc.M211609200] [PMID: 12496283]

[59] Tazoe H, Otomo Y, Kaji I, Tanaka R, Karaki SI, Kuwahara A. Roles of short-chain fatty acids receptors, GPR41 and GPR43 on colonic functions. J Physiol Pharmacol 2008; 59 (Suppl. 2): 251-62. [PMID: 18812643]

[60] Topping DL, Clifton PM. Short-chain fatty acids and human colonic function: roles of resistant starch and nonstarch polysaccharides. Physiol Rev 2001; 81(3): 1031-64.
[http://dx.doi.org/10.1152/physrev.2001.81.3.1031] [PMID: 11427691]

[61] Payne AN, Chassard C, Lacroix C. Gut microbial adaptation to dietary consumption of fructose, artificial sweeteners and sugar alcohols: implications for host–microbe interactions contributing to obesity. Obes Rev 2012; 13(9): 799-809.
[http://dx.doi.org/10.1111/j.1467-789X.2012.01009.x] [PMID: 22686435]

[62] Delzenne NM, Williams CM. Prebiotics and lipid metabolism. Curr Opin Lipidol 2002; 13(1): 61-7.
[http://dx.doi.org/10.1097/00041433-200202000-00009] [PMID: 11790964]

[63] Zocco MA, Ainora ME, Gasbarrini G, Gasbarrini A. Bacteroides thetaiotaomicron in the gut: Molecular aspects of their interaction. Dig Liver Dis 2007; 39(8): 707-12.
[http://dx.doi.org/10.1016/j.dld.2007.04.003] [PMID: 17602905]

[64] de Punder K, Pruimboom L. Stress induces endotoxemia and low-grade inflammation by increasing barrier permeability. Front Immunol 2015; 6: 223.
[http://dx.doi.org/10.3389/fimmu.2015.00223] [PMID: 26029209]

[65] Houseknecht KL, Heuvel JPV, Moya-Camarena SY, *et al.* Dietary conjugated linoleic acid normalizes impaired glucose tolerance in the Zucker diabetic fatty fa/fa rat. Biochem Biophys Res Commun 1998; 244(3): 678-82.
[http://dx.doi.org/10.1006/bbrc.1998.8303] [PMID: 9535724]

[66] Begley M, Sleator RD, Gahan CGM, Hill C. Contribution of three bile-associated loci, bsh, pva, and btlB, to gastrointestinal persistence and bile tolerance of Listeria monocytogenes. Infect Immun 2005; 73(2): 894-904.
[http://dx.doi.org/10.1128/IAI.73.2.894-904.2005] [PMID: 15664931]

[67] Martinot E, Sèdes L, Baptissart M, *et al.* Bile acids and their receptors. Mol Aspects Med 2017; 56: 2-9.
[http://dx.doi.org/10.1016/j.mam.2017.01.006] [PMID: 28153453]

[68] Parker HE, Wallis K, le Roux CW, Wong KY, Reimann F, Gribble FM. Molecular mechanisms underlying bile acid-stimulated glucagon-like peptide-1 secretion. Br J Pharmacol 2012; 165(2): 414-23.
[http://dx.doi.org/10.1111/j.1476-5381.2011.01561.x] [PMID: 21718300]

[69] Frick PG, Riedler G, Brögli H. Dose response and minimal daily requirement for vitamin K in man. J Appl Physiol 1967; 23(3): 387-9.
[http://dx.doi.org/10.1152/jappl.1967.23.3.387] [PMID: 6047959]

[70] Zhan Q, Wang R, Thakur K, *et al.* Unveiling of dietary and gut-microbiota derived B vitamins: Metabolism patterns and their synergistic functions in gut-brain homeostasis. Crit Rev Food Sci Nutr 2024; 64(13): 4046-58.
[http://dx.doi.org/10.1080/10408398.2022.2138263] [PMID: 36271691]

[71] Rowland I, Gibson G, Heinken A, *et al.* Gut microbiota functions: metabolism of nutrients and other food components. Eur J Nutr 2018; 57(1): 1-24.
[http://dx.doi.org/10.1007/s00394-017-1445-8] [PMID: 28393285]

[72] Wolf PG, Biswas A, Morales SE, Greening C, Gaskins HR. H_2 metabolism is widespread and diverse among human colonic microbes. Gut Microbes 2016; 7(3): 235-45.
[http://dx.doi.org/10.1080/19490976.2016.1182288] [PMID: 27123663]

[73] Suarez F, Furne J, Springfield J, Levitt M. Insights into human colonic physiology obtained from the study of flatus composition. Am J Physiol 1997; 272(5 Pt 1): G1028-33.
[PMID: 9176210]

[74] Christl SU, Gibson GR, Murgatroyd PR, Scheppach W, Cummings JH. Impaired hydrogen metabolism in pneumatosis cystoides intestinalis. Gastroenterology 1993; 104(2): 392-7.
[http://dx.doi.org/10.1016/0016-5085(93)90406-3] [PMID: 8425681]

[75] Dai ZL, Wu G, Zhu WY. Amino acid metabolism in intestinal bacteria: links between gut ecology and host health. Front Biosci 2011; 16(1): 1768-86.
[http://dx.doi.org/10.2741/3820] [PMID: 21196263]

[76] Davila AM, Blachier F, Gotteland M, *et al.* Re-print of Intestinal luminal nitrogen metabolism: Role of the gut microbiota and consequences for the host. Pharmacol Res 2013; 69(1): 114-26.
[http://dx.doi.org/10.1016/j.phrs.2013.01.003] [PMID: 23318949]

[77] Blachier F, Mariotti F, Huneau JF, Tomé D. Effects of amino acid-derived luminal metabolites on the colonic epithelium and physiopathological consequences. Amino Acids 2007; 33(4): 547-62.
[http://dx.doi.org/10.1007/s00726-006-0477-9] [PMID: 17146590]

CHAPTER 2

Inflammatory Bowel Diseases and Gut Microbiota

Bani Kumar Jana[1], **Mohini Singh**[1], **Tumpa Sarkar**[1], **Prativa Sadhu**[1], **Deepak Chetia**[1] and **Bhaskar Mazumder**[1,*]

[1] *Department of Pharmaceutical Sciences, Dibrugarh University, Dibrugarh-786004, Assam, India*

Abstract: Inflammatory Bowel Diseases are a type of intestinal chronic inflammation affecting the gastrointestinal tract generally developed due to environmental susceptibility, immune-mediated susceptibility, gene-mediated susceptibility, and gut microbiota. These heterogeneous complex immune disorders have two subtypes commonly known as Crohn's Disease and Ulcerative Colitis. Most studies of gut dysbiosis are concerned with various forms of IBD. The gut microbiome consists of up to 100 trillion microorganisms with about 10^{11}–10^{12} cells/ml density comprising viruses, protozoa, fungi, and most abundantly different bacterial strains. Bacteria belonging to *Firmicutes*, *Bacteroides*, *Proteus*, and *Actinomycetes* phyla are the most dominant ones in the gut microbiome and any change in the combination can cause an abundance of pathogenic bacteria. A dysbiosis in the gut environment regarding the above-mentioned bacterial and other microorganism compositions may lead to gastrointestinal inflammation leading to CD and UC. Alteration in microbiota also causes an abundance of fungi like *Candida spp.* and yeast, *Malassezia spp.* especially *M. restricta* and *M. globosa* in the gut, which has been linked to severe colitis and CD. Different drug-based therapies have been used for short-term relief of symptomatic complications in IBD for the last two decades. But to avoid the side effects due to the chronic use of conventional drugs alternative strategies such as prebiotics, probiotics, and synbiotics have evolved in the past few years as effective treatment regimens. In this chapter, the abnormalities of the gut microbiome are linked with IBD, and the mechanism of the gut microbiome associated with the disease is discussed along with the novel therapies.

Keywords: Chron's disease, Dysbiosis, Gut microbiota, Inflammatory Bowel Diseases, IBD therapy, Short-chain fatty acids, Ulcerative colitis.

* **Corresponding author Bhaskar Mazumder:** Department of Pharmaceutical Sciences, Dibrugarh University, Dibrugarh-786004, Assam, India; E-mail: bhmaz@dibru.ac.in

Sandipan Dasgupta & Moitreyee Chattopadhyay (Eds.)

INTRODUCTION

Definition and Overview

The incidence rate of Inflammatory Bowel Diseases (IBD) has been found to be progressive and emerged as a major public health challenge globally. The need for early identification is underscored by the fact that millions of individuals across the globe from developed to developing nations are impacted by IBD [1]. It is an intestinal chronic inflammation affecting the gastrointestinal tract (GIT) generally developed due to environmental susceptibility, immune-mediated susceptibility, gene-mediated susceptibility, and gut microbiota. Side-by-side etiopathogenesis of IBD depends on the consumption of plant-based or animal-based processed diets, smoking, antibiotic administration, etc [2]. In 1859, Samuel Wilks suspected microbes as a potent cause of IBD in the 19th century. These heterogeneous complex immune disorders have two subtypes commonly known as Crohn's Disease (CD) and Ulcerative Colitis (UC), which could be characterized by a disrupted mucosa structure, systemic biochemical abnormalities, and altered gut microbial composition affecting 0.3% to 0.5% people [3]. Developed countries, *viz.* North America, Australia, New Zealand, and Europe faced the highest incidents and it has also increased in developing countries *viz.* Brazil, South Korea, and China. The incidence of UC and CD was found to be 11.6 cases/lakh and 1.4 cases/lakh per year, respectively in China [4, 5]. Chronic inflammation of the colonic mucosa is observed in UC, whereas CD often involves the GI tract from the mouth to the anus and could be patchy, and transmural. Diarrhea, bloody stools, and abdominal spasms are the clinical manifestations of IBD [6]. If the gut microbial composition of healthy individuals and IBD patients is compared, prominent differences will link IBD with the gut microorganisms. Experimental IBD models using chemicals or genetic modulation abolish disease development or attenuate effectively under germ-free conditions mentioning the microbes as a major factor in IBD where any mismatches in host-microbe interactions promote the disease. The gut microbiome consists of up to 100 trillion microorganisms with about 10^{11}–10^{12} cells/ml density comprising viruses, protozoa, fungi, bacteriophage, and archaea being the most abundantly different bacterial strains [7]. It should be noted that most studies on altered gut microbiota, *i.e.*, gut dysbiosis associated it with various forms of IBD (Fig. **1**). In the gut microbiome, these microorganisms actively participate in nutritional absorption, immunity modulation, and combating pathogens and metabolize short-chain fatty acids (SCFAs) namely propionic acid, butyric acid, *etc.* which provide energy to the intestinal epithelium [8, 9]. The immunosuppressive potential of these beneficial bacteria regulates host immune cells. Immune cell interactions with pathogenic bacteria and bacterial metabolites can increase GI damage by inducing inflammatory cytokines.

Bacteria belonging to *Firmicutes* and *Bacteroides* are the most dominant ones among *Firmicutes*, *Bacteroides*, *Proteus*, and *Actinomycetes* phyla, which cumulatively comprise 90% of gut bacterial flora in healthy individuals. *Ruminicoccus*, *Lactobacillus*, *Bacillus*, *Clostridium*, and *Enterococcus* are the primary genus from *Firmicutes* phylum [10]. In the gut microbiome, pathogenic bacteria such as *Bacteroides fragilis*, *Ruminococcus torques*, *and Ruminococcus* are found with relatively higher growth rates in UC and CD, whereas the levels of beneficial bacteria *viz.* *Bifidobacterium longum*, *Faecalibacterium prausnitzii*, *Roseburia intestinalis*, and *Eubacterium rectale*, *etc.* were found to be prominently reduced [11, 12]. In CD patients, there is a rise in *Actinomyces*, *Escherichia coli*, and *Veillonella* spp. families whereas the *Coriobacteriaceae* and *Christensenellaceae* families, and *Clostridium leptum* in particular, decrease. Bacteriophages and archaea appear to be less abundant in an active disease in the human GIT [13, 14]. On the other hand, fungi like *Candida albicans* display an increased abundance but *Saccharomyces cerevisiae* has a decreased count during the pathogenesis of IBD. *Malassezia* especially *M. restricta* and *M. globosa* has also been linked to severe colitis caused by yeast in animals and the intestinal mucosa of CD patients [15]. Generally, corticosteroids, amino-salicylates, immunosuppressive, and biological agents have been used for short-term relief of symptomatic complications in IBD for the last two decades but prominent side effects like immunodeficiency and resistance of drugs have taken place. Novel therapeutic strategies *viz.* synbiotics, prebiotics, and probiotics have evolved in the past few years. Other than that, surgical therapies, gene-mediated therapies, and other related future therapies are now adopted and exposed to clinical trials [16]. In this chapter, the abnormalities of the gut microbiome linked with IBD and the mechanism associated with the disease are discussed. In a nutshell, the population, classification, and diagnosis of the GIT microbiome along with its contribution to the pathogenesis of IBD, and respective therapies were demonstrated.

Effect of Gut Microbiota on Ibd and its Mechanism

In the human body, a symbiotic relationship is consistent between a host and gut bacteria where the host provides residence and nutrients, but gut bacteria contribute by producing SCFAs and vitamins in the host [9]. Different species including bacteria, fungi, and viruses constitute the human gut microbiome where over 90% of beneficial bacteria are from diverse subspecies of a few major phyla *i.e.*, *Bacteroidetes*, *Actinobacteria*, *Firmicutes*, and *Proteobacteria*. *Ruminicoccus*, *Lactobacillus*, *Bacillus*, *Enterococcus,* and *Clostridium (Clostridium XIVa* and *IV* groups*)* are the primary genera of the *Firmicutes* phylum [10]. Existing beneficial bacteria get reduced and pathogens may increase, which could be referred to as dysbiosis. The beneficial and pathogenic bacterial imbalance between taxa causes damage to the intestinal microbial barrier [17]. Medications mostly antibiotics, diet, age, smoking, *etc.* correspond to different factors associated with dysbiosis [2, 18]. Some diagnostic factors should be taken under consideration like sample type either mucosal or fecal, sampling location either inflamed or non-inflamed sites, disease activity either active or quiescent, *etc.* An increase in *Proteobacteria* was observed in IBD patients. *Firmicutes, Clostridium leptum* namely *Faecalibacterium prausnitzii*, has also been reported to be decreased in IBD, mostly in UC patients [19, 20]. Normal anaerobic bacteria *viz. Lactobacillus*, *Bacteroides*, *Eubacterium*, *Escherichia*, and *Ruminococcus* are found to be decreased. It was hypothesized that particular enrichment of *Malassezia* namely *M. restricta* and *M. globose* can promote IBD [15]. Additionally, it has been shown that an individual's gut microbiome varies between inflammatory and noninflammatory regions. The elevated overall level of bacteria in the mucosal layer associated with IBD indicates a compromised mucosal barrier function. Most of the UC-susceptible genes correspond with mucosal barrier function. The physiological functions relate bacteria and susceptible genes in IBD by acquired immunity, bacterial recognition, and processing, autophagy, and mucosal barrier [21]. Bacteria like *Ruminococcus gnavus* and *Ruminococcus torques* increased in IBD, damaging mucins to be utilized as energy sources. Furthermore, for nutrition, gut microbiota competes with the pathogenic bacteria, and the general microbiome thus plays an antagonistic role against the pathogenic bacteria. In UC inflammation, an increase in sulfate-reducing bacteria (SRB) producing hydrogen sulfide was observed [22]. A "dysbiosis index," was shown to be associated with the clinical disease proposed by Gevers *et al.* to assess the severity of Crohn's Disease Index [23]. Hence, the simultaneous presence of the gut microorganism and host reveals that the gut microbial flora has a major role in host health and overall systemic physiology. Genetic and environmental factors are the main reasons for dysbiosis. A decrease in genes responsible for carbohydrates and amino acid metabolism initiating oxidative pathways in IBD patients raises the possibility that oxidative stress in the gut microbiota causes intestinal inflammation in IBD patients [24]. Human *Lactobacillus* produces lactobacillin thereby preventing *Listeria monocytogenes* infection [25]. An increased intestinal epithelial permeability can limit the absorption of ascorbic acid through the NF-κB pathway caused by enterotoxin from Enterotoxigenic *E. coli* (ETEC) [26]. The normal gut microbiome is considered similar to a homeostatic organ and aids in the production of SCFAs, vitamin synthesis, and energy development. Tryptophan imbalance, bile acids, SCFAs, and over 2,700 bacterial metabolites are closely linked to IBD [27].

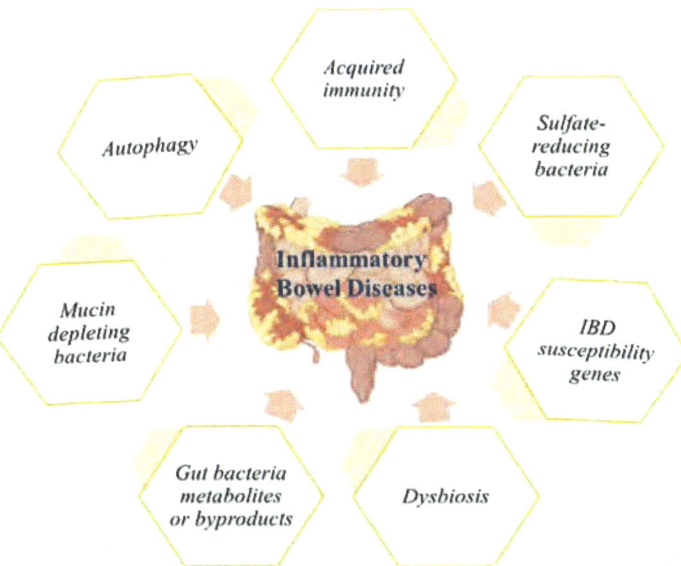

Fig. (1). Possible mechanisms of IBD associated with gut microbiome.

SCFAs promote the expansion of B cells and increase regulatory T cells (T-reg) to regulate mucosal immunity, which could activate inflammatory cytokine rush and relate SCFAs to IBD in an inversely proportional manner [28]. To be precise, butyric acid increases the quantity and efficiency of T-reg in intestinal mucosa immune cells and inhibits dendritic cells, macrophages, and neutrophils to exhibit their natural mechanism. SCFAs also activate Nucleotide-binding oligomerization domains (NOD) like receptors including three pyridine domains via G-protei--coupled receptor (GPCR-43 and GPCR-109) thereby influencing ion efflux and regulating interleukin (IL-18) to promote epithelial repair in UC [29]. SCFA depletion occurs as a result of antibiotics initiating the transition of M1 hyperreactive phenotype, producing pro-inflammatory cytokines and thereby inducing GI inflammation [30]. When cells are starving, an internal mechanism called autophagy helps break down and recycle proteins. IBD is additionally triggered by intracellular infections, which are handled by autophagy. The immune responses by T cells may influence the IBD [31]. Helper T cells (Th cells) develop inflammatory responses to protect the host from pathogens, but the development of intestinal inflammation occurs when over-activated. In the intestine, effector T cells can initiate excessive immune response, which results in intestinal mucosal injury since T-reg cells conduct limited immunosuppressive regulation [32]. Activation of Th1 and Th17 cells is generally observed in CD, while Th1 and Th2 cell interaction cause UC [33]. Under normal circumstances, both Th17 and T-reg cells are in balance but any imbalance *viz.* Th17 increase and decrease in T-regs cells indicates the occurrence of IBD. By influencing the intestinal microenvironment, the gut microbiome can encourage T cells to produce Th 17, T-reg, and other phenotypes. Garrett *et al.* reported antibiotics ameliorated spontaneous UC in mice due to a deficiency of Tbx21, which is an immune cell transcription factor required for Th1 differentiation indispensable for the acquired immune system [34]. When wild-type mice were co-housed with both Tbx21 and Recombination-activating genes deficient mice with colitis, the healthy wild mice also developed similar colitis, which can be concluded that dysbiosis is communicable also. Th17 is countered by gut bacteria from *Clostridia* and *Bacteroides* genera by balancing T-reg cell responses with anti-inflammatory cytokines management. By stimulating the 'Farnesoid X receptor' and lowering the rate of action of bile salt hydrolase in individuals with inflammatory bowel disease, bile acids have an immunomodulatory effect that leads to an unbalance amongst both primary and secondary bile acids [35]. Heineken *et al.* reported that every bacterium can synthesize 6-13 kinds of secondary bile acids. Bacterial antigenic signals *viz.* retinoic acid from *Clostridium* cluster IV and XIVa, polysaccharide A from *Bacteroides fragilis* and *Faecalibacterium prausnitzii* trigger an immune response and accumulate regulatory T cells [36]. Modified bile acids activate immune response regulators *viz.* T-regs and Th17, which promote inflammation [37]. Dietary tryptophan is also metabolized by casein and serotonin pathways and indole pathways. Biologically activated indole could be generated by bacteria from tryptophan to inhibit inflammatory cytokines induction and activate aryl hydrocarbon receptors [38]. Caspase recruitment domain-containing protein 9 (CARD9) activates the IL-22 pathway thereby promoting the recovery of colitis. The metabolic limitation of GIT bacteria cannot degrade tryptophan in the CARD9 knockout mouse model [39]. *B. thetaiotaomicron* promotes T-regs to affect the immune system in IBD patients, recapitulating impacts of gut microbiota throughout the illness while *F. prausnitzii* is an intestinal bacterium that produces butyrate, inhibits IL-6/ IL-17 and promotes 'Forkhead Box Protein P3' [40, 41]. In human colonic mucosa, *F. prausnitzii*-specific T cells (CD4 and CD8a), were found to have T-reg cell-like properties. On the other hand, *K. pneumoniae* had almost no effect on anti-inflammatory and T-reg cells rather it promoted Th1 induction in UC [42]. In a symbiotic relationship with humans, *B. fragilis* secretes outer membrane vesicles (OMVs), which are used to transfer immunological regulatory chemicals to immune cells. The OMV function activates the non-classical autophagy pathway and is strongly linked to NOD2 and *Atg16L1* genes, thereby countering IBD. The expression of NOD2 is shown in intestinal epithelial cells as well as monocytes. NOD2 overexpression in CD patients impart malfunction in antimicrobial peptide (AMP) production from Paneth cells as well as reduced production of IL-10, which is an anti-inflammatory cytokine in peripheral mononuclear cells [43].

When intestinal epithelial cells are invaded by *Klebsiella pneumoniae*, they interact with macrophages and cause the production of interleukin IL-1β and tumor necrosis factor [44]. By NOD2, *Fusobacterium nucleatum* can stimulate colonic Caspase Activation and Recruitment Domain 3 (CARD3), an inflammation modulator protein kinase. This causes the activation of the IL-17F/NF-κB signaling pathway resulting in the promotion of intestinal inflammation [45]. Another CD-susceptible gene is *Atg16L,* essential for autophagosome formation. Dendritic cells with *Atg16L1* deficiency are unable to induce T-regs cells and *Atg16L1* mutation points out deficiencies in the Tregs response to OMV [46]. It was found that genetically modified mice with increased intestinal epithelial cell expression of one of the AMPs, *i.e.*, α-defensin had reduced 'Segmented Filamentous Bacteria' (SFB) in GIT, which led to impaired Th17 formation highlighting the critical role paneth cells play in balancing of the gut microbiota and intestinal immune system [47]. The colonization of SFB in the small intestine of mice can stimulate the production of IL-17 and IL-22, hence promoting intestinal inflammation. Paneth cells, which house AMPs, exhibit abnormalities in the quantity, size, and location of their granules observed in CD [48]. *Xbp1* is another CD-susceptible gene that induces impaired autophagy in paneth cells thereby inducing chronic ileitis [49]. In SIRT1 mutant animals, Paneth cells are activated and stimulate the NF-κB pathway, causing inflammation in the ileum. Because of modifications in bile acid metabolism, SIRT1 mutant animals have a different fecal microbiome. Furthermore, compared to control mice, SIRT1 deletion animals with dysbiosis experienced more severe colitis [50]. With the Nod-like receptor (NLR) family, in particular, some research links metabolic abnormalities of intestinal epithelial cells to the gut microbiota. NLRX1 which is a mitochondria-related NLR is required for barrier function and glutamine metabolism [51, 52]. The abundance of *Veillonella* spp. and *Clostridium* spp. is high in NLRX1 deficient mice [53]. The decline in H_2S detoxification and the rise in the relative number of H_2S-producing bacteria are also associated with mitochondrial damage in CD patients. There exists a correlation between the severity of CD patients and the quantity of H_2S-producing bacteria, *Atopobium parvulum*. In the intestinal mucosa of more than 50% of individuals with CD, adherent-invasive *E. Coli* (AIEC) colonization is seen [54]. Through employing FimH and cell adhesion molecule 6, AIEC is able to get through the mucus layer and attach to intestinal epithelial cells, eventually colonizing the intestinal mucosa [55]. *Enterobacteriaceae* can drive the progression of IBD by pushing the pflB gene, which codes for pyruvate formate lyase, by utilizing soluble substances released by intestinal epithelial cells. This promotes colonization and proliferation of the bacteria [56].

GUT POPULATION AND DIAGNOSIS OF PROBIOTICS, SPECIFICALLY FOCUSING ON THE PHYLUM, FAMILY, GENUS, AND SPECIES CLASSIFICATIONS

Probiotics are defined as "live microorganisms that, when given in sufficient quantities, impart a health benefit on the host" by the 'International Scientific Association for Probiotics and Prebiotics' [57]. These non-beneficial microorganisms found in fermented foods, mostly bacteria and yeasts can be added to food products and nutritional supplements. However, not every food on the market that has a probiotic label or dietary supplement has been shown to provide health advantages. Probiotics can be recognized by their unique strain, which has an alphanumeric strain name together with the genus, species, and subspecies [58]. The seven main bacteria genera that are most frequently found in probiotic products are *Bacillus, Saccharomyces, Bifidobacterium, Enterococcus, Streptococcus,* and *Escherichia*. Prebiotics, which are usually complex carbohydrates like inulin and other fructo-oligosaccharides that microorganisms in the gastrointestinal tract need as metabolic fuel, should not be mistaken for probiotics [59]. Synbiotics are frequently defined as commercial products that contain both probiotic microbes and prebiotic carbohydrates. Furthermore, by definition, probiotics do not include compounds that are manufactured of bacteria or that contain dead microorganisms, such as proteins, and polysaccharides. Mucosal inflammation and immunological dysfunction associated with IBD can significantly change local ecosystems by impacting intestinal permeability, mucus composition and content, mucosal gene expression, cellular content, and immune signals in the gut. Additionally, these alterations have an impact on the dynamics and connection between microbial members in the gut as well as the assemblage, function, and healthy host-microbe interactions that in vulnerable individuals promote inflammation and immune activation. This section examines current data demonstrating how host factors affect the gut microbiota [57, 60]. Negative changes to the microbial ecology in the gut are known as dysbiosis and are linked to both health and illness [61]. The pathophysiology of IBD is mostly dependent on the global modification of the gut microbial ecology rather than the existence of particular genera. Previous research utilizing faecal samples revealed dysbiosis in IBD, which is typified by an increase in the phylum *Proteobacteria* and a decrease in the abundance of the phylum *Firmicutes* (such as *Faecalibacterium, Roseburia,* and *Ruminococcus*) [60]. Similar results have also been observed in mucus samples, where there is a considerable rise in the abundance of putatively aggressive bacteria, including those of the genera *Escherichia, Ruminococcus* (*R. gnavus*), and *Fusobacteria*. Compared to UC, these alterations are more noticeable in CD [60, 62]. Comparing mucus samples from CD patients to healthy controls, similar results have also been observed, showing a significant increase in the abundance of putatively aggressive bacteria like the genus *Escherichia*, the genus *Ruminococcus (R. gnavus),* and *Fusobacteria* species, and a significant decrease in the abundance of bacteria like the genera *Faecalibacterium, Coprococcus, and Roseburia* [63]. It has been claimed that in about 70% of healthy persons, fungi can be found in the GI system. They make up about 0.1% of the gut microbiome and interact with bacteria and viruses in the gut antagonistically, cooperatively, or both [64]. From the ileum to the colon, the number of fungi grows progressively and reaches its peak at the distal colon. Compared to bacteria, the variety and quantity of fungi in the GI tract are far smaller, and their composition is thought to be both diverse and unstable [65]. *Ascomycota, Basidiomycota,* and *Chytridiomycota* are the most common phyla of the human GI tract mycobiome. Other fungal genera, including *Aspergillus, Cryptococcus, Rhodotorula, Mucor*, and *Trichosporon*, are less common than the genus *Candida*. The gut bacterial community interacts with the gut virome, primarily made up of bacteriophages (phages), to affect gut homeostasis and pathogenic conditions [66, 67]. Ninety percent of viruses are eukaryotic, meaning they infect humans, plants, and animals. The remaining 10 percent are viruses that infect prokaryotic cells, such as bacteria and/or archaea [68]. In the infected cells (bacteria), phages multiply and multiply until they are discharged through cell rupture (the lytic cycle) [67]. The lytic cycle significantly influences the composition of gut bacteria and changes the ratio of bacterial strains. Conversely, certain phages transfer viral genomic information to the following host generation by directly inserting their genetic material into the genome of the infected cells.

Mapping of Gut Microbial Flora in IBD

Opportunistic infections colonize and invade the gut as a result of an imbalance in microbial homeostasis, which raises the possibility of a host immune response and encourages the onset of inflammatory bowel disease.

Fig. (**2**) is a depiction of IBD-mediated inflammation, generation of ROS, and downregulation in good bacterial flora. Determining the precise pathogens connected to the etiology of IBD is essential. It is crucial to have a thorough grasp of the many pathogenic variables in order to identify IBD early on. This study emphasizes how the gut microbiota contributes to the pathophysiology of inflammatory bowel disease and offers treatment approaches that alter the gut microbiota. Ten to one hundred trillion microorganisms, including bacteria, viruses, protozoa, and fungi, make up the human microbiota [69, 70]. Numerous aspects including nutrition, immunity, metabolism, and defence against pathogens, are significantly influenced by gut bacteria [71]. By controlling host immune cells, beneficial bacteria in GIT can have an immunosuppressive effect [72]. In order to exacerbate intestinal damage, certain pathogenic bacteria can also trigger the release of inflammatory cytokines through interactions with immune cells or their metabolites [73]. Here, we go over the harmful interactions between the microbial communities and the immune system, metabolome, and intestinal epithelium of IBD patients. We also talk about the useful approaches that microbiota-based medicines employ to treat IBD patients and provide protection from infections [71]. IBD development is largely influenced by the makeup and diversity of the gut microbiota [74]. Table **1** is a compilation of the altered gut bacterial flora in Chron's disease and ulcerative colitis, which are two major subtypes of IBD.

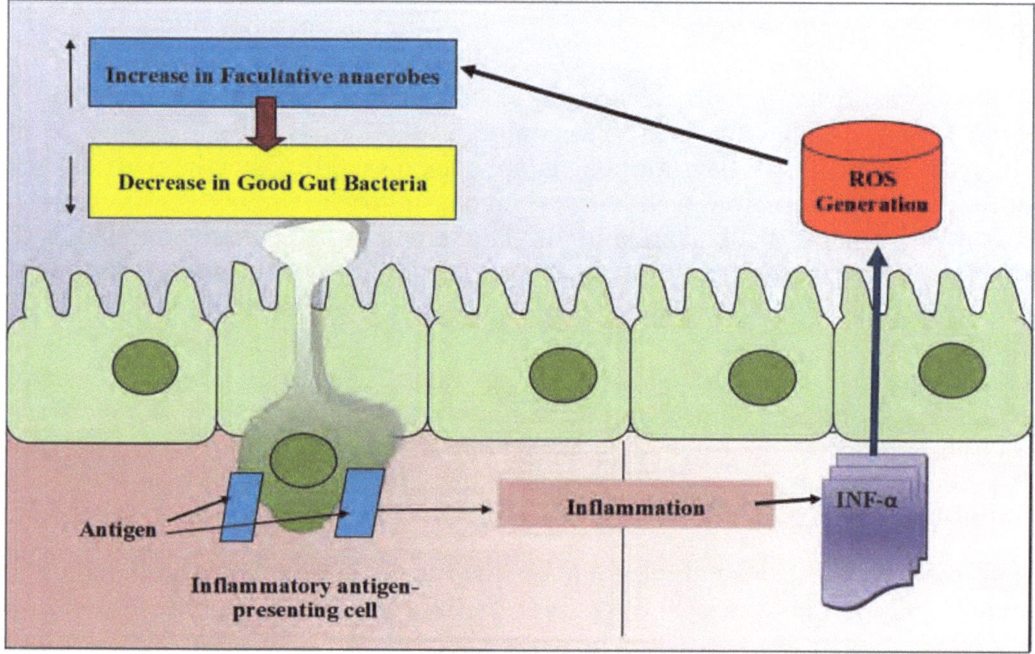

Fig. (2). Inflammation-mediated decrease in beneficial bacterial flora in IBD, A pictorial depiction of downregulation.

Table 1. The altered gut bacterial flora in Chron's disease and ulcerative colitis.

IBD Types	Gut Microbiota	Abundance	Reference
UC & CD	*Ruminococcus torques*	High proliferation	[7]
UC & CD	*Clostridium hathewayi*	High proliferation	[7]
UC & CD	*Clostidridium bolteae*	High proliferation	[7]
CD	*Clostridium leptum*	Less abundant	[13]
	Coriobacteriaceae	Less abundant	[13]
	Actinomyces	High proliferation	[13]
UC & CD	*Escherichia coli*	High proliferation	[13]

(Table 1) cont.....

IBD Types	Gut Microbiota	Abundance	Reference
CD	*Clostridium leptum*	Less abundant	[13]
UC & CD	*Ruminococcus gnavus*	High proliferation	[75]
UC & CD	*Faecalibacterium prausnitzil*	Less abundant	[76]
UC & CD	*Eubacterium rectum*	Less abundant	[13]
UC & CD	*Roseburia Intestinalis*	Less abundant	[76]
UC	*Bifidobacterium Longum*	Less abundant	[76]
	Eubacterium rectale	Less abundant	[76]
	Akkermansia muciniphilia	Less abundant	[13]

Early on in the course of IBD, the gut microbiota's makeup may alter. According to certain research, people with CD have a higher degree of dysbiosis than people with UC [77]. *Roseburia intestinalis, Eubacterium rectale, Faecalibacterium prausnitzii, Bifidobacterium longum*, and other beneficial bacteria were significantly lower in CD and UC when compared to healthy controls. The notable variations in the abundance of *Clostridium hathewayi, Clostridium bolteae*, and *Ruminococcus gnavus* indicate that a small number of strains also exhibit increased transcriptional activity [7]. Patients with CD had decreased levels of the families Christensenellaceae, *Coriobacteriaceae,* and especially *Clostridium leptum*, but increased levels of *Actinomyces spp.*, *Veillonella spp.*, and *Escherichia coli.* According to Pittayanon *et al.* (2020), there is an enrichment of *Eubacterium rectum* and a decrease in *Akkermansia muciniphila* in UC patients, but an increase in *E. coli* levels. According to a comparative analysis, the number of *Coprococcus spp.* considerably drops in CD, but the abundance of *Intestinibacter spp.* increases in both CD and UC [78]. According to Hall et al., *R. gnavus* is substantially more prevalent in IBD Patients. *R. gnavus. A. muciniphila* is a pathobiont that has been found to stimulate the growth of IBD and 'NOD-like receptor 6' (NLRP6). It is also observed to be an important modulator of *A. muciniphila* abundance. The low *Roseburia* abundance is associated with IBD-related genes, including CARD9, NOD2, ATG16L1, IRGM, and FUT2. When comparing patients with active IBD to healthy persons, the prevalence of *Blastocystis spp.* was lower in the former group. In the etiology of IBD, the immune system's genetic variations significantly influence the microbiota. There is mounting evidence linking the pathophysiology of inflammatory bowel disease to the effects of environment and genetic vulnerability on gut microbiota [75].

Bacterial Microbiota and IBD

It has been shown that gut microbes play a critical role in intestinal inflammation in people with IBD [79]. A dysbiosis was found, decreasing the count of phylum

Firmicutes and *Bacteroides*, and increasing abundances of *Gammaproteobacteria* suggesting that dysbiosis occurs in IBD [80, 81]. It has been repeatedly demonstrated that there is a decline in species and biodiversity, specifically alpha diversity, in IBD. When compared to healthy controls, patients with CD had less α diversity in their faecal microbiome. Monozygotic twins who were discordant for CD also showed similar results. According to Martinez *et al.* (2008), there was a correlation between the declining diversity and the dominating taxa's temporal instability in IBD. Even within the same patient, there is less variation between inflammatory and non-inflammatory tissues, and bacterial loads were found to be lower in inflammatory areas in CD patients [82]. According to Manichanh *et al.* (2012), CD patients had less α diversity in their faecal microbiome than healthy controls [83]. Dicksved *et al.* (2008) observed comparable results in monozygotic twins who were discordant for CD. The temporal instability of the dominating taxa in IBD was partially attributed to this decline in diversity [84]. Additionally, even within the same patient, there is less variation between inflammatory and non-inflammatory tissues, and in CD patients, the inflammatory regions show a lower bacterial burden [85]. Another clade of invasive and adherent bacteria is Fusobacteria. Germs belonging to the *Fusobacterium* primarily inhabit the gut and mouth cavities. Compared to healthy controls, patients with UC have more *Fusobacterium* species in their colonic mucosa. *Fusobacterium varium* was able to induce inflammation of the colonic mucosa in rats when given by rectal enema [86]. According to Strauss *et al.* (2011), the degree of IBD in the host is positively correlated with the invasiveness of human *Fusobacterium* bacteria. This suggests that invasive *Fusobacterium* species may have an effect on IBD pathogenesis. Furthermore, studies on colorectal cancer have shown that *Fusobacterium* species are more prevalent in the tumor than in the nearby normal tissue [87, 88]. It has been demonstrated that *Faecalibacterium prausnitzii* possesses anti-inflammatory qualities and is underrepresented [89]. In CD ileum specimens, the quantity of E. coli was substantially higher than that of *F. prausnitzii* mice's involvement in carcinogenesis [90]. Following surgery, patients with CD who have reduced mucosal abundances of *F. prausnitzii* are more prone to experience relapses [90]. On the other hand, preservation of clinical remission of UC is linked to restoration of *F. prausnitzii* following recurrence. Infection by *Helicobacter pylori* may be protective against the onset of autoimmune illnesses, such as IBD, according to epidemiological evidence in humans [91]. According to findings from laboratories, *H. pylori* can restrict inflammatory responses and induce immunological tolerance [92].

Fungal Microbiota and IBD

Fungi comprise less than 0.1 percent of all bacteria and are a tiny component of the gut microbiota [93]. Because of the existing difficulty in annotating fungi due to an inadequate fungal genome database, this may be underestimated [94]. However, target region sequencing of marker genes, including 18S rRNA and 'Internal Transcribed Spacer' has increased our knowledge of the gut microbiota [93]. In humans, the makeup of fungi varies in different bodily regions. The majority of the up to 160 species that make up the genus *Candida* are found in the urogenital tract, GIT, and buccal cavity [95, 96]. Mammals exhibit species-specific patterns of *Candida* colonization. While *C. tropicalis* is more frequent in mice, *Candida albicans*, *C. parapsilosis*, and *C. blabrata* are commonly found [94]. It was noted that fungi and gut bacteria competed with one another. Relatively long-term antibiotic usage in humans and mice can encourage fungal overgrowth and infection [95, 97]. According to these results, exposure to mould spores can cause an allergic airway to develop in the host due to fungal overgrowth in the stomach caused by antibiotics. These findings provide credence to the idea that immune-mediated illnesses are influenced by the gut microbiota. *Saccharomyces, Candida*, and *Cladosporium* were the most common genera in healthy persons [96]. It has been demonstrated that patients with IBD have significantly higher levels of *Basidiomycota, Ascomycota*, and *C. albicans* [87, 89, 98]. Nonetheless, information regarding the makeup of the mucosa's fungus has only lately begun to emerge. Liguori *et al.* assessed the fungal makeup of the gut in both healthy individuals and CD patients. Furthermore, *Xylariales* were raised in the inflamed mucosa of CD, while *Saccharomyces cerevisiae* and *Filobasidium uniguttulatum* were considerably enhanced in the non-inflamed mucosa [98]. UC patients displayed a comparatively lower diversity of fungus than CD patients did due to altered bile acid reabsorption and a decrease in the inhibition of antimicrobial peptides. Overall, these early findings imply that the pathogenic characteristic of CD may be linked to a higher fungal burden of Candida species and a changed bacterial diversity.

Viral Microbiota and IBD

As high-throughput sequencing methods continue to grow in popularity, the significance of the gut virobiota is becoming increasingly clear [99]. Prokaryotic bacteriophages and eukaryotic viruses make up the virobiota, often known as the viral component of the microbiota. Compared to the gut bacterial microbiota, they comprise a wider variety of biological entities [100, 101]. dsDNA *Caudovirales* and ssDNA *Microviridae* bacteriophages are major components of the healthy gut virome. In terms of health, gut bacteriophages exhibit significant subject variation while remaining stable over time in each individual. Although their role in the pathophysiology of the disease is still unclear, bacteriophages are thought to be involved in IBD [102]. Compared to controls, CD individuals showed a larger variability in gut microbiota. According to Norman *et al.* (2015), CD and UC patients from Boston, Chicago, and the United Kingdom have higher virome richness. Children with CD had higher levels of *Caudovirales,* a bacteriophage in intestinal tissues [102, 103]. Moreover, CD specimens visualized using electron microscopy have produced *Caudovirales* virions [104]. The emergence of additional viruses from the surrounding environment or commensal bacteria joining lytic cycles could be the cause of the bacteriophage proliferation in IBD. Changes in the makeup of bacteriophages may also affect the ecology of the bacterial microbiota in the interim. According to research, bacteriophages are the main factors influencing bacterial diversity and fitness [105]. Furthermore, bacteriophage invasion of the gut microbiome can alter the abundance of particular species of bacteria. Bacteriophages in the gastrointestinal tract facilitate the horizontal transmission of genetic elements, such as those involved in antibiotic resistance and disease pathogenesis, between bacterial populations [104]. Therefore, broad bacteriophage acquisition in IBD coupled with elevated virome richness—possibly from outside sources—could significantly alter bacterial fitness. A western diet may cause the *Caudovirales* to spread in mice, suggesting that food may have an impact on the gut virome [106].

LATEST TREATMENT APPROACHES

Here are some of the latest approaches and trends in treating IBD Table **2** and understanding the role of the microbiota (Fig. **3**):

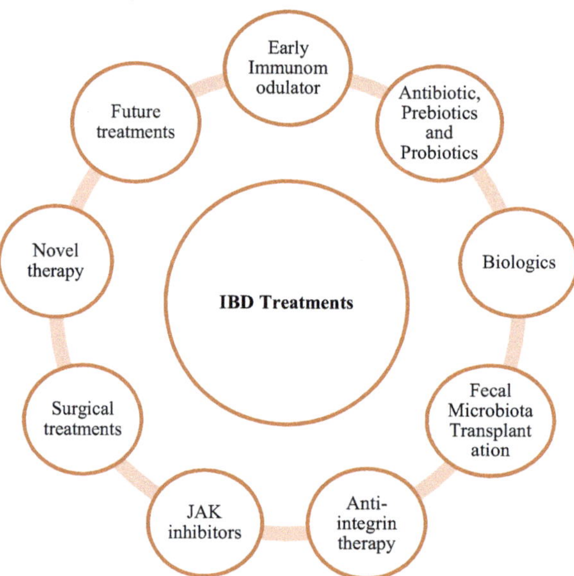

Fig. (3). Different approaches in treatment of inflammatory bowel diseases.

Table 2. Treatment approaches in treating IBD.

Treatment Type	Related Drug	Mechanism of Action	Side Effects
Early Immunomodulator	Corticosteroid (*e.g.* prednisone, prednisolone, hydrocortisone, *etc.*)	Reduce the synthesis of inflammatory cytokines and disrupt the synthesis of NF-κB.	Bone loss, infection, adrenal insufficiency, immunosuppression, hyperglycemia, etc [107, 108, 155].
Antibiotics, Prebiotics and Probiotics	Ciprofloxacin	Controlling cytokine production to modulate immunological responses	Diarrhea, enterocolitis caused by *Clostridium difficile*, and liver problems [114]
	Lactobacilli spp.	Innate immunity is a crucial component of host defense.	Gaseousness, bloating abdominal pain, and diarrhea [114]
Biologics	Adalimumab	TNF blocking mediators	Responses at the injection site [119]
	Vedolizumab	Anti-leukocyte trafficking agent	Development of lymphoma, non-melanoma skin malignancies [124]
Fecal Microbiota Transplantation	--------	The GI tract of a patient receives fecal microbiota transplanted from a healthy donor.	Moderate fever, diarrhea, constipation, and abdominal discomfort [156]
Anti-integrin therapy	Etrolizumab	Prevents leukocytes from adhering to intestinal blood arteries by blocking integrin on the surface of circulating immune cells.	Headache, arthralgia, nausea, and nasopharyngitis [145]
JAK inhibitors	Upadacitinib, filgotinib	Cytokines promote intracellular signaling by activating JAK/STAT pathway.	High cholesterol, thrombosis, serious adverse cardiovascular events, and cancer [141, 157]
Surgical treatments	-------	Ileocolectomy, partial colectomy	Wound infection at the surgical site, acute and chronic anastomotic leaks, and anastomotic strictures [153]

Early Immunomodulator

In recent years, the landscape of Inflammatory Bowel Diseases (IBD) management has witnessed a notable shift towards early immunomodulators as a pioneering approach to tackle the intricate interplay between immunological dysregulation and gut microbiota. This paradigmatic change stems from the understanding that IBD, comprising Crohn's disease and ulcerative colitis, is not solely a result of overt inflammation but involves a complex interplay of genetic susceptibility, environmental factors, and dysregulation of the immune response [114]. Salazopyrin, a salicylate compound, inadvertently became the first drug to exhibit therapeutic effects in ulcerative colitis (UC) during the late 1940s [115]. Since then, various topical and oral formulations of 5-aminosalicylic acid have been available (5-ASA). However, it is believed that their effects are mediated through prostaglandin synthesis regulation specifically pro-inflammatory cytokine downregulation [116]. While 5-ASA compounds were once the sole therapeutic option for inflammatory bowel disease, they are currently recommended primarily for mild UC patients but not for severe UC or CD patients [107, 108]. Corticosteroids (CSs) also gain appreciation as therapeutic agents in the management of inflammatory bowel disease. These compounds bind to cytoplasmic DNA receptors and cause inhibition of DNA synthesis thereby suppressing the inflammation. Initially, corticosteroids emerged as the primary treatment for IBD [109]. However, corticosteroids are effective in initiating remission, they are less suitable for sustainable therapy. Budesonide, a steroid exhibiting some degree of specificity for the intestines, presents a mitigated side effect profile compared to systemic steroids [110]. Immunomodulators *viz.* Azathioprine and 6-mercaptopurine downregulate T lymphocytes and the immune system by antagonizing purine metabolism, demonstrating a prolonged and delayed therapeutic effect [107]. Primarily suitable for maintenance therapy, these drugs are infrequently employed as standalone treatments due to inadequate efficacy and marked adverse effects like hepatotoxicity, rash, myelosuppression, skin cancer, etc [111, 112]. Methotrexate was also found beneficial for inducing and maintaining remission in CD. However, its standalone use is rare. Cyclosporine and tacrolimus are found to be used due to their neoteric efficacy and negligible side effects [113].

Antibiotics, Prebiotics, and Probiotics

During the transitional period spanning the 1980s to the early 2000s, antibiotics emerged as a pivotal component in the therapeutic arsenal for managing IBD. A plethora of antibiotics, encompassing rifaximin, clarithromycin, metronidazole, ciprofloxacin, amoxicillin, tetracyclines, and vancomycin, were systematically evaluated either in isolation or through diverse combinations. Despite the theoretical justifications underpinning their use, the outcomes of several randomized clinical trials underscored the limited efficacy of antibiotics, revealing trivial to minor benefits and an absence of prolonged effects. Consequently, antibiotics have transitioned from routine application in the treatment of UC or CD to selective deployment in specific clinical contexts, such as pouchitis treatment, perianal CD therapy, or prophylaxis for post-operative CD [114]. In the contemporary landscape of IBD management, antibiotics play a nuanced role tailored to specific clinical scenarios. Pouchitis, an inflammatory condition affecting the surgically created pouch in patients with UC, stands out as a context where antibiotics find continued utility. Moreover, antibiotics are strategically employed as adjunctive therapy in perianal CD, addressing the unique challenges posed by fistulas and abscesses in this subset of patients. Additionally, in the realm of post-operative care for CD, antibiotics are employed to mitigate the risk of disease recurrence [115]. Despite the evolving understanding of antibiotic use in IBD, research on their precise role continues to unfold. Ongoing investigations explore the intricate dynamics between antibiotics and the complex immunological landscape characterizing IBD. The delicate balance between the potential benefits and associated risks, including antimicrobial resistance and adverse effects, necessitates a judicious approach to antibiotic utilization in the context of IBD management. Parallel to antibiotic research, the exploration of prebiotics and probiotics has garnered significant attention in the scientific community. Motivated by their favorable safety profiles, these agents have been subjected to rigorous scrutiny. Notably, VSL3®, a freeze-dried lactic acid bacteria and bifidobacteria capsules by Alfasigma USA, Inc. has emerged as a noteworthy contender, demonstrating promise, particularly in pouchitis. However, the current body of evidence remains limited, and robustly establishing the consistent therapeutic benefits of prebiotics and probiotics in IBD necessitates further extensive research [116]. The journey of antibiotics in the landscape of IBD treatment reflects a dynamic interplay between theoretical justifications, empirical evidence from clinical trials, and evolving clinical practices. The contemporary paradigm emphasizes selective and targeted use in specific clinical scenarios, moving beyond the erstwhile notion of antibiotics as a routine mainstay in IBD therapy. The ongoing exploration of prebiotics and probiotics adds an additional layer to the evolving narrative of therapeutic options for IBD, holding promise but requiring further substantiation through rigorous scientific inquiry. The intricate dance between antibiotics, prebiotics, probiotics, and the complex immunological milieu in IBD forms a compelling arena for continued investigation and refinement of therapeutic strategies in the years to come [117].

Biologics

The predominant therapeutic approach for managing IBD centers around biological therapy, predominantly utilizing monoclonal antibodies designed to target specific molecules with immunomodulatory or inflammatory activities. Categorized into 4 classes depending upon their mechanisms of working, the largest and pioneering class focuses on agents directed against tumor necrosis factor (TNF), an inflammatory cytokine found in elevated concentrations in individuals with IBD. Infliximab, the first in this class, administered intravenously, has revolutionized IBD care. Subsequently, biosimilars targeting TNF have been introduced, offering a cost-effective alternative with comparable efficacy [118]. Adalimumab, a subsequent subcutaneously administered iteration of infliximab, yields similar remission rates, with only 25% of CD patients achieving remission at Week 54 and 17% of UC patients at Week 52 [118 - 120]. Clinical trials involving subsequent anti-TNF agents, like golimumab (approved solely for UC) and certolizumab (approved exclusively for CD), face challenges in achieving clinical remission or mucosal healing endpoints [121, 122]. A significant number of patients still experience failure with anti-TNF therapy, accompanied by drawbacks such as infusion reactions, opportunistic infections, and malignancy, when combined with azathioprine [123]. Vedolizumab, a distinct biological agent, acts as an anti-leukocyte trafficking agent by targeting $\alpha4\beta7$, an integrin guiding immune cell migration in GIT. Engineered for gut targeting, vedolizumab offers fewer adverse effects than anti-TNFs. However, in trials, reoccurrence rates were found in only 42% of UC individuals and 32% of CD individuals at 52 weeks [124, 125]. Ustekinumab targets the p40 subunit of IL-12 and IL-23 cytokines, used in CD [111]. Despite its targeted approach, ustekinumab achieves an overall remission rate of approximately 53% in CD and 44% in UC at the 52-week mark, with a safety profile comparable to vedolizumab [126, 127].

Fecal Microbiota Transplantation

Fecal Microbiota Transplantation (FMT) is an emerging therapeutic approach with potential implications for managing IBD. FMT emerges as a promising avenue to restore immune equilibrium within the intestinal mucosa, representing a current focal point in research. The application of FMT gains particular consideration in addressing moderate to severe cases of IBD, especially those complicated by recurrent or resistant *Clostridium difficile* infection [128, 129]. In animal models, FMT has showcased efficacy as a therapeutic intervention for IBD. In mice subjected to colitis induced by Dextran Sulfate Sodium (DSS), FMT demonstrated a suppressive effect on colon inflammation, concurrently restoring intestinal barrier functions. This beneficial impact was evident in the attenuation of colitis, characterized by a reduction in colon damage and the restoration of colon length [130]. *Bacteroides acidifaciens, Escherichia Shigella*, and *Blautia* levels were found to be decreased relatively in FMT-treated mice [131]. Additional findings by Zhang *et al.* highlighted that FMT in mice with gut dysbiosis significantly increased levels of SCFAs, crucial bacterial metabolites [132]. SCFAs play a vital role in regulating inflammatory responses and restoring immune function, suggesting that FMT could alleviate UC and CD through dysbiosis gut microbiota composition and enhancing SCFA production [133]. Progressive research is imperative to delve into the underlying mechanisms through which FMT exerts its effects, contributing to the development of more effective and targeted regimens for treating IBD [134]. In clinical studies involving patients with UC, a double-blind study explored the relationship between UC symptom remission and gut microbiota. Notably, individuals in the FMT group experiencing UC remission displayed heightened diversity of GIT microbiome, alongside an enhanced count of beneficial bacteria. Similarly, FMT demonstrated symptomatic improvements in patients with active CD, accompanied by an increase in α-diversity. These findings suggest that alterations induced by FMT in the gut microbiota composition significantly contribute to alleviating signs and symptoms associated with Inflammatory Bowel Disease [135].

Anti-integrin Therapy

In the treatment of IBD, which includes UC and CD, anti-integrin therapy has become a viable and revolutionary strategy. Integrins are a class of cell adhesion molecules that are essential for controlling inflammation and immunological responses in the gastrointestinal system. Precision medicine now has more options thanks to the development and application of biologic medicines that target particular integrins, giving IBD patients a more focused and efficient course of treatment [136]. Cell surface receptors called integrins help immune cells adhere to and migrate across inflamed gut mucosa, which in turn contributes to the persistence of chronic inflammation. The treatment objective is to stop immune cell trafficking and lower inflammation by specifically blocking these integrins, which will relieve symptoms and encourage mucosal healing [137]. α4β7 integrin is one of the main integrins addressed in anti-IBD therapy. A monoclonal antibody called vedolizumab has completely changed the way IBD is managed. It works by attaching itself to α4β7 integrin and preventing it from interacting with mucosal addressin cell adhesion molecule-1 (MAdCAM-1) [138]. The intestinal mucosa expresses the endothelial cell adhesion molecule MAdCAM-1, which aids in lymphocyte migration into the intestinal tissue. Targeted inhibition by vedolizumab obstructs this interaction, reducing immune cell infiltration and reducing inflammatory response [139]. Clinical research and real-world experience have demonstrated the efficacy of vedolizumab in inducing and maintaining remission in both Crohn's disease and ulcerative colitis. Due to its gut-selective method of action, vedolizumab has a safer profile than certain conventional medications and less chance of causing systemic immuno-suppression. Because of this customized approach, vedolizumab is now considered a valuable treatment option for people who might not respond to or tolerate other medications [140]. Apart from α4β7 integrin, α4β1 integrin is also a crucial integrin that is being highlighted for anti-IBD treatment. The novel biologic medication etrolizumab selectively targets this integrin, interfering with its capacity to connect with fibronectin and vascular cell adhesion molecule-1 (VCAM-1). By stopping immune cells from moving to the inflammatory gut tissue, etrolizumab offers an alternative method of action to vedolizumab [141]. Ontamalimab is now undergoing clinical trials; early results suggest that the drug may be able to assist individuals with IBDin going into and staying in remission. Even beyond their usefulness in achieving and maintaining remission, anti-integrin therapies contribute to the broader goal of promoting mucosal healing in IBD patients [142]. Improved long-term outcomes, fewer hospital stays, and a lower risk of complications are all associated with mucosal healing. The intestinal mucosa's healing and inflammation's cessation define it. Anti-integrin medications have demonstrated efficacy in promoting mucosal healing, thereby solidifying their position as key players in the management of inflammatory bowel disease [143]. α4β7 and α4β1 integrins are the specific targets of vedolizumab and etrolizumab, respectively. Leukocyte trafficking via α4β7 and cell adhesion via αEβ7 integrins are blocked by etolizumab (anti-β7). Large-scale phase 3 clinical trials are now being conducted to assess etrolizumab's effectiveness in the induction and maintenance of IBD patients. Abrilumab (anti-α4β7 IgG2), PN-943 (an oral, gut-restricted α4β7 antagonist peptide), AJM300 (an oral, small-molecule inhibitor of α4), and ontamalimab (anti-MAdCAM-1 IgG) are other investigational anti-integrin medicines. These treatments all provide a targeted and efficient method of adjusting immune responses in the gastrointestinal tract [144 - 146]. The advent of anti-integrin therapies has expanded the therapy possibilities for IBD patients and necessitated a re-evaluation of treatment goals and methods. Furthermore, current investigations seek to clarify the complexities of integrin biology, providing insight into possible new targets and treatment directions.

JAK Inhibitors

The development of Janus kinase (JAK) inhibitors has added a new and exciting aspect to the treatment of IBD, which encompasses diseases like ulcerative colitis and Crohn's disease. JAK inhibitors are a class of tiny compounds that specifically target and block the function of Janus kinases, which are essential elements in the signaling cascades that govern immune responses [147]. In contrast to conventional medicines, the use of JAK inhibitors in IBD represents a paradigm shift in therapeutic approaches by providing a more focused and adaptable method. The four members of the JAKs family of intracellular tyrosine protein kinases are tyrosine kinase 2 (TYK2), JAK1, JAK2, and JAK3 facilitating intracellular signaling. A lot of focus is placed on inhibiting the JAK/STAT signaling pathway in the hopes of creating new IBD treatments [148]. JAK inhibitors are the first oral IBD-targeted medication. They are tiny molecules. JAK inhibitors have a quick start of action once they enter the bloodstream and can quickly relieve symptoms. JAK inhibitors can impact several cytokine-dependent immune pathways. For instance, JAK1, JAK2, and TYK2 can influence IL-6 signaling, and JAK2 and TYK2 can also influence IL-23 signaling. In the treatment of RA, several JAK inhibitors have already received approval [149, 150]. One of these, tofacitinib inhibits JAK1 and JAK3 and was initially licensed for UC induction and maintenance therapy. In the OCTAVE Sustain study, remission rates at 52 weeks were 34.3% for 5 mg and 40.6% for 10 mg compared to 11.1% for placebo ($p < 0.0001$ for both). Patients over 65 years of age who have previously failed TNFα medications and are Asian in ethnicity are more susceptible to contracting *Herpes zoster*. The key effectiveness outcomes of CD phase 2b clinical trials did not vary statistically from placebo. JAK1 inhibitors *viz.* filgotinib and Upadacitinib can also be used. Deucravacitinib is a targeted TYK2 blocker that targets type 1 interferon, IL-12, and IL-23 in phase 2 clinical trials in CD and UC [151].

Surgical Treatments

Although there has been a great deal of progress in the medication therapy of IBD with the introduction of biologics, surgery remains a vital part of the treatment of IBD. The rate of surgery for CD has dropped from 10 to 8.8% ($P < 0.001$), while UC has declined from 7.7 to 7.5% ($P < 0.001$) [152]. According to research published in the New York State Database, the mortality rate for individuals with CD following nonselective surgery decreased in the biologics era, while it increased to 15% for patients with UC. Surgical and perioperative management still has space for development. Patients with UC are mostly at risk for severe excessive bleeding, intestinal perforation, carcinogenesis, and extremely suspected carcinogenesis [153]. Among the relative indications are the following: (1) Patients with toxic megacolon have no response to medical treatment, and early surgical surgery is recommended; patients with severe UC do not respond to aggressive medical treatment. (2) The quality of life has been significantly impacted by unfavorable drug responses or inadequate results from medical treatments. Laparoscopic resection is advised for individuals with localized ileocaecal CD who did not improve or relapsed after starting medication therapy or who favored surgery over ongoing medication therapy [154]. Surgery for a perianal Crohn's fistula can only be recommended to a limited number of patients following consultation, particularly those with complex conditions and ongoing disease activity, due to poor long-term results. According to one study, the endoscopic recurrence rate for CD patients was 85% and 73%, respectively, while the symptomatic recurrence rate was 20% and 34% at one and three years following ileocolectomy. Establishing preventive and treatment measures and keeping an eye on recurrence can be facilitated by routine post-operative endoscopic examinations.

Novel Therapy

Here are some novel and futuristic strategies in the spotlight these days to treat IBD (Table **3**):

Table 3. Neoteric and futuristic therapies and their mechanism of action in clinical trials.

Novel Therapy			
Treatment Type	**Related Active Components**	**Mechanism of Action**	**ClinicalTrial Phase**
Apheresis therapy	Granulocyte/monocyte	Taking one or more specific leukocytes out of the peripheral blood and absorbing them [158].	Phase III
Sphingosine-1-Phosphate Modulators	Amiselimod and Etrasimod	Regulation of lymphocyte egress by the interaction between S1P and S1P1 receptors [164].	Phase III
IL-12/23 Pathways	Ustekinumab	Focusing on the inflammatory mechanism mediated by IL-23 [165].	Phase II
TLI1A Inhibitor	PF-06480605	Controls mucosal immunity and is involved in immune pathways [168].	Phase IIb
Phosphodiesterase Inhibitor	Apremilast	As intracellular cAMP levels grow, inflammatory cytokine expression is reduced [169].	Phase III
IL-36 Inhibitor	Spesolimab	Encourages intestinal fibrosis and inflammation while controlling the gut immune response [170].	Phase II
Future Treatments			
Gut Microbiota Modulation	------	Activation of the AhR/IL-22 pathway [174]	-----
Stem Cell Therapy	Local Injection of Mesenchymal Stem Cells	Colonization repair [175]	Phase II
Gut-Brain Axis regulation	-------	Acetylcholine (ACh) is released at the distal end of the VN [179].	---
B Cells regulation	Belimumab	generating large amounts of IgA and IgM, which aid in maintaining the epithelial barrier [147].	Phase IIb

(Table 3) cont.....

Novel Therapy			
Treatment Type	**Related Active Components**	**Mechanism of Action**	**ClinicalTrial Phase**
ILCs regulation	Mirikizumab	IL-17 and IFN-γ increase [166].	Phase III

Apheresis Therapy

Apheresis therapy was first created in Japan to lower the local inflammatory response by separating and absorbing one or more particular leukocytes from the peripheral blood—such as granulocytes, monocytes, and activated lymphocytes. It has been revealed that adsorptive granulocyte/monocyte apheresis (GMA) is useful in bringing UC and CD patients into remission [158]. A meta-analysis showed that the incidence of adverse events linked to GMA was much lower than that of CSs, in producing clinical remission in individuals with active UC (OR = 2.23, 95% CI: 1.38–3.60) [159]. The first multicenter clinical trial in China that included GMA participants validated the drug's safety and efficacy (the overall efficacy rate of roughly 70%) and involved 34 active UC patients [160]. According to Motoya *et al.,* older IBD patients using GMA had a 46.4% reduction rate for UC with no increase in side effects. Retrospective research conducted recently revealed that following GMA treatment, over 80% of UC patients experienced clinical remission [161]. During the 52-week treatment, the rates of clinical remission and mucosal healing were 81.8 and 50%, respectively, with no significant side effects. GMA is highly well-liked among IBD sufferers [162]. Approximately 50% of patients reported feeling satisfied with the results of GMA after treatment, and 80% said they would be open to receiving this kind of care once more in the future, regardless of how the treatment went. Further research is necessary because there is less evidence to demonstrate the effectiveness of GMA therapy [163].

Sphingosine-1-Phosphate Modulators

There are five subtypes of the sphingosine-1-phosphate receptor (S1PR). They are involved in intercellular communication and other several critical processes, such as the maintenance of vascularization, cell migration, proliferation, and other cardiovascular functions. Many S1P regulators have been created to treat IBD. Ozanimod, an oral small molecule selectively modulates the S1PR1 and S1PR5 receptors by blocking receptor internalization and degradation. Thus, it maintains inflammatory bowel disease by preventing lymphocyte migration into the systemic circulation. Some S1P modulators developed and used in clinical trials, such as amiselimod and etrasimod, etc [164].

Targeting IL-12/23 Pathways

Myeloid cells, such as DCs and macrophages, release IL-12, a heterodimer of p40 and p35, and IL-23, a heterodimer of p40 and p19. These molecules induce the differentiation of naïve CD4+ T cells into T-helper 1 (Th1) and T-helper 17 (Th17) cells and are crucial in the pathophysiology of inflammatory bowel disease (IBD). A completely human IgG1 monoclonal antibody called uzekinumab targets and inhibits the IL-12/23 common p40 subunit from binding to cell receptors. The long-term safety and efficacy of ustekinumab for IBD have been demonstrated by UNITI and UNIFI studies [165]. By selectively targets the IL-23, risankizumab may theoretically have fewer adverse effects than ustekinumab. Research on the effects of other biologics, such as brazikumab, guselkumab, and mirikizumab, on the IL-23 p19 subunit, also demonstrated their efficacy in reducing intestinal inflammation. A promising approach for IBD treatment was anticipated given the efficacious outcomes of the anti-IL-23 p40 and p19 monoclonal antibodies, which target the IL-23 [166].

TLI1A Inhibitor

The TNF superfamily member 15 (TNFSF15) locus is one of the strongest genetic variations linked to IBD, according to genome-wide association studies. By binding to death receptor 3, the TNFSF15 gene also known as 'TNF-like ligand 1A' (TL1A) is released following activation from antigen-presenting cells and is essential in initiating both innate and adaptive immunological pathways (DR3) [167]. Profibrotic pathways and T-cell activation are two proinflammatory outcomes of TL1A-DR3 signaling that are essential for the pathophysiology of IBD. In moderate-to-severe UC, an anti-TL1A antibody called PF-06480605 significantly improves endoscopic outcomes while also downregulating tissue Th1 and Th17 cytokine responses [168].

Phosphodiesterase Inhibitor

The breakdown of cAMP and cGMP is catalyzed by the enzymes known as phosphodiesterases (PDEs). T cells, monocytes, macrophages, and DCs all express PDE4. When PDE4 is inhibited, intracellular cAMP levels rise, which decreases expression of TNFα, IL-17, IFN-γ, and IL-23, and increases levels of regulating cytokines like IL10. As a result, the PDE4 inhibitor apremilast has been tried and proven to be successful in treating active UC [169].

IL-36 Inhibitor

In IBD, intestinal inflammation is associated with an upregulation of the IL-36 family's expression. Different gut-residing cells (lymphocytes, macrophages, and epithelium) secrete IL-36α and IL-36γ, which are then digested enzymatically by external neutrophil proteases to produce extremely potent IL-36R agonists. DCs, macrophages, and T lymphocytes are among the cells whose proinflammatory signaling is activated by ligand binding to the IL-36R complex. IBD patients may benefit from spesolimab by acting on IL-36R which is now undergoing clinical studies [170].

Treatment Approaches in the Near Future

Gut Microbiota Modulation

The host immune system, the gut microbiota, and intestinal epithelial cells have all been the subject of extensive global research in the past ten years. There is still a great deal of uncertainty surrounding the diversity and makeup of the human gut microbiota, although it is thought to be crucial for both human health and the emergence of many diseases. IBD is thought to develop because gut microbiotas are less diverse (dysbiosis) in patients than those of healthy individuals. As a result, attention is drawn to microbiome-modulation as a novel treatment strategy [171]. Their metabolism and metabolic byproducts, such as lactic acids, hydroperoxides, bacteriocins, secondary Bile Acid (BA), and short-chain fatty acids, are mostly responsible for the positive benefits. According to a meta-analysis, FMT is a safe, and effective treatment; however, further research is needed to determine its long-term efficacy and safety [172]. Due to dysbiosis-blocked transformation, the amount of conjugated primary BA in feces increases in people with IBD, although the amount of secondary BA in feces decreases. Inhibiting Th17 cell differentiation and encouraging T cell differentiation are two ways that secondary BA reduces inflammation. BA also functions to control immunological and metabolic processes, including FXR, TGR5, PXR, and VDR. Thus, targeting the BA-gut microbiota axis may represent novel approaches to the treatment of IBD [173]. In order to produce indole-related derivatives, intestinal microbes metabolize tryptophan, to bind with the 'Aryl Hydrocarbon Receptor' (AhR). This activation of the AhR/IL-22 pathway, which is essential for intestinal homeostasis, improves barrier integrity. Peripheral serotonin, a crucial gastrointestinal signaling chemical for intestinal peristalsis and motility, secretion, vasodilatation, and nutritional absorption, is produced by a different tryptophan metabolic pathway in microbes. As a result, microbes that alter tryptophan metabolism might be advantageous [174].

Stem Cell Therapy

About one-third of people with CD commonly get perianal fistulas within 20 years of diagnosis. They negatively affect life quality and do not respond well to therapy. Long-term surgical closure of the fistula is difficult and carries an increased risk of incontinence. As a result, less harmful therapies for perianal fistulas have been researched; in particular, local injection of mesenchymal stem cells has been proven to be more effective in treating perianal fistula in patients with CD [175].

Regulation of Gut-Brain Axis

The gut-brain axis is a highly complex system of bidirectional communication that is fueled by neurological, hormonal, metabolic, immunological, and microbial signals. An essential part of the autonomic nervous system and a major player in the brain-gut axis is the vagus nerve (VN). High TNFα levels in IBD are linked to blunted vagal tone, and VN stimulation offers two possible therapeutic avenues for treating IBD. Through its afferent fibers, VN stimulates the hypothalamus-pituitary-adrenal axis, which results in the release of glucocorticoids and the subsequent reduction of peripheral inflammation. Acetylcholine (ACh) release from vagus nerve endings is another mechanism that reduces inflammation. It does this by connecting to α7-nicotinic ACh receptors and preventing macrophages from releasing TNFα. Moreover, disruption of the gut-brain axis is linked to neurological and gastrointestinal disorders, and in those with IBD, it increases the chance of developing Parkinson's disease and multiple sclerosis [176].

Regulation of B Cells

Immune homeostasis depends on B cells at the intestinal mucosal surface, and individuals with IBD may benefit from treatment for their dysregulated B-cell response. Inhibition of CD40L decreases inflammatory IgG1 responses as IBD patients exhibit elevated mucosal IgG1+ plasma cells. TNF superfamily cytokine B-cell-activating factor (BAFF) is secreted by many immune cells in response to stimuli for class-switch recombination, B-cell maturation, and plasma cell and B-cell survival [177]. Since Belimumab, reduces both activated and naïve B cells and plasma cells in systemic lupus erythematosus and RA, and since BAFF is overexpressed in IBD, BAFF antagonists could help. Vedolizumab has the potential to prevent α4β7+ plasmablasts from penetrating inflamed mucosa. Furthermore, immunoglobulins inhibiting the activity of the Fcγ receptor may be a desirable strategy, albeit the exact mechanism is yet unknown [147].

Regulation of ILCs

ILCs influence the GIT epithelium, produce cytokines, and interact with the microbiota to contribute to the pathophysiology of IBD. In a normal condition, ILC3s make up the majority of intestinal ILCs; however, in an active state, ILC1s and ILC3s that produce IL-17 and IFN-γ increase, whereas ILC3s that produce

IL-22 decrease. Because of their capacity to recognize microbiota and preserve the intestinal barrier, ILC2s play a role in IBD. More investigation is needed into the mechanisms that alter the subpopulation and function of ILCs as well as how these ILCs exert their inflammatory and protective functions to create novel treatments for IBD [178] Table **3**.

CONCLUSION

Despite many advances in technologies and experimental models, the detailed etiology of IBD is still unknown. In some current studies in animal models and integration analyses across cohorts elucidating microbiome relation with IBD, the pathophysiology of IBD is discovered to a limited extent and more research in this field is required to elucidate all mechanisms or pathways of these diseases. Both human and animal models showed gut dysbiosis is complexly concerned with IBD and cannot be treated with conventional therapy because of their high adverse effects. This suggests alternative strategies such as prebiotics, probiotics, and synbiotics for effective treatment of IBD. Gut microbiota modulation, stem cell therapy, gut-brain axis regulation, B cells regulation, and Ilcs regulation may be counted as effective treatment approaches in the near future. It has also been found that in most cases, dysbiosis occurs due to the consumption of plant-based or animal-based processed diets, and improper antibiotic administration. Reduced antibiotic consumption or recommended antibiotic therapy under proper surveillance along with qualitative differences in diet will help counter dysbiosis and thereby IBD.

CONSENT FOR PUBLICATON

All authors have consented to publish the book chapter “Inflammatory Bowel Diseases And Gut Microbiota” in this book.

ACKNOWLEDGEMENTS

We are thankful to the Department of Pharmaceutical Sciences, Dibrugarh University, Dibrugarh, Assam for providing all facilities.

REFERENCES

[1] Haneishi Y, Furuya Y, Hasegawa M, Picarelli A, Rossi M, Miyamoto J. Inflammatory Bowel Diseases and Gut Microbiota. Int J Mol Sci 2023; 24(4): 3817. [http://dx.doi.org/10.3390/ijms24043817] [PMID: 36835245]

[2] Zheng L, Wen XL. Gut microbiota and inflammatory bowel disease: The current status and perspectives. World J Clin Cases 2021; 9(2): 321-33. [http://dx.doi.org/10.12998/wjcc.v9.i2.321] [PMID: 33521100]

[3] Lee M, Chang EB. Inflammatory Bowel Diseases (IBD) and the Microbiome—Searching the Crime Scene for Clues. Gastroenterology 2021; 160(2): 524-37.

[http://dx.doi.org/10.1053/j.gastro.2020.09.056] [PMID: 33253681]

[4] Ananthakrishnan AN, Kaplan GG, Ng SC. Changing Global Epidemiology of Inflammatory Bowel Diseases: Sustaining Health Care Delivery Into the 21st Century. Clin Gastroenterol Hepatol 2020; 18(6): 1252-60.
[http://dx.doi.org/10.1016/j.cgh.2020.01.028] [PMID: 32007542]

[5] Ye L, Cao Q, Cheng J. Review of inflammatory bowel disease in China. ScientificWorldJournal 2013; 2013(1): 296470.
[http://dx.doi.org/10.1155/2013/296470] [PMID: 24348149]

[6] Hendrickson BA, Gokhale R, Cho JH. Clinical aspects and pathophysiology of inflammatory bowel disease. Clin Microbiol Rev 2002; 15(1): 79-94.
[http://dx.doi.org/10.1128/CMR.15.1.79-94.2002] [PMID: 11781268]

[7] Lloyd-Price J, Arze C, Ananthakrishnan AN, *et al.* Multi-omics of the gut microbial ecosystem in inflammatory bowel diseases. Nature 2019; 569(7758): 655-62.
[http://dx.doi.org/10.1038/s41586-019-1237-9] [PMID: 31142855]

[8] Tian Z, Zhuang X, Luo M, Yin W, Xiong L. The propionic acid and butyric acid in serum but not in feces are increased in patients with diarrhea-predominant irritable bowel syndrome. BMC Gastroenterol 2020; 20(1): 73.
[http://dx.doi.org/10.1186/s12876-020-01212-3] [PMID: 32178625]

[9] den Besten G, van Eunen K, Groen AK, Venema K, Reijngoud DJ, Bakker BM. The role of short-chain fatty acids in the interplay between diet, gut microbiota, and host energy metabolism. J Lipid Res 2013; 54(9): 2325-40.
[http://dx.doi.org/10.1194/jlr.R036012] [PMID: 23821742]

[10] Rinninella E, Raoul P, Cintoni M, *et al.* What is the Healthy Gut Microbiota Composition? A Changing Ecosystem across Age, Environment, Diet, and Diseases. Microorganisms 2019; 7(1): 14.
[http://dx.doi.org/10.3390/microorganisms7010014] [PMID: 30634578]

[11] Arumugam M, Raes J, Pelletier E, *et al.* Enterotypes of the human gut microbiome. Nature 2011; 473(7346): 174-80.
[http://dx.doi.org/10.1038/nature09944] [PMID: 21508958]

[12] Wiredu Ocansey DK, Hang S, Yuan X, *et al.* The diagnostic and prognostic potential of gut bacteria in inflammatory bowel disease. Gut Microbes 2023; 15(1): 2176118.
[http://dx.doi.org/10.1080/19490976.2023.2176118] [PMID: 36794838]

[13] Pittayanon R, Lau JT, Leontiadis GI, *et al.* Differences in Gut Microbiota in Patients With vs Without Inflammatory Bowel Diseases: A Systematic Review. Gastroenterology 2020; 158(4): 930-946.e1.
[http://dx.doi.org/10.1053/j.gastro.2019.11.294] [PMID: 31812509]

[14] Qiu P, Ishimoto T, Fu L, Zhang J, Zhang Z, Liu Y. The Gut Microbiota in Inflammatory Bowel Disease. Front Cell Infect Microbiol 2022; 12: 733992.
[http://dx.doi.org/10.3389/fcimb.2022.733992] [PMID: 35273921]

[15] Kong G, Lê Cao KA, Hannan AJ. Alterations in the Gut Fungal Community in a Mouse Model of Huntington's Disease. Microbiol Spectr 2022; 10(2): e02192-21.
[http://dx.doi.org/10.1128/spectrum.02192-21] [PMID: 35262396]

[16] Cai Z, Wang S, Li J. Treatment of Inflammatory Bowel Disease: A Comprehensive Review. Front Med (Lausanne) 2021; 8: 765474.
[http://dx.doi.org/10.3389/fmed.2021.765474] [PMID: 34988090]

[17] Tong M, Li X, Wegener Parfrey L, *et al.* A modular organization of the human intestinal mucosal microbiota and its association with inflammatory bowel disease. PLoS One 2013; 8(11): e80702.
[http://dx.doi.org/10.1371/journal.pone.0080702] [PMID: 24260458]

[18] Talapko J, Včev A, Meštrović T, Pustijanac E, Jukić M, Škrlec I. Homeostasis and Dysbiosis of the Intestinal Microbiota: Comparing Hallmarks of a Healthy State with Changes in Inflammatory Bowel

Disease. Microorganisms 2022; 10(12): 2405.
[http://dx.doi.org/10.3390/microorganisms10122405] [PMID: 36557658]

[19] Sokol H, Pigneur B, Watterlot L, *et al.* *Faecalibacterium prausnitzii* is an anti-inflammatory commensal bacterium identified by gut microbiota analysis of Crohn disease patients. Proc Natl Acad Sci USA 2008; 105(43): 16731-6.
[http://dx.doi.org/10.1073/pnas.0804812105] [PMID: 18936492]

[20] Wang W, Chen L, Zhou R, *et al.* Increased proportions of Bifidobacterium and the Lactobacillus group and loss of butyrate-producing bacteria in inflammatory bowel disease. J Clin Microbiol 2014; 52(2): 398-406.
[http://dx.doi.org/10.1128/JCM.01500-13] [PMID: 24478468]

[21] Lees CW, Barrett JC, Parkes M, Satsangi J. New IBD genetics: common pathways with other diseases. Gut 2011; 60(12): 1739-53.
[http://dx.doi.org/10.1136/gut.2009.199679] [PMID: 21300624]

[22] Pitcher MCL, Beatty ER, Cummings JH. The contribution of sulphate reducing bacteria and 5-aminosalicylic acid to faecal sulphide in patients with ulcerative colitis. Gut 2000; 46(1): 64-72.
[http://dx.doi.org/10.1136/gut.46.1.64] [PMID: 10601057]

[23] Gevers D, Kugathasan S, Denson LA, *et al.* The treatment-naive microbiome in new-onset Crohn's disease. Cell Host Microbe 2014; 15(3): 382-92.
[http://dx.doi.org/10.1016/j.chom.2014.02.005] [PMID: 24629344]

[24] Morgan XC, Tickle TL, Sokol H, *et al.* Dysfunction of the intestinal microbiome in inflammatory bowel disease and treatment. Genome Biol 2012; 13(9): R79.
[http://dx.doi.org/10.1186/gb-2012-13-9-r79] [PMID: 23013615]

[25] Rolhion N, Chassaing B, Nahori MA, *et al.* A Listeria monocytogenes Bacteriocin Can Target the Commensal Prevotella copri and Modulate Intestinal Infection. Cell Host Microbe 2019; 26(5): 691-701.e5.
[http://dx.doi.org/10.1016/j.chom.2019.10.016] [PMID: 31726031]

[26] Subramenium GA, Sabui S, Marchant JS, Said HM, Subramanian VS. Enterotoxigenic *Escherichia coli* heat labile enterotoxin inhibits intestinal ascorbic acid uptake via a cAMP-dependent NF-κ--mediated pathway. Am J Physiol Gastrointest Liver Physiol 2019; 316(1): G55-63.
[http://dx.doi.org/10.1152/ajpgi.00259.2018] [PMID: 30285481]

[27] Zheng L, Wen XL, Duan SL. Role of metabolites derived from gut microbiota in inflammatory bowel disease. World J Clin Cases 2022; 10(9): 2660-77.
[http://dx.doi.org/10.12998/wjcc.v10.i9.2660] [PMID: 35434116]

[28] Bernardi F, D'Amico F, Bencardino S, *et al.* Gut Microbiota Metabolites: Unveiling Their Role in Inflammatory Bowel Diseases and Fibrosis. Pharmaceuticals (Basel) 2024; 17(3): 347.
[http://dx.doi.org/10.3390/ph17030347] [PMID: 38543132]

[29] Macia L, Tan J, Vieira AT, *et al.* Metabolite-sensing receptors GPR43 and GPR109A facilitate dietary fibre-induced gut homeostasis through regulation of the inflammasome. Nat Commun 2015; 6(1): 6734.
[http://dx.doi.org/10.1038/ncomms7734] [PMID: 25828455]

[30] Michaudel C, Sokol H. The Gut Microbiota at the Service of Immunometabolism. Cell Metab 2020; 32(4): 514-23.
[http://dx.doi.org/10.1016/j.cmet.2020.09.004] [PMID: 32946809]

[31] Qiu P, Ishimoto T, Fu L, Zhang J, Zhang Z, Liu Y. The Gut Microbiota in Inflammatory Bowel Disease. Front Cell Infect Microbiol 2022; 12: 733992.
[http://dx.doi.org/10.3389/fcimb.2022.733992] [PMID: 35273921]

[32] Sun X, He S, Lv C, *et al.* Analysis of murine and human Treg subsets in inflammatory bowel disease. Mol Med Rep 2017; 16(3): 2893-8.

[http://dx.doi.org/10.3892/mmr.2017.6912] [PMID: 28677759]

[33] Lopetuso LR, Napoli M, Rizzatti G, Gasbarrini A. The intriguing role of Rifaximin in gut barrier chronic inflammation and in the treatment of Crohn's disease. Expert Opin Investig Drugs 2018; 27(6): 543-51.
[http://dx.doi.org/10.1080/13543784.2018.1483333] [PMID: 29865875]

[34] Garrett WS, Lord GM, Punit S, *et al.* Communicable ulcerative colitis induced by T-bet deficiency in the innate immune system. Cell 2007; 131(1): 33-45.
[http://dx.doi.org/10.1016/j.cell.2007.08.017] [PMID: 17923086]

[35] Gadaleta RM, van Erpecum KJ, Oldenburg B, *et al.* Farnesoid X receptor activation inhibits inflammation and preserves the intestinal barrier in inflammatory bowel disease. Gut 2011; 60(4): 463-72.
[http://dx.doi.org/10.1136/gut.2010.212159] [PMID: 21242261]

[36] Qiu X, Zhang M, Yang X, Hong N, Yu C. Faecalibacterium prausnitzii upregulates regulatory T cells and anti-inflammatory cytokines in treating TNBS-induced colitis. J Crohn's Colitis 2013; 7(11): e558-68.
[http://dx.doi.org/10.1016/j.crohns.2013.04.002] [PMID: 23643066]

[37] Hang S, Paik D, Yao L, *et al.* Bile acid metabolites control T_H17 and T_{reg} cell differentiation. Nature 2019; 576(7785): 143-8.
[http://dx.doi.org/10.1038/s41586-019-1785-z] [PMID: 31776512]

[38] Langan D, Perkins DJ, Vogel SN, Moudgil KD. Microbiota-Derived Metabolites, Indole-3-aldehyde and Indole-3-acetic Acid, Differentially Modulate Innate Cytokines and Stromal Remodeling Processes Associated with Autoimmune Arthritis. Int J Mol Sci 2021; 22(4): 2017.
[http://dx.doi.org/10.3390/ijms22042017] [PMID: 33670600]

[39] Lamas B, Michel ML, Waldschmitt N, *et al.* Card9 mediates susceptibility to intestinal pathogens through microbiota modulation and control of bacterial virulence. Gut 2018; 67(10): 1836-44.
[http://dx.doi.org/10.1136/gutjnl-2017-314195] [PMID: 28790160]

[40] Zhou L, Zhang M, Wang Y, *et al.* Faecalibacterium prausnitzii Produces Butyrate to Maintain Th17/Treg Balance and to Ameliorate Colorectal Colitis by Inhibiting Histone Deacetylase 1. Inflamm Bowel Dis 2018; 24(9): 1926-40.
[http://dx.doi.org/10.1093/ibd/izy182] [PMID: 29796620]

[41] Hoffmann TW, Pham HP, Bridonneau C, *et al.* Microorganisms linked to inflammatory bowel disease-associated dysbiosis differentially impact host physiology in gnotobiotic mice. ISME J 2016; 10(2): 460-77.
[http://dx.doi.org/10.1038/ismej.2015.127] [PMID: 26218241]

[42] Godefroy E, Alameddine J, Montassier E, *et al.* Expression of CCR6 and CXCR6 by Gut-Derived $CD4^+/CD8\alpha^+$ T-Regulatory Cells, Which Are Decreased in Blood Samples From Patients With Inflammatory Bowel Diseases. Gastroenterology 2018; 155(4): 1205-17.
[http://dx.doi.org/10.1053/j.gastro.2018.06.078] [PMID: 29981781]

[43] Noguchi E, Homma Y, Kang X, Netea MG, Ma X. A Crohn's disease–associated NOD2 mutation suppresses transcription of human IL10 by inhibiting activity of the nuclear ribonucleoprotein hnRNP-A1. Nat Immunol 2009; 10(5): 471-9.
[http://dx.doi.org/10.1038/ni.1722] [PMID: 19349988]

[44] Read E, Curtis MA, Neves JF. The role of oral bacteria in inflammatory bowel disease. Nat Rev Gastroenterol Hepatol 2021; 18(10): 731-42.
[http://dx.doi.org/10.1038/s41575-021-00488-4] [PMID: 34400822]

[45] Chen Y, Chen Y, Cao P, Su W, Zhan N, Dong W. *Fusobacterium nucleatum* facilitates ulcerative colitis through activating IL□17F signaling to NF□κB via the upregulation of CARD3 expression. J Pathol 2020; 250(2): 170-82.
[http://dx.doi.org/10.1002/path.5358] [PMID: 31610014]

[46] Chu H, Khosravi A, Kusumawardhani IP, Kwon AHK, Vasconcelos AC, Cunha LD, *et al.* Gene-microbiota interactions contribute to the pathogenesis of inflammatory bowel disease. Science 1979; 352(6289): 1116-20.

[47] Salzman NH, Hung K, Haribhai D, *et al.* Enteric defensins are essential regulators of intestinal microbial ecology. Nat Immunol 2010; 11(1): 76-82.
[http://dx.doi.org/10.1038/ni.1825] [PMID: 19855381]

[48] Lin L, Zhang J. Role of intestinal microbiota and metabolites on gut homeostasis and human diseases. BMC Immunol 2017; 18(1): 2.
[http://dx.doi.org/10.1186/s12865-016-0187-3] [PMID: 28061847]

[49] Adolph TE, Tomczak MF, Niederreiter L, *et al.* Paneth cells as a site of origin for intestinal inflammation. Nature 2013; 503(7475): 272-6.
[http://dx.doi.org/10.1038/nature12599] [PMID: 24089213]

[50] Wellman AS, Metukuri MR, Kazgan N, *et al.* Intestinal Epithelial Sirtuin 1 Regulates Intestinal Inflammation During Aging in Mice by Altering the Intestinal Microbiota. Gastroenterology 2017; 153(3): 772-86.
[http://dx.doi.org/10.1053/j.gastro.2017.05.022] [PMID: 28552621]

[51] Rodrigues e-Lacerda R, Fang H, Robin N, Bhatwa A, Marko DM, Schertzer JD. Microbiota and Nod-like receptors balance inflammation and metabolism during obesity and diabetes. Biomed J 2023; 46(5): 100610.
[http://dx.doi.org/10.1016/j.bj.2023.100610] [PMID: 37263539]

[52] Snäkä T, Fasel N. Behind the Scenes: Nod-Like Receptor X1 Controls Inflammation and Metabolism. Front Cell Infect Microbiol 2020; 10: 609812.
[http://dx.doi.org/10.3389/fcimb.2020.609812] [PMID: 33344269]

[53] Leber A, Hontecillas R, Tubau-Juni N, Zoccoli-Rodriguez V, Abedi V, Bassaganya-Riera J. NLRX1 Modulates Immunometabolic Mechanisms Controlling the Host–Gut Microbiota Interactions during Inflammatory Bowel Disease. Front Immunol 2018; 9: 363.
[http://dx.doi.org/10.3389/fimmu.2018.00363] [PMID: 29535731]

[54] Shawki A, McCole DF. Mechanisms of Intestinal Epithelial Barrier Dysfunction by Adherent-Invasive *Escherichia coli.* Cell Mol Gastroenterol Hepatol 2017; 3(1): 41-50.
[http://dx.doi.org/10.1016/j.jcmgh.2016.10.004] [PMID: 28174756]

[55] Palmela C, Chevarin C, Xu Z, *et al.* Adherent-invasive *Escherichia coli* in inflammatory bowel disease. Gut 2018; 67(3): 574-87.
[http://dx.doi.org/10.1136/gutjnl-2017-314903] [PMID: 29141957]

[56] Anderson CJ, Medina CB, Barron BJ, *et al.* Microbes exploit death-induced nutrient release by gut epithelial cells. Nature 2021; 596(7871): 262-7.
[http://dx.doi.org/10.1038/s41586-021-03785-9] [PMID: 34349263]

[57] Pandey KR, Naik SR, Vakil BV. Probiotics, prebiotics and synbiotics- a review. J Food Sci Technol 2015; 52(12): 7577-87.
[http://dx.doi.org/10.1007/s13197-015-1921-1] [PMID: 26604335]

[58] Andrews JM, Tan M. Probiotics in luminal gastroenterology: the current state of play. Intern Med J 2012; 42(12): 1287-91.
[http://dx.doi.org/10.1111/imj.12015] [PMID: 23252997]

[59] Abrams SA, Griffin IJ, Hawthorne KM, *et al.* A combination of prebiotic short- and long-chain inulin-type fructans enhances calcium absorption and bone mineralization in young adolescents. Am J Clin Nutr 2005; 82(2): 471-6.
[http://dx.doi.org/10.1093/ajcn/82.2.471] [PMID: 16087995]

[60] Nishino K, Nishida A, Inoue R, *et al.* Analysis of endoscopic brush samples identified mucosa-associated dysbiosis in inflammatory bowel disease. J Gastroenterol 2018; 53(1): 95-106.

[http://dx.doi.org/10.1007/s00535-017-1384-4] [PMID: 28852861]

[61] Sartor RB. Microbial influences in inflammatory bowel diseases. Gastroenterology 2008; 134(2): 577-94.
[http://dx.doi.org/10.1053/j.gastro.2007.11.059] [PMID: 18242222]

[62] Willing BP, Dicksved J, Halfvarson J, *et al.* A pyrosequencing study in twins shows that gastrointestinal microbial profiles vary with inflammatory bowel disease phenotypes. Gastroenterology 2010; 139(6): 1844-1854.e1.
[http://dx.doi.org/10.1053/j.gastro.2010.08.049] [PMID: 20816835]

[63] Sartor RB, Wu GD. Roles for Intestinal Bacteria, Viruses, and Fungi in Pathogenesis of Inflammatory Bowel Diseases and Therapeutic Approaches. Gastroenterology 2017; 152(2): 327-339.e4.
[http://dx.doi.org/10.1053/j.gastro.2016.10.012] [PMID: 27769810]

[64] Sheehan D, Moran C, Shanahan F. The microbiota in inflammatory bowel disease. J Gastroenterol 2015; 50(5): 495-507.
[http://dx.doi.org/10.1007/s00535-015-1064-1] [PMID: 25808229]

[65] Cui L, Morris A, Ghedin E. The human mycobiome in health and disease. Genome Med 2013; 5(7): 63.
[http://dx.doi.org/10.1186/gm467] [PMID: 23899327]

[66] Tisza MJ, Buck CB. A catalog of tens of thousands of viruses from human metagenomes reveals hidden associations with chronic diseases. Proc Natl Acad Sci USA 2021; 118(23): e2023202118.
[http://dx.doi.org/10.1073/pnas.2023202118] [PMID: 34083435]

[67] Norman JM, Handley SA, Baldridge MT, *et al.* Disease-specific alterations in the enteric virome in inflammatory bowel disease. Cell 2015; 160(3): 447-60.
[http://dx.doi.org/10.1016/j.cell.2015.01.002] [PMID: 25619688]

[68] Maronek M, Link R, Ambro L, Gardlik R. Phages and Their Role in Gastrointestinal Disease: Focus on Inflammatory Bowel Disease. Cells 2020; 9(4): 1013.
[http://dx.doi.org/10.3390/cells9041013] [PMID: 32325706]

[69] Mukhopadhya I, Hansen R, Meharg C, *et al.* The fungal microbiota of de-novo paediatric inflammatory bowel disease. Microbes Infect 2015; 17(4): 304-10.
[http://dx.doi.org/10.1016/j.micinf.2014.12.001] [PMID: 25522934]

[70] Marchesi JR, Adams DH, Fava F, *et al.* The gut microbiota and host health: a new clinical frontier. Gut 2016; 65(2): 330-9.
[http://dx.doi.org/10.1136/gutjnl-2015-309990] [PMID: 26338727]

[71] Wilson ID, Nicholson JK. Gut microbiome interactions with drug metabolism, efficacy, and toxicity. Transl Res 2017; 179: 204-22.
[http://dx.doi.org/10.1016/j.trsl.2016.08.002] [PMID: 27591027]

[72] Allen-Vercoe E, Coburn B. A Microbiota-Derived Metabolite Augments Cancer Immunotherapy Responses in Mice. Cancer Cell 2020; 38(4): 452-3.
[http://dx.doi.org/10.1016/j.ccell.2020.09.005] [PMID: 32976777]

[73] Stappenbeck TS, Virgin HW. Accounting for reciprocal host–microbiome interactions in experimental science. Nature 2016; 534(7606): 191-9.
[http://dx.doi.org/10.1038/nature18285] [PMID: 27279212]

[74] Lavelle A, Hoffmann TW, Pham HP, Langella P, Guédon E, Sokol H. Baseline microbiota composition modulates antibiotic-mediated effects on the gut microbiota and host. Microbiome 2019; 7(1): 111.
[http://dx.doi.org/10.1186/s40168-019-0725-3] [PMID: 31375137]

[75] Hall AB, Yassour M, Sauk J, *et al.* A novel Ruminococcus gnavus clade enriched in inflammatory bowel disease patients. Genome Med 2017; 9(1): 103.
[http://dx.doi.org/10.1186/s13073-017-0490-5] [PMID: 29183332]

[76] Vich Vila A, Imhann F, Collij V, *et al.* Gut microbiota composition and functional changes in inflammatory bowel disease and irritable bowel syndrome. Sci Transl Med 2018; 10(472): eaap8914. [http://dx.doi.org/10.1126/scitranslmed.aap8914] [PMID: 30567928]

[77] Kriss M, Hazleton KZ, Nusbacher NM, Martin CG, Lozupone CA. Low diversity gut microbiota dysbiosis: drivers, functional implications and recovery. Curr Opin Microbiol 2018; 44: 34-40. [http://dx.doi.org/10.1016/j.mib.2018.07.003] [PMID: 30036705]

[78] Forbes JD, Chen C, Knox NC, *et al.* A comparative study of the gut microbiota in immune-mediated inflammatory diseases—does a common dysbiosis exist? Microbiome 2018; 6(1): 221. [http://dx.doi.org/10.1186/s40168-018-0603-4] [PMID: 30545401]

[79] Tamboli CP, Neut C, Desreumaux P, Colombel JF. Dysbiosis in inflammatory bowel disease. Gut 2004; 53(1): 1-4. [http://dx.doi.org/10.1136/gut.53.1.1] [PMID: 14684564]

[80] Putignani L, Del Chierico F, Vernocchi P, Cicala M, Cucchiara S, Dallapiccola B. Gut Microbiota Dysbiosis as Risk and Premorbid Factors of IBD and IBS Along the Childhood–Adulthood Transition. Inflamm Bowel Dis 2016; 22(2): 487-504. [http://dx.doi.org/10.1097/MIB.0000000000000602] [PMID: 26588090]

[81] Frank DN, Robertson CE, Hamm CM, *et al.* Disease phenotype and genotype are associated with shifts in intestinal-associated microbiota in inflammatory bowel diseases. Inflamm Bowel Dis 2011; 17(1): 179-84. [http://dx.doi.org/10.1002/ibd.21339] [PMID: 20839241]

[82] Martinez C, Antolin M, Santos J, *et al.* Unstable composition of the fecal microbiota in ulcerative colitis during clinical remission. Am J Gastroenterol 2008; 103(3): 643-8. [http://dx.doi.org/10.1111/j.1572-0241.2007.01592.x] [PMID: 18341488]

[83] Manichanh C, Borruel N, Casellas F, Guarner F. The gut microbiota in IBD. Nat Rev Gastroenterol Hepatol 2012; 9(10): 599-608. [http://dx.doi.org/10.1038/nrgastro.2012.152] [PMID: 22907164]

[84] Dicksved J, Halfvarson J, Rosenquist M, *et al.* Molecular analysis of the gut microbiota of identical twins with Crohn's disease. ISME J 2008; 2(7): 716-27. [http://dx.doi.org/10.1038/ismej.2008.37] [PMID: 18401439]

[85] Sepehri S, Kotlowski R, Bernstein CN, Krause DO. Microbial diversity of inflamed and noninflamed gut biopsy tissues in inflammatory bowel disease. Inflamm Bowel Dis 2007; 13(6): 675-83. [http://dx.doi.org/10.1002/ibd.20101] [PMID: 17262808]

[86] Ohkusa T, Kato K, Terao S, *et al.* Newly developed antibiotic combination therapy for ulcerative colitis: a double-blind placebo-controlled multicenter trial. Am J Gastroenterol 2010; 105(8): 1820-9. [http://dx.doi.org/10.1038/ajg.2010.84] [PMID: 20216533]

[87] Castellarin M, Warren RL, Freeman JD, *et al. Fusobacterium nucleatum* infection is prevalent in human colorectal carcinoma. Genome Res 2012; 22(2): 299-306. [http://dx.doi.org/10.1101/gr.126516.111] [PMID: 22009989]

[88] Strauss J, Kaplan GG, Beck PL, *et al.* Invasive potential of gut mucosa-derived fusobacterium nucleatum positively correlates with IBD status of the host. Inflamm Bowel Dis 2011; 17(9): 1971-8. [http://dx.doi.org/10.1002/ibd.21606] [PMID: 21830275]

[89] Sokol H, Leducq V, Aschard H, *et al.* Fungal microbiota dysbiosis in IBD. Gut 2017; 66(6): 1039-48. [http://dx.doi.org/10.1136/gutjnl-2015-310746] [PMID: 26843508]

[90] Willing B, Halfvarson J, Dicksved J, *et al.* Twin studies reveal specific imbalances in the mucosa-associated microbiota of patients with ileal Crohn's disease. Inflamm Bowel Dis 2009; 15(5): 653-60. [http://dx.doi.org/10.1002/ibd.20783] [PMID: 19023901]

[91] Papamichael K, Konstantopoulos P, Mantzaris GJ. *Helicobacter pylori* infection and inflammatory

bowel disease: Is there a link? World J Gastroenterol 2014; 20(21): 6374-85.
[http://dx.doi.org/10.3748/wjg.v20.i21.6374] [PMID: 24914359]

[92] Rokkas T, Gisbert JP, Niv Y, O'Morain C. The association between *Helicobacter pylori* infection and inflammatory bowel disease based on meta□analysis. United European Gastroenterol J 2015; 3(6): 539-50.
[http://dx.doi.org/10.1177/2050640615580889] [PMID: 26668747]

[93] Qin J, Li R, Raes J, *et al.* A human gut microbial gene catalogue established by metagenomic sequencing. Nature 2010; 464(7285): 59-65.
[http://dx.doi.org/10.1038/nature08821] [PMID: 20203603]

[94] Underhill DM, Iliev ID. The mycobiota: interactions between commensal fungi and the host immune system. Nat Rev Immunol 2014; 14(6): 405-16.
[http://dx.doi.org/10.1038/nri3684] [PMID: 24854590]

[95] Dollive S, Chen YY, Grunberg S, *et al.* Fungi of the murine gut: episodic variation and proliferation during antibiotic treatment. PLoS One 2013; 8(8): e71806.
[http://dx.doi.org/10.1371/journal.pone.0071806] [PMID: 23977147]

[96] Hoffmann C, Dollive S, Grunberg S, *et al.* Archaea and fungi of the human gut microbiome: correlations with diet and bacterial residents. PLoS One 2013; 8(6): e66019.
[http://dx.doi.org/10.1371/journal.pone.0066019] [PMID: 23799070]

[97] Noverr MC, Noggle RM, Toews GB, Huffnagle GB. Role of antibiotics and fungal microbiota in driving pulmonary allergic responses. Infect Immun 2004; 72(9): 4996-5003.
[http://dx.doi.org/10.1128/IAI.72.9.4996-5003.2004] [PMID: 15321991]

[98] Liguori G, Lamas B, Richard ML, *et al.* Fungal Dysbiosis in Mucosa-associated Microbiota of Crohn's Disease Patients. J Crohn's Colitis 2016; 10(3): 296-305.
[http://dx.doi.org/10.1093/ecco-jcc/jjv209] [PMID: 26574491]

[99] Virgin HW. The virome in mammalian physiology and disease. Cell 2014; 157(1): 142-50.
[http://dx.doi.org/10.1016/j.cell.2014.02.032] [PMID: 24679532]

[100] Lecuit M, Eloit M. The human virome: new tools and concepts. Trends Microbiol 2013; 21(10): 510-5.
[http://dx.doi.org/10.1016/j.tim.2013.07.001] [PMID: 23906500]

[101] Ogilvie LA, Jones BV. The human gut virome: a multifaceted majority. Front Microbiol 2015; 6: 918.
[http://dx.doi.org/10.3389/fmicb.2015.00918] [PMID: 26441861]

[102] Pérez-Brocal V, García-López R, Vázquez-Castellanos JF, *et al.* Study of the viral and microbial communities associated with Crohn's disease: a metagenomic approach. Clin Transl Gastroenterol 2013; 4(6): e36.
[http://dx.doi.org/10.1038/ctg.2013.9] [PMID: 23760301]

[103] Wagner J, Maksimovic J, Farries G, *et al.* Bacteriophages in gut samples from pediatric Crohn's disease patients: metagenomic analysis using 454 pyrosequencing. Inflamm Bowel Dis 2013; 19(8): 1598-608.
[http://dx.doi.org/10.1097/MIB.0b013e318292477c] [PMID: 23749273]

[104] Lepage P, Colombet J, Marteau P, Sime-Ngando T, Doré J, Leclerc M. Dysbiosis in inflammatory bowel disease: a role for bacteriophages? Gut 2008; 57(3): 424-5.
[http://dx.doi.org/10.1136/gut.2007.134668] [PMID: 18268057]

[105] Brüssow H, Canchaya C, Hardt WD. Phages and the evolution of bacterial pathogens: from genomic rearrangements to lysogenic conversion. Microbiol Mol Biol Rev 2004; 68(3): 560-602.
[http://dx.doi.org/10.1128/MMBR.68.3.560-602.2004] [PMID: 15353570]

[106] Maiques E, Úbeda C, Campoy S, *et al.* β-lactam antibiotics induce the SOS response and horizontal transfer of virulence factors in *Staphylococcus aureus.* J Bacteriol 2006; 188(7): 2726-9.
[http://dx.doi.org/10.1128/JB.188.7.2726-2729.2006] [PMID: 16547063]

[107] Lichtenstein GR, Loftus EV, Isaacs KL, Regueiro MD, Gerson LB, Sands BE. ACG Clinical Guideline: Management of Crohn's Disease in Adults. Am J Gastroenterol 2018; 113(4): 481-517. [http://dx.doi.org/10.1038/ajg.2018.27] [PMID: 29610508]

[108] Rubin DT, Ananthakrishnan AN, Siegel CA, Sauer BG, Long MD. ACG Clinical Guideline: Ulcerative Colitis in Adults. Am J Gastroenterol 2019; 114(3): 384-413. [http://dx.doi.org/10.14309/ajg.0000000000000152] [PMID: 30840605]

[109] Ho GT, Chiam P, Drummond H, Loane J, Arnott IDR, Satsangi J. The efficacy of corticosteroid therapy in inflammatory bowel disease: analysis of a 5□year UK inception cohort. Aliment Pharmacol Ther 2006; 24(2): 319-30. [http://dx.doi.org/10.1111/j.1365-2036.2006.02974.x] [PMID: 16842459]

[110] Kuenzig ME, Rezaie A, Seow CH, *et al.* Budesonide for maintenance of remission in Crohn's disease. Cochrane Libr 2014; 2020(4): CD002913. [http://dx.doi.org/10.1002/14651858.CD002913.pub3] [PMID: 25141071]

[111] Neurath MF. Current and emerging therapeutic targets for IBD. Nat Rev Gastroenterol Hepatol 2017; 14(5): 269-78. [http://dx.doi.org/10.1038/nrgastro.2016.208] [PMID: 28144028]

[112] Chande N, Patton PH, Tsoulis DJ, Thomas BS, MacDonald JK. Azathioprine or 6-mercaptopurine for maintenance of remission in Crohn's disease. Cochrane Libr 2015; 2016(5): CD000067. [http://dx.doi.org/10.1002/14651858.CD000067.pub3] [PMID: 26517527]

[113] Feagan BG, Rochon J, Fedorak RN, *et al.* Methotrexate for the treatment of Crohn's disease. N Engl J Med 1995; 332(5): 292-7. [http://dx.doi.org/10.1056/NEJM199502023320503] [PMID: 7816064]

[114] Ledder O, Turner D. Antibiotics in IBD: Still a Role in the Biological Era? Inflamm Bowel Dis 2018; 24(8): 1676-88. [http://dx.doi.org/10.1093/ibd/izy067] [PMID: 29722812]

[115] Townsend CM, Parker CE, MacDonald JK, *et al.* Antibiotics for induction and maintenance of remission in Crohn's disease. Cochrane Libr 2019; 2(2): CD012730. [http://dx.doi.org/10.1002/14651858.CD012730.pub2] [PMID: 30731030]

[116] Naseer M, Poola S, Ali S, Samiullah S, Tahan V. Prebiotics and Probiotics in Inflammatory Bowel Disease: Where are we now and where are we going? Curr Clin Pharmacol 2020; 15(3): 216-33. [http://dx.doi.org/10.2174/22123938MTA1pMTY42] [PMID: 32164516]

[117] Ortigão R, Pimentel-Nunes P, Dinis-Ribeiro M, Libânio D. Gastrointestinal Microbiome – What We Need to Know in Clinical Practice. GE Port J Gastroenterol 2020; 27(5): 336-51. [http://dx.doi.org/10.1159/000505036] [PMID: 32999906]

[118] Hanauer SB, Feagan BG, Lichtenstein GR, *et al.* Maintenance infliximab for Crohn's disease: the ACCENT I randomised trial. Lancet 2002; 359(9317): 1541-9. [http://dx.doi.org/10.1016/S0140-6736(02)08512-4] [PMID: 12047962]

[119] Sandborn WJ, Hanauer SB, Rutgeerts P, *et al.* Adalimumab for maintenance treatment of Crohn's disease: results of the CLASSIC II trial. Gut 2007; 56(9): 1232-9. [http://dx.doi.org/10.1136/gut.2006.106781] [PMID: 17299059]

[120] Colombel JF, Sandborn WJ, Rutgeerts P, *et al.* Adalimumab for maintenance of clinical response and remission in patients with Crohn's disease: the CHARM trial. Gastroenterology 2007; 132(1): 52-65. [http://dx.doi.org/10.1053/j.gastro.2006.11.041] [PMID: 17241859]

[121] Sandborn WJ, Feagan BG, Marano C, *et al.* Subcutaneous golimumab maintains clinical response in patients with moderate-to-severe ulcerative colitis. Gastroenterology 2014; 146(1): 96-109.e1. [http://dx.doi.org/10.1053/j.gastro.2013.06.010] [PMID: 23770005]

[122] Schreiber S, Khaliq-Kareemi M, Lawrance IC, *et al.* Maintenance therapy with certolizumab pegol for

Crohn's disease. N Engl J Med 2007; 357(3): 239-50.
[http://dx.doi.org/10.1056/NEJMoa062897] [PMID: 17634459]

[123] Colombel JF, Sandborn WJ, Reinisch W, *et al.* Infliximab, azathioprine, or combination therapy for Crohn's disease. N Engl J Med 2010; 362(15): 1383-95.
[http://dx.doi.org/10.1056/NEJMoa0904492] [PMID: 20393175]

[124] Feagan BG, Rutgeerts P, Sands BE, *et al.* Vedolizumab as induction and maintenance therapy for ulcerative colitis. N Engl J Med 2013; 369(8): 699-710.
[http://dx.doi.org/10.1056/NEJMoa1215734] [PMID: 23964932]

[125] Sands BE, Sandborn WJ, Van Assche G, *et al.* Vedolizumab as Induction and Maintenance Therapy for Crohn's Disease in Patients Naïve to or Who Have Failed Tumor Necrosis Factor Antagonist Therapy. Inflamm Bowel Dis 2017; 23(1): 97-106.
[http://dx.doi.org/10.1097/MIB.0000000000000979] [PMID: 27930408]

[126] Feagan BG, Sandborn WJ, Gasink C, *et al.* Ustekinumab as Induction and Maintenance Therapy for Crohn's Disease. N Engl J Med 2016; 375(20): 1946-60.
[http://dx.doi.org/10.1056/NEJMoa1602773] [PMID: 27959607]

[127] Sands BE, Sandborn WJ, Panaccione R, *et al.* Ustekinumab as Induction and Maintenance Therapy for Ulcerative Colitis. N Engl J Med 2019; 381(13): 1201-14.
[http://dx.doi.org/10.1056/NEJMoa1900750] [PMID: 31553833]

[128] Nishida A, Imaeda H, Ohno M, *et al.* Efficacy and safety of single fecal microbiota transplantation for Japanese patients with mild to moderately active ulcerative colitis. J Gastroenterol 2017; 52(4): 476-82.
[http://dx.doi.org/10.1007/s00535-016-1271-4] [PMID: 27730312]

[129] Goyal A, Yeh A, Bush BR, *et al.* Safety, Clinical Response, and Microbiome Findings Following Fecal Microbiota Transplant in Children With Inflammatory Bowel Disease. Inflamm Bowel Dis 2018; 24(2): 410-21.
[http://dx.doi.org/10.1093/ibd/izx035] [PMID: 29361092]

[130] Wen X, Wang HG, Zhang MN, Zhang MH, Wang H, Yang XZ. Fecal microbiota transplantation ameliorates experimental colitis *via* gut microbiota and T-cell modulation. World J Gastroenterol 2021; 27(21): 2834-49.
[http://dx.doi.org/10.3748/wjg.v27.i21.2834] [PMID: 34135557]

[131] Zhang W, Zou G, Li B, *et al.* Fecal Microbiota Transplantation (FMT) Alleviates Experimental Colitis in Mice by Gut Microbiota Regulation. J Microbiol Biotechnol 2020; 30(8): 1132-41.
[http://dx.doi.org/10.4014/jmb.2002.02044] [PMID: 32423189]

[132] Maslowski KM, Vieira AT, Ng A, *et al.* Regulation of inflammatory responses by gut microbiota and chemoattractant receptor GPR43. Nature 2009; 461(7268): 1282-6.
[http://dx.doi.org/10.1038/nature08530] [PMID: 19865172]

[133] Caruso R, Lo BC, Núñez G. Host–microbiota interactions in inflammatory bowel disease. Nat Rev Immunol 2020; 20(7): 411-26.
[http://dx.doi.org/10.1038/s41577-019-0268-7] [PMID: 32005980]

[134] Paramsothy S, Nielsen S, Kamm MA, *et al.* Specific Bacteria and Metabolites Associated With Response to Fecal Microbiota Transplantation in Patients With Ulcerative Colitis. Gastroenterology 2019; 156(5): 1440-1454.e2.
[http://dx.doi.org/10.1053/j.gastro.2018.12.001] [PMID: 30529583]

[135] Vaughn BP, Vatanen T, Allegretti JR, *et al.* Increased Intestinal Microbial Diversity Following Fecal Microbiota Transplant for Active Crohn's Disease. Inflamm Bowel Dis 2016; 22(9): 2182-90.
[http://dx.doi.org/10.1097/MIB.0000000000000893] [PMID: 27542133]

[136] Park SC, Jeen YT. Anti-integrin therapy for inflammatory bowel disease. World J Gastroenterol 2018; 24(17): 1868-80.

[http://dx.doi.org/10.3748/wjg.v24.i17.1868] [PMID: 29740202]

[137] Zundler S, Becker E, Weidinger C, Siegmund B. Anti-Adhesion Therapies in Inflammatory Bowel Disease—Molecular and Clinical Aspects. Front Immunol 2017; 8: 891. [http://dx.doi.org/10.3389/fimmu.2017.00891] [PMID: 28804488]

[138] Soler D, Chapman T, Yang LL, Wyant T, Egan R, Fedyk ER. The binding specificity and selective antagonism of vedolizumab, an anti-$\alpha_4\beta_7$ integrin therapeutic antibody in development for inflammatory bowel diseases. J Pharmacol Exp Ther 2009; 330(3): 864-75. [http://dx.doi.org/10.1124/jpet.109.153973] [PMID: 19509315]

[139] Gubatan J, Keyashian K, Rubin SJS, Wang J, Buckman C, Sinha S. Anti-Integrins for the Treatment of Inflammatory Bowel Disease: Current Evidence and Perspectives. Clin Exp Gastroenterol 2021; 14: 333-42. [http://dx.doi.org/10.2147/CEG.S293272] [PMID: 34466013]

[140] Loftus EV Jr, Feagan BG, Panaccione R, *et al.* Long□term safety of vedolizumab for inflammatory bowel disease. Aliment Pharmacol Ther 2020; 52(8): 1353-65. [http://dx.doi.org/10.1111/apt.16060] [PMID: 32876349]

[141] Sandborn WJ, Vermeire S, Tyrrell H, *et al.* Etrolizumab for the Treatment of Ulcerative Colitis and Crohn's Disease: An Overview of the Phase 3 Clinical Program. Adv Ther 2020; 37(7): 3417-31. [http://dx.doi.org/10.1007/s12325-020-01366-2] [PMID: 32445184]

[142] Reinisch W, Sandborn WJ, Danese S, *et al.* Long-term Safety and Efficacy of the Anti-MAdCAM-1 Monoclonal Antibody Ontamalimab [SHP647] for the Treatment of Ulcerative Colitis: The Open-label Study TURANDOT II. J Crohn's Colitis 2021; 15(6): 938-49. [http://dx.doi.org/10.1093/ecco-jcc/jjab023] [PMID: 33599720]

[143] Noman M, Ferrante M, Bisschops R, *et al.* Vedolizumab Induces Long-term Mucosal Healing in Patients With Crohn's Disease and Ulcerative Colitis. J Crohn's Colitis 2017; 11(9): 1085-9. [http://dx.doi.org/10.1093/ecco-jcc/jjx048] [PMID: 28369329]

[144] Sugiura T, Kageyama S, Andou A, *et al.* Oral treatment with a novel small molecule alpha 4 integrin antagonist, AJM300, prevents the development of experimental colitis in mice. J Crohn's Colitis 2013; 7(11): e533-42. [http://dx.doi.org/10.1016/j.crohns.2013.03.014] [PMID: 23623333]

[145] Hibi T, Motoya S, Ashida T, *et al.* Efficacy and safety of abrilumab, an $\alpha4\beta7$ integrin inhibitor, in Japanese patients with moderate-to-severe ulcerative colitis: a phase II study. Intest Res 2019; 17(3): 375-86. [http://dx.doi.org/10.5217/ir.2018.00141] [PMID: 30739435]

[146] Sandborn WJ, Lee SD, Tarabar D, *et al.* Phase II evaluation of anti-MAdCAM antibody PF-00547659 in the treatment of Crohn's disease: report of the OPERA study. Gut 2018; 67(10): 1824-35. [http://dx.doi.org/10.1136/gutjnl-2016-313457] [PMID: 28982740]

[147] Higashiyama M, Hokari R. New and Emerging Treatments for Inflammatory Bowel Disease. Digestion 2023; 104(1): 74-81. [http://dx.doi.org/10.1159/000527422] [PMID: 36366823]

[148] Dudek P, Fabisiak A, Zatorski H, Malecka-Wojciesko E, Talar-Wojnarowska R. Efficacy, Safety and Future Perspectives of JAK Inhibitors in the IBD Treatment. J Clin Med 2021; 10(23): 5660. [http://dx.doi.org/10.3390/jcm10235660] [PMID: 34884361]

[149] Danese S, Peyrin-Biroulet L. Selective Tyrosine Kinase 2 Inhibition for Treatment of Inflammatory Bowel Disease: New Hope on the Rise. Inflamm Bowel Dis 2021; 27(12): 2023-30. [http://dx.doi.org/10.1093/ibd/izab135] [PMID: 34089259]

[150] De Vries LCS, Ghiboub M, van Hamersveld PHP, *et al.* Tyrosine Kinase 2 Signalling Drives Pathogenic T cells in Colitis. J Crohn's Colitis 2021; 15(4): 617-30. [http://dx.doi.org/10.1093/ecco-jcc/jjaa199] [PMID: 33005945]

[151] Sandborn WJ, Ghosh S, Panes J, *et al.* Efficacy of Upadacitinib in a Randomized Trial of Patients With Active Ulcerative Colitis. Gastroenterology 2020; 158(8): 2139-2149.e14. [http://dx.doi.org/10.1053/j.gastro.2020.02.030] [PMID: 32092309]

[152] Alsoud D, Verstockt B, Fiocchi C, Vermeire S. Breaking the therapeutic ceiling in drug development in ulcerative colitis. Lancet Gastroenterol Hepatol 2021; 6(7): 589-95. [http://dx.doi.org/10.1016/S2468-1253(21)00065-0] [PMID: 34019798]

[153] Shen B, Kochhar G, Hull TL. Bridging Medical and Surgical Treatment of Inflammatory Bowel Disease: The Role of Interventional IBD. Am J Gastroenterol 2019; 114(4): 539-40. [http://dx.doi.org/10.1038/s41395-018-0416-x] [PMID: 30464306]

[154] Biondi A, Zoccali M, Costa S, Troci A, Contessini-Avesani E, Fichera A. Surgical treatment of ulcerative colitis in the biologic therapy era. World J Gastroenterol 2012; 18(16): 1861-70. [http://dx.doi.org/10.3748/wjg.v18.i16.1861] [PMID: 22563165]

[155] Svartz N. The treatment of 124 cases of ulcerative colitis with salazopyrine and attempts of desensibilization in cases of hypersensitiveness to sulfa. Acta Med Scand 1948; 130(S206) (Suppl. 206): 465-72. [http://dx.doi.org/10.1111/j.0954-6820.1948.tb12083.x] [PMID: 18881171]

[156] Colman RJ, Rubin DT. Fecal microbiota transplantation as therapy for inflammatory bowel disease: A systematic review and meta-analysis. J Crohn's Colitis 2014; 8(12): 1569-81. [http://dx.doi.org/10.1016/j.crohns.2014.08.006] [PMID: 25223604]

[157] Feagan BG, Danese S, Loftus EV Jr, *et al.* Filgotinib as induction and maintenance therapy for ulcerative colitis (SELECTION): a phase 2b/3 double-blind, randomised, placebo-controlled trial. Lancet 2021; 397(10292): 2372-84. [http://dx.doi.org/10.1016/S0140-6736(21)00666-8] [PMID: 34090625]

[158] Naganuma M, Yokoyama Y, Motoya S, *et al.* Efficacy of apheresis as maintenance therapy for patients with ulcerative colitis in an open-label prospective multicenter randomised controlled trial. J Gastroenterol 2020; 55(4): 390-400. [http://dx.doi.org/10.1007/s00535-019-01651-0] [PMID: 31811562]

[159] Yoshino T, Nakase H, Minami N, *et al.* Efficacy and safety of granulocyte and monocyte adsorption apheresis for ulcerative colitis: A meta-analysis. Dig Liver Dis 2014; 46(3): 219-26. [http://dx.doi.org/10.1016/j.dld.2013.10.011] [PMID: 24268950]

[160] Lai YM, Yao WY, He Y, *et al.* Adsorptive Granulocyte and Monocyte Apheresis in the Treatment of Ulcerative Colitis: The First Multicenter Study in China. Gut Liver 2017; 11(2): 216-25. [http://dx.doi.org/10.5009/gnl15408] [PMID: 27843131]

[161] Motoya S, Tanaka H, Shibuya T, *et al.* Safety and effectiveness of granulocyte and monocyte adsorptive apheresis in patients with inflammatory bowel disease in special situations: a multicentre cohort study. BMC Gastroenterol 2019; 19(1): 196. [http://dx.doi.org/10.1186/s12876-019-1110-1] [PMID: 31752695]

[162] Fukuchi T, Nakase H, Ubukata S, *et al.* Therapeutic effect of intensive granulocyte and monocyte adsorption apheresis combined with thiopurines for steroid- and biologics-naïve Japanese patients with early-diagnosed Crohn's disease. BMC Gastroenterol 2014; 14(1): 124. [http://dx.doi.org/10.1186/1471-230X-14-124] [PMID: 25015328]

[163] Rodríguez-Lago I, Benítez JM, García-Sánchez V, *et al.* Granulocyte and monocyte apheresis in inflammatory bowel disease: The patients' point of view. Gastroenterol Hepatol 2018; 41(7): 423-31. [http://dx.doi.org/10.1016/j.gastrohep.2018.04.007] [PMID: 29739692]

[164] Verstockt B, Vetrano S, Salas A, *et al.* Sphingosine 1-phosphate modulation and immune cell trafficking in inflammatory bowel disease. Nat Rev Gastroenterol Hepatol 2022; 19(6): 351-66. [http://dx.doi.org/10.1038/s41575-021-00574-7] [PMID: 35165437]

[165] Moschen AR, Tilg H, Raine T. IL-12, IL-23 and IL-17 in IBD: immunobiology and therapeutic

targeting. Nat Rev Gastroenterol Hepatol 2019; 16(3): 185-96.
[http://dx.doi.org/10.1038/s41575-018-0084-8] [PMID: 30478416]

[166] Zhou C, Wu D, Jawale C, *et al.* Divergent functions of IL-17-family cytokines in DSS colitis: Insights from a naturally-occurring human mutation in IL-17F. Cytokine 2021; 148: 155715.
[http://dx.doi.org/10.1016/j.cyto.2021.155715] [PMID: 34587561]

[167] Siakavellas SI, Bamias G. Tumor Necrosis Factor–like Cytokine TL1A and Its Receptors DR3 and DcR3. Inflamm Bowel Dis 2015; 21(10): 1.
[http://dx.doi.org/10.1097/MIB.0000000000000492] [PMID: 26099067]

[168] Furfaro F, Alfarone L, Gilardi D, *et al.* TL1A: A New Potential Target in the Treatment of Inflammatory Bowel Disease. Curr Drug Targets 2021; 22(7): 760-9.
[http://dx.doi.org/10.2174/1389450122999210120205607] [PMID: 33475057]

[169] Danese S, Neurath MF, Kopoń A, *et al.* Effects of Apremilast, an Oral Inhibitor of Phosphodiesterase 4, in a Randomized Trial of Patients With Active Ulcerative Colitis. Clin Gastroenterol Hepatol 2020; 18(11): 2526-2534.e9.
[http://dx.doi.org/10.1016/j.cgh.2019.12.032] [PMID: 31926340]

[170] Neufert C, Neurath MF, Atreya R. Rationale for IL-36 receptor antibodies in ulcerative colitis. Expert Opin Biol Ther 2020; 20(4): 339-42.
[http://dx.doi.org/10.1080/14712598.2020.1695775] [PMID: 31773994]

[171] Amoroso C, Perillo F, Strati F, Fantini M, Caprioli F, Facciotti F. The Role of Gut Microbiota Biomodulators on Mucosal Immunity and Intestinal Inflammation. Cells 2020; 9(5): 1234.
[http://dx.doi.org/10.3390/cells9051234] [PMID: 32429359]

[172] Tan XY, Xie YJ, Liu XL, Li XY, Jia B. A Systematic Review and Meta-Analysis of Randomized Controlled Trials of Fecal Microbiota Transplantation for the Treatment of Inflammatory Bowel Disease. Evid Based Complement Alternat Med 2022; 2022: 1-14.
[http://dx.doi.org/10.1155/2022/8266793] [PMID: 35795291]

[173] Yang M, Gu Y, Li L, *et al.* Bile Acid–Gut Microbiota Axis in Inflammatory Bowel Disease: From Bench to Bedside. Nutrients 2021; 13(9): 3143.
[http://dx.doi.org/10.3390/nu13093143] [PMID: 34579027]

[174] Agus A, Planchais J, Sokol H. Gut Microbiota Regulation of Tryptophan Metabolism in Health and Disease. Cell Host Microbe 2018; 23(6): 716-24.
[http://dx.doi.org/10.1016/j.chom.2018.05.003] [PMID: 29902437]

[175] Cao Y, Su Q, Zhang B, Shen F, Li S. Efficacy of stem cells therapy for Crohn's fistula: a meta-analysis and systematic review. Stem Cell Res Ther 2021; 12(1): 32.
[http://dx.doi.org/10.1186/s13287-020-02095-7] [PMID: 33413661]

[176] Bonaz B. Is-there a place for vagus nerve stimulation in inflammatory bowel diseases? Bioelectron Med 2018; 4(1): 4.
[http://dx.doi.org/10.1186/s42234-018-0004-9] [PMID: 32232080]

[177] Castro-Dopico T, Colombel JF, Mehandru S. Targeting B cells for inflammatory bowel disease treatment: back to the future. Curr Opin Pharmacol 2020; 55: 90-8.
[http://dx.doi.org/10.1016/j.coph.2020.10.002] [PMID: 33166872]

[178] Saez A, Gomez-Bris R, Herrero-Fernandez B, Mingorance C, Rius C, Gonzalez-Granado JM. Innate Lymphoid Cells in Intestinal Homeostasis and Inflammatory Bowel Disease. Int J Mol Sci 2021; 22(14): 7618.
[http://dx.doi.org/10.3390/ijms22147618] [PMID: 34299236]

[179] Günther C, Rothhammer V, Karow M, Neurath M, Winner B. The Gut-Brain Axis in Inflammatory Bowel Disease—Current and Future Perspectives. Int J Mol Sci 2021; 22(16): 8870.
[http://dx.doi.org/10.3390/ijms22168870] [PMID: 34445575]

CHAPTER 3

Obesity and the Gut Microbiome

Soumyadeep Chattopadhyay[1], Rudradeep Hazra[1], Arijit Mallick[1], Sakuntala Gayen[1] and **Souvik Roy[1,*]**

[1] *Department of Pharmaceutical Technology, NSHM Knowledge Campus, Kolkata-Group of Institutions, 124, B. L. Saha Road, Tara Park, Behala, Kolkata, West Bengal-700053, India*

Abstract: The gut microbiota (GM) comprises a complicated community of bacteria within the human intestinal tract. Nutrient absorption, immune reaction, energy metabolism, and various other physiological functions are all greatly impacted by the extensive and dynamic population of microbes found in the human gut. Scientific study indicates that a disorder in the configuration and role of the gut microbiota known as dysbiosis plays a major part in the development of inflammation leading to the development of obesity and illnesses associated with it like metabolic syndrome, non-alcoholic fatty liver, and the development of type 2 diabetes mellitus and cancer. There is a common interactive relationship between the microbiota in the gut with all the organs in the body including the brain. Food addiction along with dysfunctional eating patterns reflect changes in the interrelationship between the brain- gut-microbiota (BGM), along with a tipping point in this balance towards hedonistic pathways that result in obesity. Research supports the belief that the pathophysiology of obesity is influenced by bidirectional transmission in the gut-brain axis (GBA), which is assisted by the immune system, neurological, endocrine, and metabolic mechanisms. This study discusses the roles played by the gut microbiota in promoting obesity, the comorbidities that go along with it, and how microbial manipulation can assist in avoiding or alleviating weight gain and related comorbidities. It also encompasses the various strategies used to address the issue, including diet modifications to address individual microflora or the use of probiotics, prebiotics, synbiotics, and fecal microbiota transplants (FMT).

Keywords: Brain-gut microbiota (BGM), Diet modification,endocrine regulation, Fecal microbiota transplants (FMT), Food addiction, Gut-brain axis (GBA), Gut microbiota, Hedonistic pathways, Microbial dysbiosis.

INTRODUCTION

The incidence of obesity, a complicated metabolic disease spurred on by an array of genetic and nongenetic causes, is increasing rapidly in both developed and

* **Corresponding author Souvik Roy:** Department of Pharmaceutical Technology, NSHM Knowledge Campus, Kolkata-Group of Institutions, 124, B. L. Saha Road, Tara Park, Behala, Kolkata, West Bengal-700053, India; E-mail: souvikroy35@gmail.com

Sandipan Dasgupta & Moitreyee Chattopadhyay (Eds.)

developing nations. Though the exact definition varies by nation, the World Health Organization (WHO) describes the condition of obesity as having a body mass index (BMI) of more than thirty. Based on comprehensive studies all over the world, approximately 35% of the community is considered to have body mass more than BMI, and 11% are obese [1]. Besides its outward manifestations, obesity has been linked with metabolic issues such as deposition of fat and glucose, oxidative stress, chronic inflammation, and an increased risk of several ailments, including cancer, type 2 diabetes, and cardiovascular disorders [2]. Within the gut resides a community of symbiotic microbes known as the gut microbiota, which can number up to 100 trillion and is ten times more numerous than all the cells in the body. The bacterial genome that comprises the gut microbiota, or microbiome, influences nutrition uptake, energy management, and fat accumulation whose imbalance can lead to obesity. To sustain its robust population, the gut microbiota relies on a supply of deceased cells for nutrients, along with mucus secreted by the gut and undigested remnants from the diet that are inaccessible to the human body for absorption [3, 4].

The gut microbiota among human beings is a complicated and constantly changing ecological system that has developed with its host and makes up about one kilogram of total body weight. The idea that the communities of microbes that live in our stomachs work similarly to an organ and affect several facets of human health by way of immunological, metabolic, and endocrine processes is becoming a growing consensus. A significant portion of gut bacteria remains unculturable, thus impeding our comprehension of this microbiota due to technical limitations. In the 1980s, Pace and colleagues pioneered a novel culture-independent approach for bacterial identification, centered on sequencing the 16S rRNA gene. The implementation of 16S ribosomal RNA (rRNA)-based, culture-independent molecular techniques in the 1990s included competitive PCR, real-time PCR, fluorescent in situ hybridization, and denaturing/temperature gradient gel electrophoresis, supported the understanding that *Bacteroidetes and Firmicutes* bacteria are most prevalent in the gut microbiome of human [5]. In addition to producing various biologically active compounds such as SCFAs and vitamins, the dynamic gut microbiota can generate both potentially harmful substances like neurotoxins, carcinogens, and immunotoxins, as well as beneficial compounds such as antioxidants, pain relievers, and anti-inflammatory agents [6]. Obesity is often classified into two main types: visceral and subcutaneous. A known biomarker for obesity is an elevated *Firmicutes/Bacteroidetes* ratio. But in cases of extreme obesity, there is a positive link between the relative abundance of *Firmicutes* and indicators of brown adipocytes in subcutaneous adipose tissue as opposed to visceral adipose tissue. This implies that browning of white adipose tissue may assist the maintenance of a healthy obesity pattern, suggesting a potential benefit of a larger relative abundance of *Firmicutes* for subcutaneous obesity [7]. Thus, the maintenance of the body's metabolism and energy equilibrium relies on the presence of a healthy gut flora. Metabolic complications and elevated central appetite could originate from an imbalance in the gut flora, which might lead to obesity [8]. Moreover, obesity is recognized to hurt the quality of life and increase the likelihood of experiencing psychological conditions such as depression and anxiety disorders. The gut-brain axis (GBA), which serves as a shorthand for the bidirectional connection that exists between the gut microbiome and the brain, is mediated by immunological, endocrine, and neurological pathways [9, 10]. Signals from the central nervous system regulate several gastrointestinal processes, such as the mucus transition and secretion of fluid motility. These signals are transmitted along the autonomic nervous system *via* the hypothalamic-pituitary-adrenal (HPA) axis [11]. Recent research has linked obesity to the gut microbiota due to its influence on hormones regulating appetite, such as ghrelin, leptin (LEP), and glucagon-like peptide 1 (GLP-1). Furthermore, studies have shown that modifying eating behaviors and appetite heavily depends on the gut-brain axis's neuronal connection with the vagus nerve. A unique approach to obesity management involves targeting the gut-microbiot--brain axis, as it plays a crucial role in regulating behaviors and physiological processes associated with obesity. Fecal microbiota transplantation and probiotic, prebiotic, and synbiotic supplements constitute some of the GBA-based therapies [12].

THE GI TRACT AND IT'S MICROBIOME

The Development and Robustness of the Gut Microbiome

While there may be limited bacterial translocation through the placental circulation contributing to a basic microbiota before birth, fetuses are commonly believed to be devoid of microbes while in the womb [13]. An infant's gut rapidly gets colonized by germs on delivery from the mother as well as from the surroundings. Breastfeeding compared to antibiotic therapy, delivery method (cesarean section vs vaginal delivery), and hygiene in the environment all affect the makeup of this microbiota. The host's genotype, growth modifications to the gut environment, and the consumption of solid foods represent a few of the factors that impact these microbiotas during the first few years of life [14]. Around the age of three, a more robust and intricate community that is similar to the adult microbiota develops. The "core microbiome," consisting of a vast array of shared microbial genes, illustrates the evolutionary convergence among diverse bacterial species [15].

The Diversity and Functions of the Microbiota in the Gut

The microbiome of the gastrointestinal tract plays vital roles that the human body alone cannot fulfill, leading to a mutually beneficial relationship. It is indispensable for nourishing normal gastrointestinal and immune functions, as well as for efficient nutrient digestion. The microbiota, for example, facilitates the fermentation of indigestible food components, the synthesis of vital vitamins and micronutrients, the metabolism of dietary toxins and carcinogens, the conversion of cholesterol and bile acids, the promotion of immune system maturation, the regulation of intestinal blood vessel formation, the growth and differentiation of intestinal cells, and the defense against enteric pathogens [16]. Moreover, dysbiosis which is an imbalance in the consistency of the gut microbiome has been connected to immunological problems, increased vulnerability to infections, and more recently several non-intestinal illnesses, including diabetes, obesity, liver disease, and even neurological issues [17].

Eubiotic Gut Microbiota

Eubiosis refers to a state of balanced and harmonious gut microbiota. In an eubiotic environment, diverse beneficial bacteria, such as *Bacteroides* and *Firmicutes*, coexist in a symbiotic relationship with the host. These microbes support several physiological processes, such as the modulation of the immune system, nutrient absorption, digestion, and the synthesis of certain vitamins [18]. A well-balanced eubiotic gut microbiota is associated with overall health, proper metabolism, and protection against pathogenic invaders. Factors like a diverse diet, prebiotics, and a healthy lifestyle contribute to maintaining eubiosis [19].

Dysbiotic Gut Microbiota

Dysbiosis refers to an imbalance or disruption in the gut microbiota composition. This imbalance may result from various factors, such as antibiotic use, poor dietary choices, stress, or infections. Dysbiosis can lead to a reduction in beneficial bacteria, an overgrowth of harmful microorganisms, and alterations in microbial diversity [20]. Dysbiotic gut microbiota is associated with various health issues, including gastrointestinal disorders, inflammation, metabolic disorders, and a compromised immune system. Imbalances in the gut microbiota have also been linked to conditions like irritable bowel syndrome (IBS), inflammatory bowel disease (IBD), and obesity [21].

Firmicutes, Bacteroides, Proteus, Actinomycetes, Fusobacteria, and Verrucomicrobia make up the majority of the typical human gut microbiota. The biodegradation of polysaccharides, the production of short-chain fatty acids, the enrichment of specific lipopolysaccharides, and the synthesis of vitamins and essential amino acids constitute the primary roles of a healthy gut microbiome [22]. The gut microbiota and humans have a reciprocal advantage because they perform vital functions that the human body cannot perform. The microbiota breaks down indigestible food components, breaks toxins and carcinogens, processes lipids and bile acids, promotes immune system development, and guards against intestinal pathogens. Therefore, sustaining healthy GI and immunological systems as well as effective nutrition digestion depends on the gut bacteria [23].

Link between Dysbiosis and Obesity

Modifications in the gut microbiota's constitution may play a major role in the emergence of obesity. Ley *et al.* 2016) found that in an obese mouse model without leptin (ob/ob mice), there was a significant increase in *Firmicutes* levels and a drop in the abundance of the *Bacteroidetes* phylum with their 16S rRNA gene sequencing research [24]. Some months later, Turnbaugh, working with the same team, used shotgun metagenomics sequencing to confirm that the bacterial DNA from the cecum of obese mice had a higher ratio of *Firmicutes* to *Bacteroidetes* than that of their slender, healthy counterparts [25]. Furthermore, in comparison to control mice, the cecal microbial population of ob/ob animals showed elevated amounts of *Archaea.* These changes in bacterial abundance have spurred additional research into the dynamics of gut microbiota in human individuals and different obesity models. As a result, further research on obesity has linked lower levels of *Bifidobacteria* to higher concentrations of some bacteria, such as *Sphingomonas* or *Halomonas* [26, 27].

Although healthy people often have diverse gut microbiota, those who are obese or have high levels of adiposity, insulin resistance, or dyslipidemia frequently have low counts of bacterial genes in their gut microbiota. A lower percentage of *Bacteroidetes* and higher concentrations of *Firmicutes* are commonly linked to obesity. As an example, people who have a *Firmicutes/Bacteroidetes* ratio of greater than or equal to one are twenty-three percent more likely to be overweight than people who have a ratio of less than one [28]. *Fecalibacterium prausnitzii*, one of the most prevalent bacteria in the *Firmicutes phylum* in the healthy human gut, is diminished in obesity, despite a rise in *Firmicutes* such as *Clostridium*, *Lactobacillus*, or *Ruminococcus* when compared with the fecal samples of obese individuals compared to their lean counterparts, Million and colleagues found lower levels of *Lactobacillus paracasei (L. paracasei)* and *Akkermansia muciniphila (A. muciniphila)*, along with higher levels of *Lactobacillus reuteri* (*L. reuteri) and Lactobacillus gasseri (L. gasseri)*. Furthermore, different species of *Lactobacillus* and *Clostridium* have been associated with varied levels of insulin resistance in females [29]. The quantity of *Lactobacillus* has shown favorable connections with both fasting glucose and glycated hemoglobin (HbA1c) levels, while *Clostridium* is negatively connected with these measures. All of these results point to a particular role of gut bacteria in the development of obesity [30].

THE GUT-BRAIN MICROBIOTA AXIS (GBMA)

The scientific concept behind the term "gut-microbiota-brain axis" involves the exchange of information in both directions through a complex network linking the gut microbial population with the brain. It is essential for maintaining the equilibrium of the gastrointestinal and central nervous systems (CNS) [31]. A complicated community consisting of millions of micro-organisms in the gut microbiome that significantly impacts normal physiological functions and the host's susceptibility to disease. Hosting over a hundred bacterial species and possessing approximately 200 times more genes than the human genome, it predominantly consists of bacteria but also includes protozoa, viruses, archaea, and fungi. The continually changing structure of the gut microbiome influences human health and can be influenced by host factors like age and genetics in addition to environmental factors like nutrition [32]. The gut microbiome serves a variety of operations, such as maintaining intestinal integrity, forming mucus, promoting intestinal epithelial cell regeneration, and facilitating the production of short-chain fatty acids (SCFAs). It is capable of interpreting and regulating an extensive variety of environmental signals, impacting multiple areas of the body, and it's additionally essential for the early stages of innate immune maturation. Acting as a mediator between the host and the environment, the gut microbiota has the potential to significantly influence human health. Variations in beneficial microbes can influence health in significant ways and may have a role in the pathophysiology of some diseases. The microbiota's makeup can also be altered by variables like nutrition, disease, drug use, and infections [33].

Brain and Gut Neurological Connections

The digestive system and the cognitive system are physically linked *via* nerve fibers. The autonomic nervous system (ANS) and the vagus nerve are the two main neural networks implicated. While the ANS controls the gut and the enteric nervous system (ENS), the vagus nerve mediates communication between the gut and the brain stem [34]. The gut glial cells, submucosal ganglia, and myenteric ganglia that comprise the Enteric Nervous System (ENS) are included in the first tier. Prevertebral ganglia are involved in the second layer and are essential for peripheral visceral reflex responses. The third tier consists of the nucleus tractus solitarius (NTS) and the dorsal motor nucleus of the vagus nerve, which are housed in the brain stem and spinal cord, respectively. These structures project and receive signals from the vagus nerve's efferent and afferent fibers. The cerebral cortex and subcortical regions like the thalamus and basal ganglia send neuron impulses to the medulla and pontine nuclei, which are located in the fourth tier of the brain. Gut tissue-based receptors are important players in the afferent pathway. Mechanoreceptors are in charge of recognizing changes in intestine volume, whilst chemoreceptors are vital for sensing chemical stimuli including hormones and neurotransmitters. Subsequently, the vagus nerve transmits signals from these gut receptors to the central nervous system (CNS). Notably, the gut microbiota influences these receptors themselves. Metabolites generated by gut bacteria, like short-chain fatty acids (SCFAs), are detected by chemoreceptors known as enteroendocrine cells [35]. (EECs), causing calcium signaling that can be sent to certain vagus nerve fibers in the intestinal epithelium. Signals that travel downward from the central nervous system to the visceral organs and tissues are carried by the vagus nerve. It also affects how the immune system and regular metabolism are controlled. These routes reaching the gut may affect the gut environment, which would then have a big impact on the gut microbiome [36].

Brain and Gut in Conduit with the Endocrine System

The gut microbiome affects numerous neuroendocrine processes in the brain, including the hypothalamus-pituitary-adrenal (HPA) axis. This system may impact behaviors related to learning, memory, sexual and social interactions, stress regulation, eating patterns, and obesity [37, 38]. Direct synthesis of tryptophan, neurotransmitters, and some SCFAs particularly propionic and butyric acids, can penetrate the bloodstream and alter the brain directly as well as immunologically, particularly by microglia maturation, catecholamine generation, and glucose metabolism, resulting in alterations in behavior and physiology [39]. It instantly encourages the release of glucagon-like peptide 1 (GLP-1), initiates the secretion of peptide YY (PYY) as described in Fig. (**1**), and indirectly influences the release of ghrelin by activating certain G protein-coupled receptors. These systems are involved in controlling appetite, hunger, and satiety as well as eating habits [40].

GBA in Combination with Obesity

In 1983, Wostmann and colleagues were among the first researchers to demonstrate the role of gut microbiome on host obesity by studying germ-free (GF) animals raised in sterile isolators without bacteria [41]. Their findings showed that GF rodents required thirty percent more calories to sustain their body weight compared to conventionally raised ones. Later studies revealed that the introduction of intestinal bacteria from conventionally bred mice to germ-free mice resulted in the development of adipose tissue in the recipients, which led to increased levels of fat and insulin resistance even in the absence of a reduced diet [42].

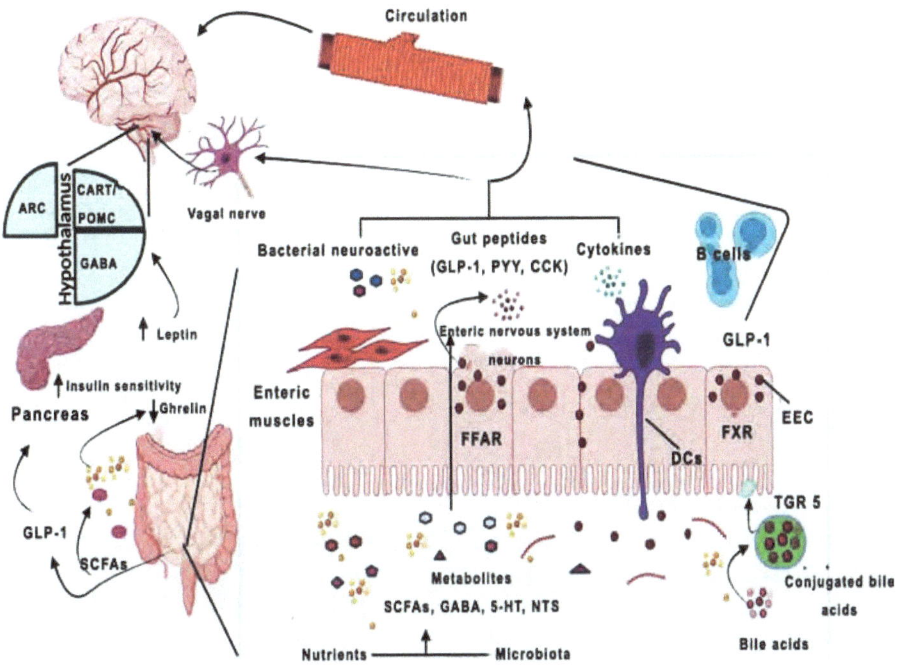

Fig. (1). The relationship between the gut-brain axis and obesity.

Dietary nutrients are converted by intestinal microorganisms into metabolites, which include serotonin (5-HT), γ-aminobutyric acid (GABA), short-chain fatty acids (SCFAs), and other neurotransmitters. These substances either directly stimulate the vagus nerve and regulate appetite, or they indirectly influence these functions through immune-neuroendocrine pathways. Enteroendocrine cells (EECs) are activated by metabolites obtained from microbes, which in turn causes the release of gut hormones like cholecystokinin (CCK), peptide YY (PYY), and glucagon-like peptide-1 (GLP-1). These hormones influence hunger and energy balance regulation in the hypothalamus by sending signals to the brain through the vagus nerve and circulation. Furthermore, farnesoid X receptor (FXR) and Takeda G-protein-coupled receptor 5 (TGR5) receptors can be activated by gut microorganisms, which raises GLP-1 production and affects insulin sensitivity and glucose tolerance. In addition to potentially influencing the synthesis of ghrelin and leptin, microbial metabolites can also cause inflammation by releasing lipopolysaccharide (LPS), which in turn can activate immunological responses.

MECHANISM OF GUT-MICROBIOTA-INDUCED OBESITY

Energy Consumption

In animal experiments, it was observed that germ-free mice colonized with the "obese microbiota" exhibited a significant increase in total body fat compared to those colonized with the "lean microbiota," even when their food intake and weight remained unchanged [43]. These findings suggest that the gut microbiota of obese individuals is better able to absorb energy from food. Obese hosts exhibited higher lipid absorption, according to a multiomics study. The genes that regulate lipid absorption were downregulated in germ-free mice after *Clostridium* colonization. Consequently, obese patient's gut bacteria could promote energy absorption, leading to an excessive buildup of energy and a rise in weight gain [44].

Core Appetite

The peptides glucagon-like peptide-1 (GLP-1), pancreatic polypeptide, and peptide YY are involved in information transmission along the gut-brain axis. The gut secretes two anorexigenic hormones: pancreatic polypeptide and peptide YY [45]. In addition to delaying stomach emptying and lowering glucagon levels, GLP-1 also boosts insulin synthesis and suppresses hunger. Research has shown that GLP-1 and peptide YY levels are typically lower in obese people [46]. Furthermore, data suggests that the gut microbiome and its byproducts support gut contentment. The short-term modulation of gut satiety spurred on by bacterial growth may interact with the long-term brain neuropeptide energy circuits that control appetite [47].

Accumulation of Fat

In a research study conducted in 2004, the researchers demonstrated the ability of the gut microbiome to regulate fat storage. This regulation is associated with increased expression levels of two essential transcription factors that support the hepatic production of fat: SREBP-1 (sterol regulatory element-binding protein) and ChREBP (carbohydrate response element binding protein) [48]. The gut microbiota elevates serum glucose levels and improves the host's intestinal absorption of glucose, which in turn upregulates SREBP-1 and ChREBP. Hepatic cells metabolize triglycerides before transporting them into the bloodstream with the aid of lipoprotein lipase (LPL) [49]. In a mouse model of obesity caused by a high-fat diet, Aronsson *et al.* found that *L. paracasei* controlled ANGPTL4, which is an important regulator of fat storage. *L. paracasei* may stimulate peroxisomal proliferator-activated receptors α and γ resulting in the synthesis of ANGPTL4. Because ANGPTL4 inhibits LPL function, less fat is stored [50, 51]. Mice colonized with *L. paracasei* were found to resist obesity induced by a high-fat diet. Additionally, *L. paracasei* inhibits the Akt/mTOR pathway in vitro, indicating its involvement in diverse intracellular lipid accumulation regulatory mechanisms [52].

Persistent Inflammation

Metabolic diseases such as obesity are often associated with chronic or persistent inflammation [53]. According to studies, the intestinal barrier is breached by the gut microbiome and its metabolized products, which affects the liver and adipose tissue and causes persistent inflammation [54]. In obesity-related adipose tissue inflammation, there is an elevated expression of lipopolysaccharide (LPS), an endotoxin. Binding of LPS to immune cells' Toll-like receptor 4, sets off a chain reaction that causes inflammation in the gut [55]. Additionally, gut bacteria can help prevent intestinal barrier dysfunction induced by a high-fat diet by blocking cannabinoid receptor type 1. Activation of the endocannabinoid system, a key regulator of fat formation in the gut and fat cells, may lead to increased hunger and food intake [56].

Antibiotics

Antibiotics are recognized for their ability to change the composition of the microbiota. While short-term antibiotic treatment is associated with rapid recovery, repeated antibiotic disturbances may lead to widespread consequences [57]. Recent studies in mice have shown that weight gain occurs only with early exposure to antibiotics. Mice given a low dose of penicillin at birth gained more weight than those given the same medication after weaning. Importantly, these effects persisted in adult mice for weeks following the discontinuation of antibiotic therapy, suggesting that even brief disruptions in early life can have long-lasting effects [58, 59].

DISORDERS ASSOCIATED WITH OBESITY

The pathophysiology of obesity often coincides with an imbalance characterized by a relative increase in *Firmicutes* relative to *Bacteroidetes*. Due to the non-digestible polysaccharides produced by *Firmicutes*, there can be a greater production of metabolites, which sets the host at risk for enhanced energy extraction and thus higher weight gain ultimately leading to obesity and diseases associated with it [60].

Type 2 Diabetes Mellitus

Type 2 diabetes is characterized by insulin resistance, oxidative stress, chronic low-grade inflammation, dysregulated lipid and glucose metabolism, and dysfunction of pancreatic beta cells. Individuals with type 2 diabetes often have higher levels of blood lipopolysaccharides (LPS) due to increased intestinal permeability [61, 62]. LPS triggers systemic inflammation, leading to impaired insulin function and subsequent insulin resistance in peripheral organs as described in Fig. (**2**). Research suggests that the numerous bacterial species within the gut microbiota could play a significant role in the breakdown of glucose [63]. Additionally, metformin a commonly prescribed medication for diabetes mellitus, can enhance the population of bacteria involved in producing short-chain fatty acids (SCFAs) and *Akkermansia muciniphila*, a derivative member of the *Verrucomicrobia* genus responsible for mucus breakdown [64, 65].

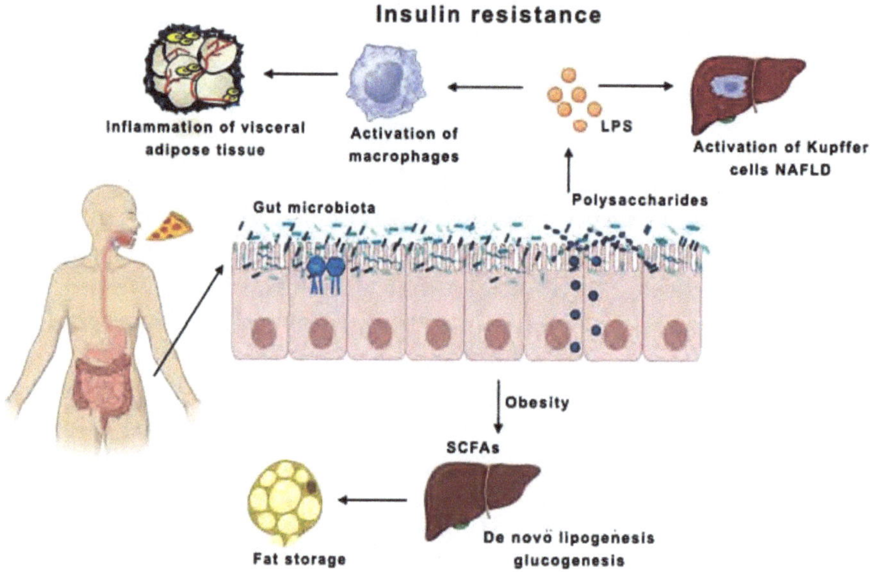

Fig. (2). Mechanisms by which gut microbiota influences human metabolism, leading to obesity and insulin resistance.

Persistent bacterial translocation resulting from heightened intestinal permeability can instigate systemic inflammation, prompting the infiltration of macrophages into visceral adipose tissue and activation of hepatic Kupffer cells, ultimately leading to insulin resistance. Short-chain fatty acids help restore intestinal permeability and modify de novo lipogenesis and gluconeogenesis by reducing the production of free fatty acids from visceral adipose tissue.

Gut Microbiota in Relation with Metabolic Syndrome

Metabolic syndrome is characterized by cardiovascular and type 2 diabetes risk factors including hyperglycemia, dyslipidemia, hypertension, and central obesity. Research suggests that aside from insulin resistance and inflammation, oxidized linoleic acid derivatives may contribute to its onset. Certain gut microbiota, like *Oscillospira* and *Coriobacteriaceae*, are associated with better metabolic health in overweight adults [66]. Intermittent fasting for eight weeks improves gut microbiota, increases short-chain fatty acids, and reduces systemic LPS levels, correlating with improved cardiovascular risk factors. Dietary and lifestyle changes lead to a favorable shift in gut microbiota composition, reducing the *Prevotella/Bacteroides* ratio and increasing *Akkermansia muciniphila* and *Faecalibacterium prausnitzii*, crucial SCFA producers, in metabolic syndrome patients [67].

Nonalcoholic Fatty Liver Disease (NAFLD) and Gut Microbiome

Fat buildup in the liver is the hallmark of nonalcoholic fatty liver disease (NAFLD), a chronic liver ailment, ranging from steatosis to nonalcoholic steatohepatitis (NASH), which can progress to fibrosis and cirrhosis as described in Fig. (**3**) [68, 69]. Several factors, including genetic susceptibility (*e.g.*, PNPLA3 polymorphisms), inflammation, gut permeability, choline metabolism, and obesity, contribute to NAFLD development and are influenced by gut microbiota interactions [70]. Changes in gut dysbiosis observed in children with NAFLD may result from heightened carbohydrate oxidation compared to healthy children. Additionally, systemic inflammation has been associated with NAFLD progression, supported by research findings [71, 72].

The involvement of the gut microbiome in the development of NAFLD is significant. Dysbiosis in the gut leads to heightened intestinal permeability, enhanced extraction of dietary energy, changes in microbial metabolites such as SCFAs, BAs, TMA, and ethanol, and an increase in microbial endotoxins.

Cancer and Gut Microbiome

Obesity may raise the chance of acquiring several cancers, including hematological malignancies, endometrial, breast, cervical, ovarian, colon, and rectum, according to a recent investigation [73]. Furthermore, obesity is associated with higher mortality rates and poorer cancer outcomes, making it a significant and avoidable risk factor for cancer development [74]. However, many weight loss interventions are ineffective in the long term, prompting greater focus on strategies for weight loss maintenance. Future approaches to preventing cancer and managing weight are likely to heavily involve the gut microbiota due to its close relationship with energy balance and metabolism [75].

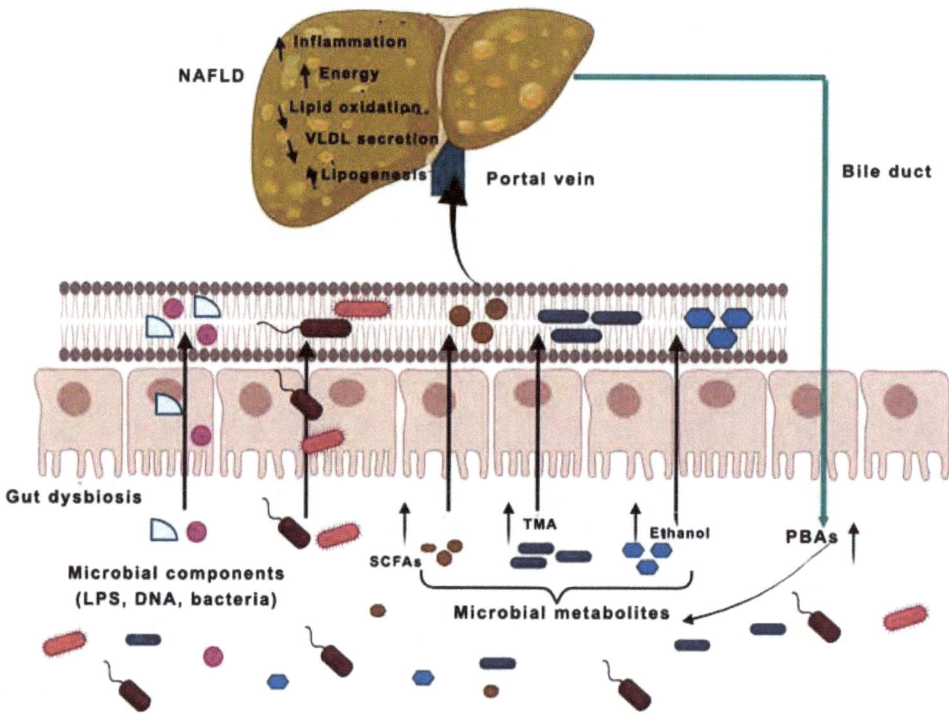

Fig. (3). The correlation between obesity and the onset of non-alcoholic fatty liver disease.

INTERVENTIONS TARGETING GUT MICROBIAL OBESITY

Probiotics, prebiotics, synbiotics, fecal microbiota transplantation (FMT), and other therapies are utilized for microbial management to prevent weight gain and associated comorbidities. The success of these treatments relies heavily on understanding the dynamic changes and composition of the resident microbiota over time [76].

Probiotics and Prebiotics

As per the World Health Organization and the Food and Agriculture Organization, probiotics are defined as "live microorganisms that, when administered in adequate amounts, confer a beneficial health effect on the host"

[77]. Probiotics have long been used in agriculture for promoting growth. Nonetheless, much research has suggested that they may be useful in treating fat-related problems and associated metabolic abnormalities in both human and animal models [78]. Probiotics have effectively lowered body fat mass, boosted glucose homeostasis, and enhanced lipid profiles in animal models of obesity, especially *Lactobacillus* strains. Although human research is limited, recent studies suggest that *Lactobacillus gasseri* may aid overweight individuals in improving postprandial blood lipid responses, reducing body weight, and decreasing abdominal obesity. In a clinical study, it has been proved that the administration of *Lactobacillus plantarum* in animals and *Lactobacillus gasseri* in both humans and animals was associated with weight reduction [79, 80].

Prebiotics are substances composed of non-digestible polysaccharides that selectively stimulate the growth and activity of one or a limited number of microbial genera/species in the gut microbiota, conferring health benefits to the host [81]. Inulin and various forms of fructooligosaccharides and galactooligosaccharides represent some of the most comprehensively investigated prebiotic compounds to date. A wealth of research, particularly in animal models, has illuminated their profound influence on the gut microbiota's composition. These prebiotics selectively foster the proliferation of health-promoting bacterial genera, notably *Bifidobacterium* and *Lactobacillus*. Such microbial modulation has been consistently linked to favorable metabolic outcomes, including significant reductions in body weight, adipose tissue mass, and the size of individual adipocytes. Additionally, these effects are often accompanied by decreased storage of fatty acids, attenuation of caloric intake, and a marked reduction in sensations of hunger. These findings underscore the potential of these prebiotics to modulate metabolic health through targeted alterations in gut microbiota dynamics [82].

Fecal Microbiota Transplantation (FMT)

Fecal microbiota transplantation (FMT) represents a pioneering therapeutic strategy that involves altering the gut microbiota of a patient to achieve specific health benefits, particularly for managing diabetes and metabolic syndrome (MS). This approach entails the introduction of microbiota-derived from the feces of a healthy donor into the gastrointestinal tract (GIT) of an individual suffering from microbiota dysbiosis [83]. FMT can be administered through various modalities, including nasal or rectal delivery *via* colonoscopy, oral administration through the upper gastrointestinal (UGI) tract, and encapsulated forms targeting the lower gastrointestinal (LGI) tract.

The efficacy of FMT was first highlighted in 1983 in cases of recurrent *Clostridium difficile* (*C. difficile*) infections, a condition unresponsive to conventional antibiotic therapy [84]. Today, FMT is the standard of care for treating *C. difficile*-associated diarrhea when standard antibiotic regimens fail. This technique is recognized for its potential to restore microbial diversity, an essential factor for maintaining gut homeostasis. Emerging evidence also suggests that FMT could be leveraged as a promising intervention for addressing obesity by reestablishing a balanced gut microbiome [85].

Therapy Employing Bacterial Consortiums

An alternative to FMT would be Bacterial Consortium Therapy (BCT), specifically designed medicinal combinations derived from clonally isolated bacteria to elicit specific immune responses. Using BCT, a particular intestinal environment could be modulated [85]. A recent study using BCT as a stand-in for FMT revealed full recovery and outcomes similar to those of FMT. Based upon varying degrees or kinds of dysbiosis, bacterial consortiums can be precisely defined and manufactured. In this manner, patient safety is enhanced because the bacterial amalgamation can be regulated for undesirable microorganisms. BCT might be a safer option in this situation a different way to control intestinal dysbiosis than FMT [86].

Modifications in the Iatrogenic Gut Microbiota

The altered gut microbiota following bariatric surgery is yet another subject of growing attention. Zhang *et al.* carried out a research showing that post-gastric bypass patients had significantly lower *Firmicutes* than both normal-weight and obese people [87]. In a similar vein, before Roux-en-Y gastric bypass (RYGB) surgery, Furet *et al.* found that obese persons had larger baseline *Firmicutes* to *Bacteroidetes* ratios; however, this ratio declined after three and six months of the procedure as the patients lost weight [88]. The gut microbiome of people who have recovered from RYGB does not have an acidic stomach; instead, it has distinct features that allow probiotics to more easily modify it. At three months, a randomized experiment with Lactobacillus probiotic supplements following RYGB showed that the treatment group had lost 9% more weight than the placebo group [89].

Gut Microbiota Therapies and Modifications: Positive and Negative Aspects

The most commonly recognized and safest microorganisms employed as probiotics belong to the genera *Lactobacillus* and *Bifidobacterium*. Other spore-forming bacterial genera, including *Streptococcus*, *Enterococcus*, and *Bacillus*, have also been utilized for probiotic purposes. Despite the well-documented benefits associated with probiotics, significant concerns persist regarding their long-term usage and the incorporation of probiotics into protein-enriched foods [90]. According to scientific discourse, the most alarming adverse effect linked to probiotic administration is bacterial translocation, a phenomenon that may precipitate severe conditions such as endocarditis, sepsis, and bacteremia. In this context, a pivotal study conducted by Cannon *et al.* involving approximately 200 individuals aged 53 years and older provided critical insights. Their *in vitro* investigations demonstrated that probiotic infections could be effectively managed through antibiotic monotherapy. However, the findings raised concerns regarding a marked reduction in sensitivity to vancomycin, cefazolin, and ciprofloxacin, particularly in infections caused by *Lactobacillus* species [91].

CLINICAL TRIALS

Table **1** represents the clinical trials exploring interventions and outcomes related to obesity caused by the modification in the gut microbiome.

Table 1. Clinical trials investigating interventions and outcomes in obesity resulting from alterations in the gut microbiome [92].

NCT No.	Patients No	Status	Intervention	Outcomes
NCT02741518	22	Completed	This is encapsulated, pre-screened fecal material.	Increased short-chain fatty acids will result from fecal microbiota transplantation, raising levels of the metabolic regulator GLP-1.
NCT05607745	54	NA	Fecal transplantation is administered *via* gastroscopy in a volume of 100–150 ml, with a 2:1 ratio compared to placebo transplantation. Every participant in the FMT and placebo groups receives the same guidance regarding a healthy diet.	An alteration in HOMA-IR in both research groups at weeks 12 and 52, and maybe more in the FMT group than in the placebo group.
NCT03727321	68	Completed	Combination Product: Fecal Microbial Dietary Supplement: Fiber and Cellulose	Insulin sensitivity Assessment, health-related quality of life (HRQL): EQ-5D Index
NCT05076656	22	Completed	Lactobacillus fermentum D3+FMT	a. Changes in HOMA-IR, b. Changes in glucose metabolism
NCT04594954	110	Completed	Dietary Supplement: Diet Other: FMT Other: Physical Activity	The proportion of patients achieving ≤ 5%of the weight loss in kg from baseline.

(Table 1) cont.....

NCT No.	Patients No	Status	Intervention	Outcomes
NCT02970877	48	NA	Biological: Fecal filtrate derived from 150 g stool obtained from healthy, lean donors	Change in Insulin Resistance compared to baseline
NCT06030999	150	Active, not recruiting	Dietary Supplement: Study product A(2g) +Study product B(2g)	Change of Weight in Kg by in body S10 from baseline to 10 weeks
NCT01718418	21	Completed	Intrinsic non-digestible carbohydrates combined with a probiotic supplement blend	Variations in the concentration of risk markers in the blood, measured after consuming a breakfast meal.
NCT01978691	225	Completed	*Bifidobacterium animalis* ssp. lactis 420 as probiotic bacteria, Polydextrose as a prebiotic	Changes in waist, BMI, change in inflammatory markers, change in lipopolysaccharides concentration, and soluble CD14, Change blood pressure.
NCT03773900	19	Completed	Kiotransine (chitin-glucan from aspergillus niger)	Fecal SCFA by GC-FID,change from baseline fecal polyunsaturated fatty acids by fame quantification. fecal albumin, zonulin, and calprotectin is analysed.
NCT01656681	130	Completed	A tablet containing 400 mg tetrahydro iso-alpha acids, 3 times a day.	Weight loss maintenance until 64 weeks.
NCT05009615	30	Completed	Dietary Supplement:	Body weight, body fat percentage, Anthropometry, and Insulin resistance, blood lipids are analyzed.
NCT05807204	20	Completed	Multi-ingredient of L-histidine, L-serine, L-carnosine and N-Acetylcysteine in powder form	a. Changes in visceral adiposity,hepatic Steatosis,BMI are analysed b. Change in biomarkers of oxidative stress.

CHALLENGES AND FUTURE PROSPECTIVE

An extensive body of evidence derived from both human and animal studieshas unequivocally highlighted the critical role of gut microbiota in the etiology and progression of obesity. The manipulation of this intricate microbial ecosystem through various interventions—ranging from dietary modifications, the administration of probiotics and prebiotics, and the strategic use of antibiotics, to surgical interventions—has been shown to exert significant influence over body weight regulation and metabolic homeostasis [93]. The relationship between dietary intake and gut microbial signaling is profoundly complex, with these signals exerting considerable effects on inflammatory mediators and gut-derived satiety hormones. Such signals, in turn, interface with central regulatory mechanisms in the brain. Disruption of these homeostatic pathways often shifts the balance towards hedonic reward-driven systems while simultaneously impairing inhibitory controls, thereby fostering an increased propensity for the consumption of energy-dense, hyper-palatable foods. This cyclical process exacerbates gut dysbiosis and perpetuates metabolic dysfunctions [94].

A formidable challenge that continues to impede progress in the field of gut microbiota research is the lack of uniformity and reproducibility in scientific observations. This inconsistency arises largely from variations in dietary practices among study populations, differences in sample collection methodologies, discrepancies in storage protocols, and the heterogeneity of sequencing and analytical techniques employed across studies. The adoption of standardized methodologies for sample handling, sequencing, and data analysis would significantly enhance the reliability and comparability of findings in this field. Furthermore, the integration of cutting-edge omics technologies, such as transcriptomics, proteomics, metabolomics, and metagenomics, offers a promising avenue to unravel the functional and metabolic roles of microbial communities in unprecedented detail [95].

Future research must broaden its scope to encompass the underexplored contributions of other components of the gut microbiome, including fungi, viruses, and archaea, to the development and progression of obesity and its associated metabolic complications. The gut microbiota is hypothesized to modulate energy balance and metabolism through multiple mechanisms, including the regulation of dietary energy extraction, the modulation of fat storage pathways, the enhancement of lipogenesis, and the promotion of fatty acid oxidation. These processes collectively underscore the integral role of the microbiome in metabolic health and disease [96].

Emerging therapeutic strategies aimed at reshaping the gut microbiome to combat obesity include bariatric surgical procedures, fecal microbiota transplantation, and the administration of functional microbial interventions such as probiotics, prebiotics, and synbiotics, as well as tailored dietary interventions. While these approaches have demonstrated considerable potential, the long-term efficacy, safety, and applicability of such treatments remain to be thoroughly validated through rigorous, large-scale clinical investigations [97].

CONCLUSION

The intricate interplay between obesity and the gut microbiome (GM) is a focal point in contemporary biomedical research, highlighting the profound influence of gut bacteria on human health. The gut microbiota, a complex community of trillions of microorganisms residing in the intestinal tract, is crucial for nutrient absorption, immune response, and energy metabolism. Dysbiosis, an imbalance in the gut microbiota, is implicated in the pathogenesis of obesity and related metabolic disorders, including metabolic syndrome, non-alcoholic fatty liver disease (NAFLD), type 2 diabetes, and certain cancers. The research underscores a bidirectional relationship between the gut-brain axis (GBA) and obesity, where the gut microbiota communicates with the brain through neural, endocrine, and immune pathways. This gut-brain communication affects food addiction and dysfunctional eating patterns, contributing to obesity through hedonistic pathways. The microbiota's influence on appetite-regulating hormones such as ghrelin, leptin, and GLP-1 is significant, as it modulates feeding behavior and energy balance.

Obesity is associated with a distinct microbial signature, characterized by a higher Firmicutes/Bacteroidetes ratio and decreased microbial diversity. This dysbiotic state fosters metabolic imbalances, promotes fat accumulation, and exacerbates inflammation. Key findings include the elevated presence of Firmicutes in obese individuals and the protective role of certain bacteria, such as Akkermansia muciniphila, in maintaining metabolic health. Therapeutic strategies targeting the gut microbiota are promising in managing obesity. These include dietary modifications to enhance microbial diversity, probiotics, prebiotics, synbiotics, and fecal microbiota transplants (FMT). These interventions aim to restore eubiosis, the state of a balanced gut microbiota, to improve metabolic health and reduce obesity-related comorbidities. In conclusion, the gut microbiome plays a pivotal role in obesity through its impact on metabolism, immune function, and the gut-brain axis. Understanding the mechanisms underlying this relationship opens avenues for novel treatments that manipulate the microbiota to combat obesity and its associated disorders. The dynamic nature of the gut microbiota and its responsiveness to dietary and environmental changes provide a promising frontier for therapeutic interventions aimed at restoring metabolic balance and improving overall health.

ACKNOWLEDGEMENTS

The authors are highly grateful to NSHM Knowledge Campus, Kolkata for their continuous support and encouragement.

REFERENCES

[1] Biener A, Cawley J, Meyerhoefer C. The high and rising costs of obesity to the US health care system. J Gen Intern Med 2017; 32(S1) (Suppl. 1): 6-8.
[http://dx.doi.org/10.1007/s11606-016-3968-8] [PMID: 28271429]

[2] Mayer EA, Bradesi S, Chang L, Spiegel BMR, Bueller JA, Naliboff BD. Functional GI disorders: from animal models to drug development. Gut 2008; 57(3): 384-404.
[http://dx.doi.org/10.1136/gut.2006.101675] [PMID: 17965064]

[3] Mancini MC, de Melo ME. The burden of obesity in the current world and the new treatments available: focus on liraglutide 3.0 mg. Diabetol Metab Syndr 2017; 9(1): 44.
[http://dx.doi.org/10.1186/s13098-017-0242-0] [PMID: 28580018]

[4] Onaolapo AY, Onaolapo OJ. Food additives, food and the concept of 'food addiction': Is stimulation of the brain reward circuit by food sufficient to trigger addiction? Pathophysiology 2018; 25(4): 263-76.
[http://dx.doi.org/10.1016/j.pathophys.2018.04.002] [PMID: 29673924]

[5] Yu M, Jia H, Zhou C, *et al.* Variations in gut microbiota and fecal metabolic phenotype associated with depression by 16S rRNA gene sequencing and LC/MS-based metabolomics. J Pharm Biomed Anal 2017; 138: 231-9.
[http://dx.doi.org/10.1016/j.jpba.2017.02.008] [PMID: 28219800]

[6] He F, Zhai J, Zhang L, *et al.* Variations in gut microbiota and fecal metabolic phenotype associated with Fenbendazole and Ivermectin Tablets by 16S rRNA gene sequencing and LC/MS-based metabolomics in Amur tiger. Biochem Biophys Res Commun 2018; 499(3): 447-53.
[http://dx.doi.org/10.1016/j.bbrc.2018.03.158] [PMID: 29596832]

[7] Hill JO. Understanding and addressing the epidemic of obesity: an energy balance perspective. Endocr Rev 2006; 27(7): 750-61.
[http://dx.doi.org/10.1210/er.2006-0032] [PMID: 17122359]

[8] Zhang Y, Liu J, Yao J, *et al.* Obesity: Pathophysiology and Intervention. Nutrients 2014; 6(11): 5153-83.
[http://dx.doi.org/10.3390/nu6115153] [PMID: 25412152]

[9] Osadchiy V, Martin CR, Mayer EA. The gut–brain axis and the microbiome: Mechanisms and clinical implications. Clin Gastroenterol Hepatol 2019; 17(2): 322-32.
[http://dx.doi.org/10.1016/j.cgh.2018.10.002] [PMID: 30292888]

[10] Cong X, Henderson WA, Graf J, McGrath JM. Early life experience and gut microbiome: The brain-gut-Microbiota signaling system. Adv Neonatal Care 2015; 15(5): 314-23.
[http://dx.doi.org/10.1097/ANC.0000000000000191] [PMID: 26240939]

[11] Bliss ES, Whiteside E. The gut-brain axis, the human gut Microbiota and their integration in the development of obesity. Front Physiol 2018; 9: 900.
[http://dx.doi.org/10.3389/fphys.2018.00900] [PMID: 30050464]

[12] Torres-Fuentes C, Schellekens H, Dinan TG, Cryan JF. The microbiota–gut–brain axis in obesity. Lancet Gastroenterol Hepatol 2017; 2(10): 747-56.
[http://dx.doi.org/10.1016/S2468-1253(17)30147-4] [PMID: 28844808]

[13] Keita , Söderholm JD. The intestinal barrier and its regulation by neuroimmune factors. Neuro gastroenterol Motil 2010; 22(7): 718-33.
[http://dx.doi.org/10.1111/j.1365-2982.2010.01498.x] [PMID: 20377785]

[14] Guyenet SJ, Schwartz MW. Clinical review: Regulation of food intake, energy balance, and body fat mass: implications for the pathogenesis and treatment of obesity. J Clin Endocrinol Metab 2012; 97(3): 745-55.
[http://dx.doi.org/10.1210/jc.2011-2525] [PMID: 22238401]

[15] Miyamoto J, Igarashi M, Watanabe K, *et al.* Gut microbiota confers host resistance to obesity by metabolizing dietary polyunsaturated fatty acids. Nat Commun 2019; 10(1): 4007. [http://dx.doi.org/10.1038/s41467-019-11978-0] [PMID: 31488836]

[16] Heymsfield SB, Wadden TA. Mechanisms, pathophysiology, and management of obesity. N Engl J Med 2017; 376(3): 254-66. [http://dx.doi.org/10.1056/NEJMra1514009] [PMID: 28099824]

[17] Moreira CG, Russell R, Mishra AA, *et al.* Bacterial adrenergic sensors regulate virulence of Enteric pathogens in the gut. MBio 2016; 7(3): e00826-16. [http://dx.doi.org/10.1128/mBio.00826-16] [PMID: 27273829]

[18] Rosenbaum M, Knight R, Leibel RL. The gut microbiota in human energy homeostasis and obesity. Trends Endocrinol Metab 2015; 26(9): 493-501. [http://dx.doi.org/10.1016/j.tem.2015.07.002] [PMID: 26257300]

[19] Gagliardi A, Totino V, Cacciotti F, *et al.* Rebuilding the gut Microbiota ecosystem. Int J Environ Res Public Health 2018; 15(8): 1679. [http://dx.doi.org/10.3390/ijerph15081679] [PMID: 30087270]

[20] Stice E, Yokum S, Burger KS, Epstein LH, Small DM. Youth at risk for obesity show greater activation of striatal and somatosensory regions to food. J Neurosci 2011; 31(12): 4360-6. [http://dx.doi.org/10.1523/JNEUROSCI.6604-10.2011] [PMID: 21430137]

[21] Dalile B, Van Oudenhove L, Vervliet B, Verbeke K. The role of short-chain fatty acids in microbiota–gut–brain communication. Nat Rev Gastroenterol Hepatol 2019; 16(8): 461-78. [http://dx.doi.org/10.1038/s41575-019-0157-3] [PMID: 31123355]

[22] Gearhardt AN, Grilo CM, DiLeone RJ, Brownell KD, Potenza MN. Can food be addictive? Public health and policy implications. Addiction 2011; 106(7): 1208-12. [http://dx.doi.org/10.1111/j.1360-0443.2010.03301.x] [PMID: 21635588]

[23] Ley RE, Bäckhed F, Turnbaugh P, Lozupone CA, Knight RD, Gordon JI. Obesity alters gut microbial ecology. Proc Natl Acad Sci USA 2005; 102(31): 11070-5. [http://dx.doi.org/10.1073/pnas.0504978102] [PMID: 16033867]

[24] Turnbaugh PJ, Ley RE, Mahowald MA, Magrini V, Mardis ER, Gordon JI. An obesity-associated gut microbiome with increased capacity for energy harvest. Nature 2006; 444(7122): 1027-31. [http://dx.doi.org/10.1038/nature05414] [PMID: 17183312]

[25] Waldram A, Holmes E, Wang Y, *et al.* Top-down systems biology modeling of host metabotype-microbiome associations in obese rodents. J Proteome Res 2009; 8(5): 2361-75. [http://dx.doi.org/10.1021/pr8009885] [PMID: 19275195]

[26] Cani PD, Moens de Hase E, Van Hul M. Gut Microbiota and host metabolism: From proof of concept to therapeutic intervention. Microorganisms 2021; 9(6): 1302. [http://dx.doi.org/10.3390/microorganisms9061302] [PMID: 34203876]

[27] Karlsson FH, Tremaroli V, Nookaew I, *et al.* Gut metagenome in European women with normal, impaired and diabetic glucose control. Nature 2013; 498(7452): 99-103. [http://dx.doi.org/10.1038/nature12198] [PMID: 23719380]

[28] David LA, Maurice CF, Carmody RN, *et al.* Diet rapidly and reproducibly alters the human gut microbiome. Nature 2014; 505(7484): 559-63. [http://dx.doi.org/10.1038/nature12820] [PMID: 24336217]

[29] DeGruttola AK, Low D, Mizoguchi A, Mizoguchi E. Current understanding of dysbiosis in disease in human and animal models. Inflamm Bowel Dis 2016; 22(5): 1137-50. [http://dx.doi.org/10.1097/MIB.0000000000000750] [PMID: 27070911]

[30] Lal S, Kirkup AJ, Brunsden AM, Thompson DG, Grundy D. Vagal afferent responses to fatty acids of different chain length in the rat. Am J Physiol Gastrointest Liver Physiol 2001; 281(4): G907-15.

[http://dx.doi.org/10.1152/ajpgi.2001.281.4.G907] [PMID: 11557510]

[31] Christiansen AM, DeKloet AD, Ulrich-Lai YM, Herman JP. "Snacking" causes long term attenuation of HPA axis stress responses and enhancement of brain FosB/deltaFosB expression in rats. Physiol Behav 2011; 103(1): 111-6.
[http://dx.doi.org/10.1016/j.physbeh.2011.01.015] [PMID: 21262247]

[32] Ochoa-Repáraz J, Kasper LH. The second brain: Is the gut Microbiota a link between obesity and central nervous system disorders? Curr Obes Rep 2016; 5(1): 51-64.
[http://dx.doi.org/10.1007/s13679-016-0191-1] [PMID: 26865085]

[33] Karra E, Chandarana K, Batterham RL. The role of peptide YY in appetite regulation and obesity. J Physiol 2009; 587(1): 19-25.
[http://dx.doi.org/10.1113/jphysiol.2008.164269] [PMID: 19064614]

[34] Buhmann H, le Roux CW, Bueter M. The gut–brain axis in obesity. Best Pract Res Clin Gastroenterol 2014; 28(4): 559-71.
[http://dx.doi.org/10.1016/j.bpg.2014.07.003] [PMID: 25194175]

[35] Houlden A, Goldrick M, Brough D, *et al.* Brain injury induces specific changes in the caecal microbiota of mice *via* altered autonomic activity and mucoprotein production. Brain Behav Immun 2016; 57: 10-20.
[http://dx.doi.org/10.1016/j.bbi.2016.04.003] [PMID: 27060191]

[36] Gomes AC, Hoffmann C, Mota JF. The human gut microbiota: Metabolism and perspective in obesity. Gut Microbes 2018; 9(4): 1-18.
[http://dx.doi.org/10.1080/19490976.2018.1465157] [PMID: 29667480]

[37] Dave M, Higgins PD, Middha S, Rioux KP. The human gut microbiome: current knowledge, challenges, and future directions. Transl Res 2012; 160(4): 246-57.
[http://dx.doi.org/10.1016/j.trsl.2012.05.003] [PMID: 22683238]

[38] de la Cuesta-Zuluaga J, Kelley ST, Chen Y, *et al.* Age- and sex-dependent patterns of gut microbial diversity in human adults. mSystems 2019; 4(4): e00261-19.
[http://dx.doi.org/10.1128/mSystems.00261-19] [PMID: 31098397]

[39] Cryan JF, O'Mahony SM. The microbiome-gut-brain axis: from bowel to behavior. Neurogastroenterol Motil 2011; 23(3): 187-92.
[http://dx.doi.org/10.1111/j.1365-2982.2010.01664.x] [PMID: 21303428]

[40] Saltiel AR, Olefsky JM. Inflammatory mechanisms linking obesity and metabolic disease. J Clin Invest 2017; 127(1): 1-4.
[http://dx.doi.org/10.1172/JCI92035] [PMID: 28045402]

[41] Caricilli A, Saad M. The role of gut microbiota on insulin resistance. Nutrients 2013; 5(3): 829-51.
[http://dx.doi.org/10.3390/nu5030829] [PMID: 23482058]

[42] Tolhurst G, Heffron H, Lam YS, *et al.* Short-chain fatty acids stimulate glucagon-like peptide-1 secretion *via* the G-protein-coupled receptor FFAR2. Diabetes 2012; 61(2): 364-71.
[http://dx.doi.org/10.2337/db11-1019] [PMID: 22190648]

[43] Earthman CP, Beckman LM, Masodkar K, Sibley SD. The link between obesity and low circulating 25-hydroxyvitamin D concentrations: considerations and implications. Int J Obes 2012; 36(3): 387-96.
[http://dx.doi.org/10.1038/ijo.2011.119] [PMID: 21694701]

[44] Heijtz RD, Wang S, Anuar F, *et al.* Normal gut microbiota modulates brain development and behavior. Proc Natl Acad Sci USA 2011; 108(7): 3047-52.
[http://dx.doi.org/10.1073/pnas.1010529108] [PMID: 21282636]

[45] Maslowski KM, Vieira AT, Ng A, *et al.* Regulation of inflammatory responses by gut microbiota and chemoattractant receptor GPR43. Nature 2009; 461(7268): 1282-6.
[http://dx.doi.org/10.1038/nature08530] [PMID: 19865172]

[46] Wimalawansa SJ. Associations of vitamin D with insulin resistance, obesity, type 2 diabetes, and metabolic syndrome. J Steroid Biochem Mol Biol 2018; 175: 177-89. [http://dx.doi.org/10.1016/j.jsbmb.2016.09.017] [PMID: 27662816]

[47] Gomes CC, Passos TS, Morais AHA. Vitamin A status improvement in obesity: Findings and perspectives using encapsulation techniques. Nutrients 2021; 13(6): 1921. [http://dx.doi.org/10.3390/nu13061921] [PMID: 34204998]

[48] Thoen RU, Barther NN, Schemitt E, *et al.* Zinc supplementation reduces diet-induced obesity and improves insulin sensitivity in rats. Appl Physiol Nutr Metab 2019; 44(6): 580-6. [http://dx.doi.org/10.1139/apnm-2018-0519] [PMID: 30339765]

[49] Eslick S, Thompson C, Berthon B, Wood L. Short-chain fatty acids as anti-inflammatory agents in overweight and obesity: a systematic review and meta-analysis. Nutr Rev 2022; 80(4): 838-56. [http://dx.doi.org/10.1093/nutrit/nuab059] [PMID: 34472619]

[50] McLoughlin RF, Berthon BS, Jensen ME, Baines KJ, Wood LG. Short-chain fatty acids, prebiotics, synbiotics, and systemic inflammation: a systematic review and meta-analysis. Am J Clin Nutr 2017; 106(3): 930-45. [http://dx.doi.org/10.3945/ajcn.117.156265] [PMID: 28793992]

[51] Bailey LC, Forrest CB, Zhang P, Richards TM, Livshits A, DeRusso PA. Association of antibiotics in infancy with early childhood obesity. JAMA Pediatr 2014; 168(11): 1063-9. [http://dx.doi.org/10.1001/jamapediatrics.2014.1539] [PMID: 25265089]

[52] Boulangé CL, Neves AL, Chilloux J, Nicholson JK, Dumas ME. Impact of the gut microbiota on inflammation, obesity, and metabolic disease. Genome Med 2016; 8(1): 42. [http://dx.doi.org/10.1186/s13073-016-0303-2] [PMID: 27098727]

[53] Gearhardt AN, Corbin WR, Brownell KD. Food Addiction. J Addict Med 2009; 3(1): 1-7. [http://dx.doi.org/10.1097/ADM.0b013e318193c993] [PMID: 21768996]

[54] Perry RJ, Peng L, Barry NA, *et al.* Acetate mediates a microbiome–brain–β-cell axis to promote metabolic syndrome. Nature 2016; 534(7606): 213-7. [http://dx.doi.org/10.1038/nature18309] [PMID: 27279214]

[55] Tseng CH, Wu CY. The gut microbiome in obesity. J Formos Med Assoc 2019; 118 (Suppl. 1): S3-9. [http://dx.doi.org/10.1016/j.jfma.2018.07.009] [PMID: 30057153]

[56] Volkow ND, Wang GJ, Tomasi D, Baler RD. The addictive dimensionality of obesity. Biol Psychiatry 2013; 73(9): 811-8. [http://dx.doi.org/10.1016/j.biopsych.2012.12.020] [PMID: 23374642]

[57] Sircana A, Framarin L, Leone N, *et al.* Altered gut Microbiota in type 2 diabetes: Just a coincidence? Curr Diab Rep 2018; 18(10): 98. [http://dx.doi.org/10.1007/s11892-018-1057-6] [PMID: 30215149]

[58] Larsen N, Vogensen FK, van den Berg FWJ, *et al.* Gut microbiota in human adults with type 2 diabetes differs from non-diabetic adults. PLoS One 2010; 5(2): e9085. [http://dx.doi.org/10.1371/journal.pone.0009085] [PMID: 20140211]

[59] Fernandes J, Su W, Rahat-Rozenbloom S, Wolever TMS, Comelli EM. Adiposity, gut microbiota and faecal short chain fatty acids are linked in adult humans. Nutr Diabetes 2014; 4(6): e121-1. [http://dx.doi.org/10.1038/nutd.2014.23] [PMID: 24979150]

[60] Zhu L, Baker SS, Gill C, *et al.* Characterization of gut microbiomes in nonalcoholic steatohepatitis (NASH) patients: a connection between endogenous alcohol and NASH. Hepatology 2013; 57(2): 601-9. [http://dx.doi.org/10.1002/hep.26093] [PMID: 23055155]

[61] Younossi ZM, Blissett D, Blissett R, *et al.* The economic and clinical burden of nonalcoholic fatty liver disease in the United States and Europe. Hepatology 2016; 64(5): 1577-86.

[http://dx.doi.org/10.1002/hep.28785] [PMID: 27543837]

[62] Yun Y, Kim HN, Lee E, *et al.* Fecal and blood microbiota profiles and presence of nonalcoholic fatty liver disease in obese versus lean subjects. PLoS One 2019; 14(3): e0213692.
[http://dx.doi.org/10.1371/journal.pone.0213692] [PMID: 30870486]

[63] Bendor CD, Bardugo A, Pinhas-Hamiel O, Afek A, Twig G. Cardiovascular morbidity, diabetes and cancer risk among children and adolescents with severe obesity. Cardiovasc Diabetol 2020; 19(1): 79.
[http://dx.doi.org/10.1186/s12933-020-01052-1] [PMID: 32534575]

[64] Saklayen MG. The global epidemic of the metabolic syndrome. Curr Hypertens Rep 2018; 20(2): 12.
[http://dx.doi.org/10.1007/s11906-018-0812-z] [PMID: 29480368]

[65] Zhao L. The gut microbiota and obesity: from correlation to causality. Nat Rev Microbiol 2013; 11(9): 639-47.
[http://dx.doi.org/10.1038/nrmicro3089] [PMID: 23912213]

[66] Nicolucci AC, Hume MP, Martínez I, Mayengbam S, Walter J, Reimer RA. Prebiotics reduce body fat and alter intestinal Microbiota in children who are overweight or with obesity. Gastroenterology 2017; 153(3): 711-22.
[http://dx.doi.org/10.1053/j.gastro.2017.05.055] [PMID: 28596023]

[67] Badgeley A, Anwar H, Modi K, Murphy P, Lakshmikuttyamma A. Effect of probiotics and gut microbiota on anti-cancer drugs: Mechanistic perspectives. Biochim Biophys Acta Rev Cancer 2021; 1875(1): 188494.
[http://dx.doi.org/10.1016/j.bbcan.2020.188494] [PMID: 33346129]

[68] Schulte EM, Gearhardt AN. Associations of food addiction in a sample recruited to be nationally representative of the United States. Eur Eat Disord Rev 2018; 26(2): 112-9.
[http://dx.doi.org/10.1002/erv.2575] [PMID: 29266583]

[69] Cani PD, Lecourt E, Dewulf EM, *et al.* Gut microbiota fermentation of prebiotics increases satietogenic and incretin gut peptide production with consequences for appetite sensation and glucose response after a meal. Am J Clin Nutr 2009; 90(5): 1236-43.
[http://dx.doi.org/10.3945/ajcn.2009.28095] [PMID: 19776140]

[70] Eichen DM, Lent MR, Goldbacher E, Foster GD. Exploration of "Food Addiction" in overweight and obese treatment-seeking adults. Appetite 2013; 67: 22-4.
[http://dx.doi.org/10.1016/j.appet.2013.03.008] [PMID: 23535004]

[71] Faith JJ, Guruge JL, Charbonneau M, *et al.* The long-term stability of the human gut microbiota. Science 2013; 341(6141): 1237439.
[http://dx.doi.org/10.1126/science.1237439] [PMID: 23828941]

[72] Li M, Liang P, Li Z, *et al.* Fecal microbiota transplantation and bacterial consortium transplantation have comparable effects on the re-establishment of mucosal barrier function in mice with intestinal dysbiosis. Front Microbiol 2015; 6: 692.
[http://dx.doi.org/10.3389/fmicb.2015.00692] [PMID: 26217323]

[73] Lee P, Yacyshyn BR, Yacyshyn MB. Gut microbiota and obesity: An opportunity to alter obesity through faecal microbiota transplant (FMT). Diabetes Obes Metab 2019; 21(3): 479-90.
[http://dx.doi.org/10.1111/dom.13561] [PMID: 30328245]

[74] Edrisi F, Salehi M, Ahmadi A, Fararoei M, Rusta F, Mahmoodianfard S. Effects of supplementation with rice husk powder and rice bran on inflammatory factors in overweight and obese adults following an energy-restricted diet: a randomized controlled trial. Eur J Nutr 2018; 57(2): 833-43.
[http://dx.doi.org/10.1007/s00394-017-1555-3] [PMID: 29063186]

[75] Sharpton SR, Maraj B, Harding-Theobald E, Vittinghoff E, Terrault NA. Gut microbiome–targeted therapies in nonalcoholic fatty liver disease: a systematic review, meta-analysis, and meta-regression. Am J Clin Nutr 2019; 110(1): 139-49.
[http://dx.doi.org/10.1093/ajcn/nqz042] [PMID: 31124558]

[76] Owaga E, Hsieh RH, Mugendi B, Masuku S, Shih CK, Chang JS. Th17 cells as potential probiotic therapeutic targets in inflammatory bowel diseases. Int J Mol Sci 2015; 16(9): 20841-58. [http://dx.doi.org/10.3390/ijms160920841] [PMID: 26340622]

[77] Wirth KM, Sheka AC, Kizy S, *et al.* Bariatric surgery is associated with decreased progression of nonalcoholic fatty liver disease to cirrhosis: A retrospective cohort analysis. Ann Surg 2020; 272(1): 32-9. [http://dx.doi.org/10.1097/SLA.0000000000003871] [PMID: 32224733]

[78] Ley RE, Turnbaugh PJ, Klein S, Gordon JI. Human gut microbes associated with obesity. Nature 2006; 444(7122): 1022-3. [http://dx.doi.org/10.1038/4441022a] [PMID: 17183309]

[79] Stachowicz N, Kiersztan A. The role of gut microbiota in the pathogenesis of obesity and diabetes. Postepy Hig Med Dosw 2013; 67: 288-303. [http://dx.doi.org/10.5604/17322693.1044746] [PMID: 23619228]

[80] Steward T, Mestre-Bach G, Vintró-Alcaraz C, *et al.* Food addiction and impaired executive functions in women with obesity. Eur Eat Disord Rev 2018; 26(6): 574-84. [http://dx.doi.org/10.1002/erv.2636] [PMID: 30159982]

[81] Pagliai G, Russo E, Niccolai E, *et al.* Influence of a 3-month low-calorie Mediterranean diet compared to the vegetarian diet on human gut microbiota and SCFA: the CARDIVEG Study. Eur J Nutr 2020; 59(5): 2011-24. [http://dx.doi.org/10.1007/s00394-019-02050-0] [PMID: 31292752]

[82] Sidhu SRK, Kok CW, Kunasegaran T, Ramadas A. Effect of plant-based diets on gut Microbiota: A systematic review of interventional studies. Nutrients 2023; 15(6): 1510. [http://dx.doi.org/10.3390/nu15061510] [PMID: 36986240]

[83] Sasidharan Pillai S, Gagnon CA, Foster C, Ashraf AP. Exploring the gut Microbiota: Key insights into its role in obesity, metabolic syndrome, and type 2 diabetes. J Clin Endocrinol Metab 2024; 109(11): 2709-19. [http://dx.doi.org/10.1210/clinem/dgae499] [PMID: 39040013]

[84] Peng LJ, Chen YP, Qu F, Zhong Y, Jiang ZS. Correlation of gut Microbiota with children obesity and weight loss. Indian J Microbiol 2024; 64(1): 82-91. [http://dx.doi.org/10.1007/s12088-023-01088-3] [PMID: 38468732]

[85] Cani PD, Van Hul M. Gut microbiota in overweight and obesity: crosstalk with adipose tissue. Nat Rev Gastroenterol Hepatol 2024; 21(3): 164-83. [http://dx.doi.org/10.1038/s41575-023-00867-z] [PMID: 38066102]

[86] Li H, Wang XK, Tang M, *et al. Bacteroides thetaiotaomicron* ameliorates mouse hepatic steatosis through regulating gut microbial composition, gut-liver folate and unsaturated fatty acids metabolism. Gut Microbes 2024; 16(1): 2304159. [http://dx.doi.org/10.1080/19490976.2024.2304159] [PMID: 38277137]

[87] Horvath A, Zukauskaite K, Hazia O, Balazs I, Stadlbauer V. Human gut microbiome: Therapeutic opportunities for metabolic syndrome—Hype or hope? Endocrinol Diabetes Metab 2024; 7(1): e436. [http://dx.doi.org/10.1002/edm2.436] [PMID: 37771199]

[88] Li H, Zhang L, Li J, *et al.* Resistant starch intake facilitates weight loss in humans by reshaping the gut microbiota. Nat Metab 2024; 6(3): 578-97. [http://dx.doi.org/10.1038/s42255-024-00988-y] [PMID: 38409604]

[89] Fan S, Zhang Z, Zhao Y, *et al.* Recent advances in targeted manipulation of the gut microbiome by prebiotics: from taxonomic composition to metabolic function. Curr Opin Food Sci 2023; 49(100959): 100959. [http://dx.doi.org/10.1016/j.cofs.2022.100959]

[90] Qiu B, Liang J, Li C. Effects of fecal microbiota transplantation in metabolic syndrome. 2023; 18(7):

e0288718.

[91] Minkoff NZ, Aslam S, Medina M, *et al.* Fecal microbiota transplantation for the treatment of recurrent Clostridioides difficile (Clostridium difficile). Cochrane Database Syst Rev 2023; 4(4): CD013871. [PMID: 37096495]

[92] Clinicaltrials.gov. Definitions. 2020. Available from: https://clinicaltrials.gov/

[93] Młynarska E, Jakubowska P, Frąk W, *et al.* Associations of Microbiota and nutrition with cognitive impairment in diseases. Nutrients 2024; 16(20): 3570. [http://dx.doi.org/10.3390/nu16203570] [PMID: 39458564]

[94] Cunningham M, Vinderola G, Charalampopoulos D, Lebeer S, Sanders ME, Grimaldi R. Applying probiotics and prebiotics in new delivery formats – is the clinical evidence transferable? Trends Food Sci Technol 2021; 112: 495-506. [http://dx.doi.org/10.1016/j.tifs.2021.04.009]

[95] Bäckhed F, Fraser CM, Ringel Y, *et al.* Defining a healthy human gut microbiome: current concepts, future directions, and clinical applications. Cell Host Microbe 2012; 12(5): 611-22. [http://dx.doi.org/10.1016/j.chom.2012.10.012] [PMID: 23159051]

[96] Cunningham M, Vinderola G, Charalampopoulos D, Lebeer S, Sanders ME, Grimaldi R. Applying probiotics and prebiotics in new delivery formats – is the clinical evidence transferable? Trends Food Sci Technol 2021; 112: 495-506. [http://dx.doi.org/10.1016/j.tifs.2021.04.009]

[97] Lutter M, Nestler EJ. Homeostatic and hedonic signals interact in the regulation of food intake. J Nutr 2009; 139(3): 629-32. [http://dx.doi.org/10.3945/jn.108.097618] [PMID: 19176746]

CHAPTER 4

Cardiovascular Diseases and Gut Microbial Metabolites

Sabir Hussain[1], **Priyakshi Chutia**[1] and **Sailendra Kumar Mahanta**[1,*]

[1] *Department of Pharmacology, School of Pharmacy, The Assam Kaziranga University, Jorhat-785006, Assam, India*

Abstract: Cardiovascular diseases (CVDs) continue to be the world's leading cause of death, and their aetiology is influenced by a complex interaction of lifestyle, environmental, and genetic variables. There is growing evidence that the billions of microorganisms and their metabolites that make up the gut microbiota may be crucial in regulating cardiovascular health. This chapter sheds insight on the possible mechanisms of action and therapeutic consequences of the complex link between gut microbial metabolites and cardiovascular disorders.

The gut microbiota produces a wide range of metabolites, including lipopolysaccharides (LPS), bile acids, trimethylamine N-oxide (TMAO), and short-chain fatty acids (SCFAs), by fermenting food substrates. These metabolites have the ability to affect a number of physiological processes that are important for cardiovascular health, including inflammation, lipid metabolism, endothelial function, and blood pressure management. They can also have systemic effects.

Certain gut microbial metabolites have been linked in recent research to the pathophysiology of heart failure, hypertension, atherosclerosis, and other CVDs. For example, a greater risk of atherosclerosis and severe cardiovascular events has been linked to elevated levels of TMAO, whereas the anti-inflammatory and potential atherogenic properties of SCFAs may offer cardioprotective advantages. Comprehending the function of gut microbiota metabolites in cardiovascular well-being presents opportunities for the creation of innovative treatment approaches and tailored therapies. Using dietary changes, prebiotics, probiotics, or microbial-based treatments to target the gut microbiota may present novel strategies for managing and preventing CVD. However, further research is warranted to elucidate the complex interactions between gut microbial metabolites, host physiology, and cardiovascular outcomes, paving the way for more effective strategies to combat CVDs in the future.

Keywords: Atherosclerosis, Bile, Hypertension, Inflammation, Lipids, LPS, Metabolites, Microbiota, Prevention, Probiotics, Prebiotics.

* **Corresponding author Sailendra Kumar Mahanta:** Department of Pharmacology, School of Pharmacy, The Assam Kaziranga University, Jorhat-785006, Assam, India; E-mails: sailendra04@gmail.com, sailendrakumar@kzu.ac.in

Sandipan Dasgupta & Moitreyee Chattopadhyay (Eds.)

INTRODUCTION TO CARDIOVASCULAR DISEASES AND GUT MICROBIAL METABOLITES

Cardiovascular diseases (CVDs) contribute to morbidity and death globally and constitute a substantial global health burden. These ailments cover a wide range of conditions that affect the heart and blood vessels, including coronary artery disease, heart failure, peripheral artery disease, and stroke. Despite advances in medical management, CVDs continue to pose substantial challenges to public health systems and individuals alike [1].

Recent years have seen an increase in interest in the function of gut bacteria in cardiovascular health and disease. Trillions of bacteria that live in the gastrointestinal system make up the gut microbiota, which is essential for regulating several physiological processes and preserving host homeostasis. Notably, interactions between gut microbial communities and host metabolism have garnered significant attention, with mounting evidence suggesting a link between gut microbiota dysbiosis and the development of cardiovascular diseases [2].

The intricate relationship between gut microbiota and cardiovascular health underscores the pivotal role of microbial metabolites in shaping physiological processes. Through the synthesis of various metabolites, gut bacteria exert profound effects on host biology, particularly in modulating immunological responses, metabolic homeostasis, and vascular function. This symbiotic interplay between the gut microbiota and the host extends beyond mere digestion; it serves as a dynamic nexus where dietary substrates and host-derived compounds converge to generate a diverse array of bioactive molecules.

The microbial metabolites produced by the fermentation of dietary fibres, proteins, and other nutrients are at the forefront of this interplay. Acetate, propionate, and butyrate are examples of short-chain fatty acids (SCFAs), which are important metabolites generated by gut bacteria when dietary fibres are broken down. SCFAs play multifaceted roles in cardiovascular health, exerting anti-inflammatory effects, enhancing insulin sensitivity, and influencing lipid metabolism. Moreover, these metabolites have been shown to regulate blood pressure and endothelial function, thereby impacting vascular health and reducing the risk of cardiovascular diseases.

Beyond SCFAs, gut microbial metabolism also yields a plethora of bioactive compounds with diverse physiological functions. Trimethylamine-N-oxide (TMAO), for example, has attracted a lot of interest since it is linked to cardiovascular events and atherosclerosis. It is produced by microorganisms that metabolise dietary choline, phosphatidylcholine, and carnitine. Elevated levels of

TMAO have been linked to increased platelet aggregation, promotion of foam cell formation, and impairment of reverse cholesterol transport, all of which contribute to the progression of cardiovascular pathology.

Conversely, certain microbial metabolites exhibit cardioprotective properties and contribute to the maintenance of cardiovascular homeostasis. For example, bile acids, which are mostly produced in the liver and then altered by gut microbes, are essential for the absorption of lipids and the metabolism of cholesterol. Certain bile acids, such as ursodeoxycholic acid and lithocholic acid, have been shown in recent research to have a part in lowering the development of atherosclerotic plaque, enhancing endothelial function, and decreasing inflammation. The regulation of host immune responses highlights the reciprocal link between gut microbiota and cardiovascular health. Secondary bile acids (SBAs) and other microbial metabolites control the development and activity of immune cells, such as macrophages and T regulatory cells, to provide immunomodulatory effects. By modulating the balance between pro-inflammatory and anti-inflammatory signaling pathways, these metabolites influence the progression of cardiovascular diseases, such as atherosclerosis and hypertension. Moreover, the metabolic activity of gut bacteria can directly impact systemic metabolism, thereby influencing cardiovascular risk factors such as dyslipidemia, insulin resistance, and obesity. The development of metabolic illnesses and cardiovascular diseases has been linked to dysbiosis, which is typified by changes in the makeup and functionality of the gut microbiota. Restoration of microbial balance through dietary interventions, probiotics, or fecal microbiota transplantation represents a promising therapeutic approach for ameliorating cardiovascular risk factors and improving overall health outcomes [3].

This chapter aims to provide an overview of the relationship between cardiovascular diseases and gut microbial metabolites.

THE GUT-HEART AXIS: LINKING GUT MICROBIOTA AND CARDIOVASCULAR HEALTH

The gut-heart axis serves as a conceptual framework to explain the complex relationship between gut microbiota and cardiovascular health, which is becoming widely acknowledged as a basic component of human physiology. This axis represents a bidirectional communication system between the gut microbiota and the cardiovascular system, wherein changes in gut microbial composition and activity can profoundly influence cardiovascular function and vice versa. Understanding this axis can help prevent and treat cardiovascular diseases (CVD), which continue to be the world's leading cause of morbidity and death. The gut microbiota, comprising trillions of microorganisms inhabiting the gastrointestinal tract, plays a crucial role in maintaining host homeostasis and health. Some of the microorganisms found in the human gut and their association with cardiovascular diseases are shown in Table **1**.

Table 1. Gut microbiota alterations linked to cardiovascular diseases [4].

<table>
<tr><th>Cardiovascular Diseases</th><th>Microbial Presence (Decrease)</th><th>Microbial Presence (Increase)</th></tr>
<tr><td rowspan="5">Atherosclerosis and coronary artery disease</td><td>Bacteroides and Prevotella</td><td>Streptococcus and Escherichia</td></tr>
<tr><td>Bacteroides and Prevotella</td><td>Order Lactobacillales</td></tr>
<tr><td>Roseburia and Eubacterium</td><td>Collinsella</td></tr>
<tr><td>Clostridium, Faecalibacterium</td><td>Prevotella</td></tr>
<tr><td>Burkholderia, Corynebacterium and Sediminibacterium, Comamonadaceae, Oxalobacteraceae, Rhodospirillaceae, Bradyrhizobiaceae and Burkholderiaceae</td><td>Curvibacter, unclassified Burkholderiales, Propionibacterium, Ralstonia</td></tr>
<tr><td rowspan="2">Hypertension</td><td>Roseburia spp., Faecalibacterium prausnitzii,</td><td>Klebsiella spp., Streptococcus spp., and Parabacteroides merdae</td></tr>
<tr><td>Butyrate-producing bacteria Odoribacter</td><td>-</td></tr>
<tr><td rowspan="4">Heart failure</td><td>Blautia, Collinsella, uncl. Erysipelotrichaceae and uncl. Ruminococcaceae</td><td>-</td></tr>
<tr><td>-</td><td>Campylobacter, Shigella, Salmonella, Yersinia enterocolitica,</td></tr>
<tr><td>Faecalibacterium</td><td>Lactobacillus</td></tr>
<tr><td>Faecalibacterium prausnitzii</td><td>Ruminococcus gnavus</td></tr>
<tr><td>Atrial fibrillation</td><td>Faecalibacterium, Alistipes, Oscillibacter, and Bilophila</td><td>Ruminococcus, Streptococcus, and Enterococcus,</td></tr>
</table>

Emerging evidence suggests that alterations in the composition and function of gut microbes, known as dysbiosis, may contribute to the development and progression of CVD. Dysbiosis may be brought on by a number of things, such as antibiotic usage, dietary habits, and lifestyle choices. It has also been linked to a number of important pathophysiological processes for CVD, such as insulin resistance, dyslipidemia, endothelial dysfunction, and systemic inflammation. Endothelial dysfunction, characterized by impaired vascular function and increased vascular permeability, is a hallmark feature of early-stage atherosclerosis and an independent predictor of cardiovascular events. Several studies have demonstrated a link between gut dysbiosis and endothelial dysfunction, highlighting the potential role of gut microbiota in modulating vascular health. Dysbiotic gut microbiota may promote endothelial dysfunction through multiple mechanisms, including the production of pro-inflammatory cytokines, alteration of nitric oxide bioavailability, and generation of microbial metabolites with vasoactive properties.

Gut microbiota also has a vital role in lipid metabolism, another important element of cardiovascular health. Dysbiosis has been linked to changes in lipid metabolism, which can result in dyslipidemia, which is characterised by decreased levels of high-density lipoprotein cholesterol (HDL-C) and raised levels of triglycerides and low-density lipoprotein cholesterol (LDL-C). The formation of lipid-laden plaques in the artery wall is a hallmark of atherosclerosis, a chronic inflammatory disease that is exacerbated by these lipid abnormalities. The relevance of gut microbiota in lipid metabolism and cardiovascular risk is further highlighted by the involvement of gut microbial metabolites, such as trimethylamine N-oxide (TMAO) and short-chain fatty acids (SCFAs), in dyslipidemia and atherosclerosis. A prevalent characteristic of numerous chronic illnesses, such as cardiovascular disease (CVD), is systemic inflammation. New research indicates that intestinal dysbiosis may be linked to systemic inflammation by means of immune cell activation, microbial product translocation across the intestinal barrier, and dysregulation of inflammatory signalling pathways. Chronic low-grade inflammation promotes endothelial dysfunction, insulin resistance, and atherosclerosis, thus linking gut dysbiosis to the pathogenesis of CVD.

The identification of specific microbial signatures associated with CVD outcomes holds promise for the development of microbiome-focused preventative and treatment approaches. Researchers have been able to uncover microbial taxa and functional pathways linked to cardiovascular risk by characterising gut microbial populations in health and illness thanks to recent advancements in high-throughput sequencing methods. For example, studies have identified specific bacterial taxa, such as *Prevotella copri* and *Collinsella aerofaciens*, that are enriched in individuals with atherosclerosis and heart failure, suggesting a potential role in disease pathogenesis.

Microbial metabolites, such as TMAO and SCFAs, represent attractive targets for therapeutic intervention due to their direct involvement in CVD pathophysiology. Strategies aimed at modulating gut microbial metabolism, such as dietary interventions, probiotics, and microbial-targeted therapies, have shown promise in preclinical and clinical studies for reducing cardiovascular risk factors and improving outcomes. For instance, dietary interventions targeting TMAO production, such as reducing dietary intake of choline and carnitine-rich foods, have been shown to decrease plasma TMAO levels and attenuate atherosclerosis progression in animal models [5, 6].

ROLE OF GUT MICROBIAL METABOLITES IN CARDIOVASCULAR DISEASES

Researchers have been able to uncover microbial taxa and functional pathways linked to cardiovascular risk by characterising gut microbial populations in health and illness thanks to recent advancements in high-throughput sequencing methods. This chapter examines the impact of certain gut microbial metabolites, such as bile acids, derivatives of amino acids, short-chain fatty acids (SCFAs), and others, on various aspects of cardiovascular health and illness.

Short-Chain Fatty Acids (SCFAs) and Cardiovascular Health

The microbial metabolites known as short-chain fatty acids (SCFAs), which comprise butyrate, propionate, and acetate, are important for preserving cardiovascular health. The fermentation of food fibres is the primary source of these SCFAs, which emphasises the symbiotic connection between host physiology, gut microbiota, and nutrition. The multifaceted effects of SCFAs on various aspects of cardiovascular function underscore their significance as key mediators in the gut-heart axis.

Their anti-inflammatory qualities are one of the important ways that SCFAs support cardiovascular health. SCFAs have been demonstrated to influence the formation of regulatory T cells (Tregs) and prevent the production of pro-inflammatory cytokines, therefore modulating immunological responses. By dampening excessive inflammation, SCFAs help to mitigate endothelial dysfunction, atherosclerosis, and other inflammatory processes implicated in cardiovascular diseases. Furthermore, the maintenance of a balanced immune response by SCFAs contributes to overall cardiovascular homeostasis.

Apart from their anti-inflammatory properties, SCFAs are essential in controlling the metabolism of fat and glucose, two major factors that determine the risk of cardiovascular disease. Research has indicated that SCFAs impact lipid metabolism by encouraging fatty acid oxidation and preventing lipogenesis in hepatocytes and adipocytes. Additionally, SCFAs improve peripheral tissue glucose utilisation and insulin sensitivity, which improves glycemic management and lowers the risk of metabolic diseases including type 2 diabetes and obesity. By modulating lipid and glucose metabolism, SCFAs exert protective effects against dyslipidemia, insulin resistance, and metabolic syndrome, all of which are major risk factors for cardiovascular diseases.

Furthermore, SCFAs have been implicated in the regulation of blood pressure, another critical determinant of cardiovascular health. Through various mechanisms, including the modulation of sympathetic nervous system activity and the renin-angiotensin-aldosterone system, SCFAs can influence vascular tone and blood pressure regulation. For example, butyrate has been shown to promote vasodilation by enhancing nitric oxide production in endothelial cells, leading to reductions in blood pressure. Moreover, SCFAs may impact the gut-kidney axis by modulating renal sodium absorption and excretion, thereby influencing blood volume and arterial pressure regulation.

Importantly, SCFAs have been demonstrated to improve endothelial function, a key determinant of vascular health. Endothelial cells play a crucial role in maintaining vascular homeostasis by regulating vascular tone, inflammation, and thrombosis. Dysfunction of the endothelium, characterized by impaired vasodilation, increased oxidative stress, and pro-inflammatory activation, is a hallmark feature of cardiovascular diseases. SCFAs exert beneficial effects on endothelial function by enhancing nitric oxide production, reducing oxidative stress, and suppressing endothelial inflammation, thus preserving vascular integrity and mitigating atherosclerosis progression [7].

Bile Acids and Lipid Metabolism

As an essential part of lipid metabolism and cholesterol homeostasis, bile acids are crucial for the breakdown and assimilation of dietary fats and fat-soluble vitamins. Synthesized in the liver from cholesterol, bile acids undergo further modification within the gastrointestinal tract through interactions with gut microbiota, ultimately shaping their composition and function. Bile acids play a multifunctional role in signalling pathways beyond their conventional involvement in lipid absorption. They activate nuclear receptors such as farnesoid X receptor (FXR) and Takeda G-protein-coupled receptor 5 (TGR5), which have a significant impact on metabolic and inflammatory processes. The activation of TGR5 and FXR by bile acids initiates a cascade of physiological responses that impact various aspects of cardiovascular health. TGR5 activation, primarily by secondary bile acids, regulates energy expenditure, glucose homeostasis, and inflammatory signaling pathways. Insulin sensitivity and glucose tolerance are enhanced when TGR5 is activated because it encourages enteroendocrine cells to secrete glucagon-like peptide 1 (GLP-1). Moreover, TGR5 activation in macrophages and endothelial cells suppresses inflammation and oxidative stress, thereby attenuating atherosclerosis progression and reducing cardiovascular risk.

Similarly, FXR activation by bile acids plays a pivotal role in lipid metabolism, glucose homeostasis, and inflammation. Bile acid homeostasis is regulated by the promotion of gene expression linked to bile acid production, secretion, and transport in hepatocytes through FXR activation. Moreover, FXR activation in the intestine and adipose tissue modulates lipid metabolism by promoting fatty acid oxidation, inhibiting lipogenesis, and enhancing triglyceride clearance. Additionally, FXR activation reduces vascular inflammation and the development of atherosclerosis by preventing the production of pro-inflammatory cytokines and chemokines. Dysregulation of bile acid metabolism has been implicated in the pathogenesis of dyslipidemia and atherosclerosis, two major cardiovascular diseases with significant morbidity and mortality. Alterations in bile acid composition and circulation, resulting from dysbiosis or impaired bile acid synthesis and transport, can disrupt lipid metabolism, promote inflammation, and contribute to atherosclerosis progression. For example, decreased FXR activation due to dysregulated bile acid metabolism may lead to impaired lipid clearance, increased lipogenesis, and enhanced pro-inflammatory signaling, thereby exacerbating dyslipidemia and atherosclerosis.

Furthermore, gut microbial modulation of bile acid composition and circulation can influence cardiovascular health through multiple mechanisms. Gut bacteria play a crucial role in bile acid metabolism by deconjugating, dehydroxylating, and epimerizing primary bile acids, thereby generating secondary bile acids with distinct biological activities. Changes in gut microbial composition and function can alter bile acid pool size, composition, and signaling capacity, consequently impacting lipid metabolism, inflammation, and atherosclerosis progression.

Moreover, emerging evidence suggests that bile acids may exert direct effects on vascular function and atherosclerosis through activation of vascular receptors and modulation of endothelial function. Bile acids have been shown to regulate vascular tone, endothelial permeability, and vascular inflammation through the activation of vascular receptors, including TGR5 and FXR. Additionally, bile acids can modulate endothelial function by regulating nitric oxide production, oxidative stress, and endothelial cell proliferation and apoptosis, thereby influencing vascular integrity and atherosclerosis development [8].

Amino Acid Derivatives and Vascular Function

Amino acid derivatives produced through gut microbiota metabolism, notably trimethylamine-N-oxide (TMAO), have emerged as significant contributors to cardiovascular diseases (CVD). Made from dietary precursors like choline, phosphatidylcholine, and carnitine, TMAO is produced by gut microbial enzymes and has drawn a lot of attention due to its possible involvement in the aetiology of heart failure, stroke, and coronary artery disease (CAD). The association between elevated TMAO levels and increased cardiovascular risk has been extensively studied, revealing a compelling link between TMAO and adverse cardiovascular outcomes. Higher levels of TMAO in the blood have been shown *via* clinical studies to be independently linked to an increased risk of significant adverse cardiovascular events, such as myocardial infarction, exacerbations of heart failure, and stroke. Moreover, prospective studies have identified TMAO as a prognostic biomarker for cardiovascular morbidity and mortality, highlighting its clinical relevance as a predictive marker of cardiovascular risk.

Mechanistically, TMAO exerts detrimental effects on cardiovascular health through multiple pathways, contributing to the development and progression of atherosclerosis, a common underlying pathology in many cardiovascular diseases. TMAO has been shown to promote atherosclerosis by enhancing the formation of macrophage foam cells, the hallmark cellular phenotype of early atherosclerotic lesions. Additionally, TMAO interferes with the process of reverse cholesterol transport, impairing the removal of cholesterol from peripheral tissues and promoting its accumulation within the arterial wall. Furthermore, TMAO induces endothelial dysfunction and vascular inflammation, key pathogenic mechanisms involved in atherosclerosis progression and plaque destabilization.

The detrimental effects of TMAO on cardiovascular health extend beyond atherosclerosis, encompassing other aspects of cardiovascular physiology and pathology. TMAO has been implicated in the pathogenesis of heart failure, a complex syndrome characterized by impaired cardiac function and neurohormonal dysregulation. Elevated TMAO levels have been associated with myocardial fibrosis, ventricular remodeling, and cardiac dysfunction, contributing to the development and progression of heart failure. Moreover, TMAO has been implicated in the pathophysiology of stroke, a devastating neurological condition resulting from cerebrovascular events. TMAO-mediated endothelial dysfunction and vascular inflammation may predispose individuals to cerebrovascular events, exacerbating the risk of stroke.

The identification of TMAO as a modifiable risk factor for cardiovascular diseases has spurred interest in developing novel therapeutic strategies aimed at targeting its formation or downstream consequences. Interventions targeting gut microbial metabolism, such as dietary modifications, probiotics, or microbial-targeted therapies, represent potential approaches for reducing TMAO levels and mitigating cardiovascular risk. For example, dietary interventions aimed at limiting the consumption of TMAO precursors, such as red meat and eggs, may help lower circulating TMAO levels and attenuate cardiovascular risk. Similarly, strategies aimed at modulating gut microbiota composition and function, such as the administration of probiotics or prebiotics, hold promise for reducing TMAO production and improving cardiovascular outcomes [8, 9].

Other Metabolites and Cardiovascular Impact

In addition to the well-studied metabolites like short-chain fatty acids (SCFAs), bile acids, and amino acid derivatives, emerging research has highlighted the potential cardiovascular impact of other metabolites produced by gut microbes. These include polyphenols, indole derivatives, and gases such as hydrogen sulphide, each of which exerts unique effects on cardiovascular health and function.

Polyphenols, abundant in many plant-based foods, possess potent antioxidant and anti-inflammatory properties that contribute to their cardioprotective effects. These bioactive compounds have been shown to attenuate oxidative stress, reduce inflammation, and improve endothelial function, all of which are critical determinants of cardiovascular health. By scavenging free radicals and inhibiting inflammatory pathways, polyphenols help mitigate the development and progression of atherosclerosis, a chronic inflammatory condition underlying many cardiovascular diseases. Furthermore, polyphenols have been associated with improvements in lipid metabolism, blood pressure regulation, and vascular tone, further underscoring their potential as therapeutic agents for cardiovascular disorders.

Derivatives of indole, produced from the breakdown of dietary tryptophan by gut microbes, have also garnered attention for their cardiovascular effects. Indole derivatives exhibit anti-inflammatory properties and have been shown to modulate vascular tone through the activation of specific receptors, such as the aryl hydrocarbon receptor (AhR). By regulating inflammatory signaling pathways and vascular function, indole derivatives help to maintain endothelial homeostasis and prevent the development of vascular dysfunction and atherosclerosis. Moreover, indole derivatives have been implicated in the regulation of blood pressure and may offer potential therapeutic targets for hypertension and related cardiovascular conditions.

Hydrogen sulphide (H_2S), a gas produced by gut microbes during the fermentation of sulfur-containing amino acids, exerts diverse effects on cardiovascular physiology. Despite its characteristic odor, H_2S serves as a crucial signaling molecule with vasodilator, antioxidant, and anti-inflammatory properties. H_2S promotes endothelial-dependent vasorelaxation, improves blood flow, and inhibits platelet aggregation, thereby contributing to the maintenance of vascular homeostasis and prevention of thrombotic events. Additionally, H_2S scavenges reactive oxygen species, attenuates oxidative stress, and modulates inflammatory pathways, thereby protecting against endothelial dysfunction, atherosclerosis, and cardiovascular injury.

Deciphering the effects of these diverse metabolites on cardiovascular health is essential for understanding the intricate interactions between gut microbiota and cardiovascular disorders. While much of the focus has been on SCFAs, bile acids, and amino acid derivatives, emerging evidence suggests that polyphenols, indole derivatives, and hydrogen sulphide also play critical roles in cardiovascular physiology and pathology. Further research is needed to elucidate the mechanisms underlying the cardiovascular effects of these metabolites and to explore their potential as therapeutic targets for managing cardiovascular risk and enhancing patient outcomes [9].

MECHANISMS UNDERLYING THE INFLUENCE OF GUT MICROBIAL METABOLITES ON THE CARDIOVASCULAR SYSTEM

Understanding the mechanisms by which gut microbial metabolites influence the cardiovascular system is crucial for elucidating their role in cardiovascular health and disease. This chapter examines the several ways in which these metabolites affect lipid homeostasis and metabolism, blood pressure management, vascular endothelial function, inflammation and immunological modulation, and metabolic regulation [10].

Inflammation and Immune Modulation

In the intricate interplay between gut microbial metabolites and cardiovascular health, inflammation, and immune modulation emerge as crucial players. These processes, intricately intertwined, exert profound effects on cardiovascular physiology and pathology. Among the myriad of gut microbial metabolites, short-chain fatty acids (SCFAs) stand out as key mediators in regulating inflammation and immune responses, thereby shaping cardiovascular health outcomes.

Microbial fermentation of food fibres in the gut produces SCFAs, namely acetate, propionate, and butyrate. These bioactive molecules serve as signaling molecules that interact with various cell types, including immune cells, within the intestinal mucosa and systemic circulation. SCFAs exert potent anti-inflammatory effects by modulating immune cell function and cytokine production, thus contributing to immune homeostasis and mitigating chronic inflammation.

One of the primary mechanisms through which SCFAs modulate inflammation is by inhibiting the generation of pro-inflammatory cytokines. Immune cells, particularly macrophages and dendritic cells, have been demonstrated to produce and release inflammatory mediators such as tumour necrosis factor-alpha (TNF-α), interleukin-6 (IL-6), and interleukin-1 beta (IL-1β) less frequently when SCFAs are present. By dampening the production of these pro-inflammatory cytokines, SCFAs help to attenuate the inflammatory response and prevent tissue damage associated with chronic inflammation.

Moreover, SCFAs stimulate the generation of anti-inflammatory responses in immune cells, including regulatory T cells (Tregs) and anti-inflammatory macrophages. Tregs are essential for preserving immunological tolerance and averting over-activation of the immune system. SCFAs decrease aberrant immune responses and reduce inflammation by encouraging Treg differentiation and expansion. Furthermore, SCFAs cause macrophages to polarise towards an anti-inflammatory phenotype, which is shown by a decrease in the production of pro-inflammatory cytokines and an increase in the expression of anti-inflammatory cytokines like interleukin-10 (IL-10).

By modulating the balance between pro-inflammatory and anti-inflammatory signals, SCFAs help to maintain immune homeostasis and mitigate chronic inflammation, which is a major driver of cardiovascular diseases such as atherosclerosis and hypertension. Prolonged inflammation stimulates endothelial dysfunction, vascular inflammation, and plaque formation, all of which are factors in the onset and advancement of atherosclerosis. Moreover, inflammation contributes to endothelial dysfunction, blood pressure dysregulation, and vascular remodelling in the pathogenesis of hypertension.

The prevention of cardiovascular disease and cardiovascular health are significantly impacted by the anti-inflammatory properties of SCFAs. As a substrate for the synthesis of SCFA, dietary fibre consumption has been shown in epidemiological studies to be inversely correlated with the risk of cardiovascular illnesses. Additionally, experimental studies using animal models have shown that supplementation with SCFAs or dietary fiber attenuates atherosclerosis development and improves cardiovascular outcomes [10].

Metabolic Regulation and Lipid Homeostasis

The aetiology of cardiovascular disorders including atherosclerosis and coronary artery disease is aided by metabolic dysregulation, which is defined by anomalies in lipid metabolism and cholesterol homeostasis. A growing body of research indicates that metabolites produced by gut microbes are essential for controlling lipid homeostasis and metabolic pathways, which in turn affects cardiovascular risk.

Short-chain fatty acids (SCFAs) are considered to be important regulators of energy balance and lipid metabolism among the many metabolites produced by gut microbes. In the stomach, microbial fermentation of dietary fibres yields SCFAs such as butyrate, propionate, and acetate. Systemic lipid levels and cardiovascular health are eventually impacted by the pleiotropic actions of these bioactive compounds on adipose tissue and hepatic lipid metabolism.

It has been demonstrated that SCFAs influence lipid metabolism in adipose tissue by preventing lipogenesis and encouraging fatty acid oxidation. Sterol-CoA carboxylase (ACC) and fatty acid synthase (FAS) are two important lipogenic enzymes whose expression is suppressed by SCFAs, which reduces triglyceride production and increases lipid mobilisation. Additionally, the expression of genes involved in fatty acid oxidation is enhanced by SCFAs, including carnitine palmitoyltransferase-1 (CPT-1) and peroxisome proliferator-activated receptor gamma coactivator 1-alpha (PGC-1α), which increases the use of fatty acids for energy generation.

SCFAs have comparable effects on lipid metabolism in the liver by promoting fatty acid oxidation and suppressing hepatic lipogenesis. SCFAs promote the expression of genes involved in fatty acid oxidation, such as peroxisome proliferator-activated receptor alpha (PPARα) and carnitine palmitoyltransferase-1 (CPT-1), while suppressing the expression of genes linked to lipogenic processes, such as fatty acid synthase (FAS) and sterol regulatory element-binding protein 1c (SREBP-1c). Furthermore, SCFAs improve hepatic insulin sensitivity, which in turn improves the liver's metabolism of lipids and glucose. Moreover, two microbial metabolites called bile acids and trimethylamine-N-oxide (TMAO) are essential for controlling the metabolism and transport of cholesterol, which is a key factor in the development of atherosclerosis and cardiovascular risk. The gut microbiota changes bile acids, which are produced in the liver and help the intestines absorb fats and cholesterol from food. In addition, *via* activating nuclear receptors such as the Takeda G-protein-coupled receptor 5 (TGR5) and the farnesoid X receptor (FXR), bile acids function as signalling molecules that control the metabolism of fat and glucose. The correlation between dyslipidemia and atherosclerosis and the dysregulation of bile acid metabolism underscores the significance of gut microbial control of bile acids in cardiovascular health.

Similarly, TMAO, derived from the microbial metabolism of dietary choline, phosphatidylcholine, and carnitine, has been associated with dyslipidemia and cardiovascular risk. Elevated TMAO levels have been linked to increased cardiovascular events and atherosclerosis progression. Mechanistically, TMAO disrupts cholesterol metabolism and promotes foam cell formation, endothelial dysfunction, and vascular inflammation, thereby contributing to atherosclerosis development and cardiovascular risk [10, 11].

Vascular Endothelial Function

The complex relationship between gut microbiota and cardiovascular physiology is highlighted by the significant effect of gut microbial metabolites on arterial endothelial function, a fundamental component of cardiovascular health. The monolayer of cells that lines the inside surface of blood arteries is called the endothelium, and it is essential for controlling blood flow, vascular tone, and vascular homeostasis. Prolonged oxidative stress, reduced vasodilation, and pro-inflammatory activation are signs of endothelial dysfunction, which is a common characteristic of many cardiovascular disorders, such as heart failure, atherosclerosis, and hypertension.

Short-chain fatty acids (SCFAs), generated by the microbial fermentation of dietary fibers in the gut, have emerged as key modulators of endothelial function and vascular health. SCFAs, such as acetate, propionate, and butyrate, exert beneficial effects on endothelial cell activity by stimulating the synthesis of nitric oxide (NO), a crucial vasodilator molecule. NO plays a central role in regulating vascular tone and endothelial function by promoting vasodilation, inhibiting platelet aggregation, and preventing leukocyte adhesion to the endothelium. By enhancing NO production, SCFAs improve endothelial function and maintain vascular integrity, thereby protecting against the development of cardiovascular diseases.

Moreover, SCFAs exhibit anti-inflammatory and antioxidant properties that contribute to their beneficial effects on endothelial function. SCFAs reduce endothelial inflammation and stop leukocyte infiltration into the vessel wall by suppressing the production of adhesion molecules and pro-inflammatory cytokines in endothelial cells. Additionally, SCFAs scavenge reactive oxygen species (ROS) and inhibit oxidative stress-induced endothelial dysfunction, further supporting vascular health and integrity.

Conversely, dysbiosis-induced metabolites such as trimethylamine-N-oxide (TMAO) have been implicated in the impairment of endothelial function and the pathogenesis of cardiovascular diseases. Derived from the microbial metabolism of dietary choline, phosphatidylcholine, and carnitine, TMAO has been linked to inflammation, oxidative stress, and endothelial dysfunction—all of which are factors in the initiation and advancement of atherosclerosis and the risk of cardiovascular disease.

Mechanistically, TMAO causes endothelial dysfunction, which is marked by increased oxidative stress, pro-inflammatory activation, and decreased NO bioavailability. TMAO has been shown to inhibit endothelial NO synthase (eNOS) activity and impair NO-mediated vasodilation, thereby compromising vascular function and promoting vasoconstriction. Additionally, TMAO induces endothelial oxidative stress by promoting the production of reactive oxygen species (ROS) and inhibiting antioxidant defense mechanisms, leading to endothelial dysfunction and vascular damage.

Furthermore, TMAO promotes endothelial inflammation by activating inflammatory signaling pathways and inducing the expression of adhesion molecules and pro-inflammatory cytokines in endothelial cells. Endothelial inflammation contributes to leukocyte adhesion, endothelial dysfunction, and atherosclerosis progression, thereby exacerbating cardiovascular risk [11].

Blood Pressure Regulation

The gut microbiota and their metabolites also play a role in regulating blood pressure, a major determinant of cardiovascular health. Multiple processes, such as the control of sympathetic nervous system activity, the function of the renin-angiotensin-aldosterone system, and the absorption of salt in the kidneys and gut, have all been linked to the regulation of blood pressure by SCFAs. On the other hand, *via* enhancing vascular dysfunction and changing renal salt management, dysbiosis-induced metabolites such as TMAO have been linked to hypertension [11].

Therefore, for the purpose of creating focused therapies meant to maintain cardiovascular health and prevent cardiovascular illnesses, it is crucial to comprehend the complex processes underpinning the impact of gut microbial metabolites on the circulatory system. More studies in this field might lead to the discovery of cutting-edge treatment approaches that use gut microbiota and its metabolites to lower cardiovascular risk and enhance patient outcomes.

GUT MICROBIAL DYSBIOSIS IN CARDIOVASCULAR DISEASES

Altered Microbiota Composition

Through complex interactions with host physiology and metabolism, the gut microbiota—a varied population of bacteria living in the gastrointestinal tract—has a significant impact on cardiovascular health. Many variables, such as nutrition, antibiotics, lifestyle, and host genetics, dynamically alter the makeup and function of the gut microbiota. Dysbiosis has emerged as a major player in the pathophysiology of cardiovascular illnesses. It is characterised by changes in microbial diversity, abundance of certain taxa, and disturbances in microbial metabolite synthesis.

Numerous cardiovascular diseases, including atherosclerosis, hypertension, heart failure, and stroke, are linked to microbial dysbiosis. Disturbances in the composition of gut microbiota have been noted between cardiovascular disease patients and healthy persons, indicating a possible involvement of dysbiosis in the aetiology of the illness. These alterations in microbial diversity and abundance may lead to changes in microbial metabolism and the production of bioactive metabolites that impact cardiovascular risk.

One of the key factors contributing to dysbiosis is diet, which serves as a major determinant of microbial composition and function. Dietary patterns rich in processed foods, saturated fats, and refined carbohydrates have been associated with alterations in gut microbiota composition and increased cardiovascular risk. Conversely, diets high in fiber, whole grains, fruits, and vegetables promote microbial diversity and the growth of beneficial bacteria, which may have protective effects against cardiovascular diseases. For example, the Mediterranean diet, characterized by the high intake of plant-based foods, olive oil, and fish, has been associated with a favorable gut microbiota profile and reduced cardiovascular risk.

Antibiotic use represents another important factor contributing to dysbiosis and cardiovascular risk. Antibiotics, while effective in treating bacterial infections, can indiscriminately disrupt the gut microbiota, leading to alterations in microbial diversity and composition. Dysbiosis induced by antibiotic exposure has been linked to increased susceptibility to cardiovascular diseases, possibly through mechanisms involving inflammation, oxidative stress, and dysregulation of lipid metabolism. Furthermore, repeated or prolonged antibiotic use may lead to the emergence of antibiotic-resistant bacteria, which pose additional risks to cardiovascular health.

Lifestyle variables that affect gut microbiota composition and cardiovascular risk include stress, physical exercise, and sleep habits. Frequent exercise has been demonstrated to support the growth of beneficial bacteria and microbial diversity, but poor sleep and long-term stress have been linked to dysbiosis and an increased risk of cardiovascular disease. Additionally, environmental factors such as pollution and exposure to toxins may impact microbial composition and contribute to dysbiosis-mediated cardiovascular diseases.

The mechanisms underlying the association between dysbiosis and cardiovascular diseases are multifactorial and complex. Changes in microbial metabolites caused by dysbiosis, such as bile acids, trimethylamine-N-oxide (TMAO), and short-chain fatty acids (SCFAs), may have a direct impact on cardiovascular risk factors such as endothelial function, inflammation, and lipid metabolism. Furthermore, dysbiosis-induced changes in gut barrier function and immune regulation may promote systemic inflammation and endothelial dysfunction, further exacerbating cardiovascular risk. Understanding these alterations is crucial for developing targeted interventions [12].

Implications for Cardiovascular Risk

Dysbiosis-induced alterations in gut microbial metabolites have profound implications for cardiovascular risk, contributing to the pathogenesis of various cardiovascular diseases. Trimethylamine-N-oxide (TMAO), bile acids, and short-chain fatty acids (SCFAs) are some of the major microbial metabolites linked to cardiovascular health. These compounds each have unique impacts on endothelial function, lipid metabolism, and systemic inflammation.

Trimethylamine-N-oxide (TMAO), which is produced when microbes metabolise dietary choline, phosphatidylcholine, and carnitine, has attracted a lot of interest due to its potential involvement in the pathophysiology of cardiovascular disease. Increased cardiovascular risk and unfavourable outcomes, such as myocardial infarction, heart failure, and stroke, have been linked to elevated TMAO levels. Mechanistically, TMAO promotes atherosclerosis by disrupting lipid metabolism, impairing endothelial function, and inducing vascular inflammation. TMAO interferes with cholesterol transport and metabolism, promoting the formation of foam cells and the development of atherosclerotic plaques. Additionally, TMAO induces endothelial dysfunction by inhibiting nitric oxide (NO) production and promoting oxidative stress, thereby contributing to vascular dysfunction and hypertension.

The liver produces bile acids, which are then altered by the gut microbiota and are essential for maintaining cholesterol homeostasis and lipid metabolism. Dysregulation of bile acid metabolism has been implicated in dyslipidemia and atherosclerosis, highlighting the importance of gut microbial modulation of bile acids in cardiovascular health. The effects of bile acids on lipid absorption, cholesterol production, and glucose metabolism are mediated by their interactions with nuclear receptors, including the Takeda G-protein-coupled receptor 5 (TGR5) and the farnesoid X receptor (FXR). Dysbiosis-induced alterations in bile acid composition and circulation can disrupt lipid metabolism, promote inflammation, and contribute to atherosclerosis progression. When dietary fibres are fermented by gut bacteria, short-chain fatty acids (SCFAs) are created that have a variety of consequences on cardiovascular health. By preventing lipogenesis and encouraging fatty acid oxidation in the liver and adipose tissue, SCFAs regulate lipid metabolism. Additionally, SCFAs improve endothelial function by stimulating the synthesis of nitric oxide (NO), a crucial vasodilator, and suppressing endothelial inflammation and oxidative stress. SCFAs also exert anti-inflammatory effects by inhibiting the production of pro-inflammatory cytokines and promoting the differentiation of regulatory T cells (Tregs), thereby mitigating chronic inflammation and atherosclerosis progression.

The dysregulation of microbial metabolites implicated in cardiovascular health underscores the potential for targeting the gut microbiota as a novel approach to controlling cardiovascular risk and developing new treatment strategies. Modulating the composition and activity of the gut microbiota through dietary interventions, probiotics, or microbial-targeted therapies offers promise for reducing cardiovascular risk and improving patient outcomes. Strategies aimed at restoring microbial balance, enhancing the production of beneficial metabolites, and inhibiting the synthesis of detrimental metabolites may represent innovative approaches for the prevention and treatment of cardiovascular diseases. Changing the makeup of the gut microbiota and the generation of metabolites offers a potential way to control cardiovascular risk and provide new treatment approaches [13].

THERAPEUTIC APPROACHES TARGETING GUT MICROBIAL METABOLITES IN CARDIOVASCULAR DISEASES

The relationship between gut microbiota metabolites and cardiovascular health has attracted a lot of interest lately, which has prompted the investigation of several treatment modalities. These tactics alter the composition of the gut microbiota and the synthesis of metabolites in an effort to improve outcomes and lower the risk of cardiovascular disease. In an effort to harness the gut microbiome's potential to impact cardiovascular health, scientists and medical professionals are concentrating on dietary interventions, probiotics and prebiotics, and faecal microbiota transplantation (FMT).

Dietary Interventions

Dietary modifications represent a fundamental approach to managing cardiovascular health through the manipulation of gut microbial metabolites. Foods rich in fibre, polyphenols, and omega-3 fatty acids are among the fundamental components of a diet that influence the composition of the gut microbiota and stimulate the production of metabolites that are beneficial to health. For example, short-chain fatty acids (SCFAs), which have anti-inflammatory and cardioprotective properties, are produced when gut bacteria digest fibre. Furthermore, it has been demonstrated that diets heavy in plant-based foods and low in saturated fats can lower the synthesis of toxic metabolites such as trimethylamine-N-oxide (TMAO), which lowers the risk of cardiovascular disease. The potential for improving cardiovascular outcomes through personalised dietary treatments based on an individual's microbiome profile emphasises the need for a comprehensive approach to dietary management in the prevention and treatment of cardiovascular disease [14].

Probiotics and Prebiotics

Probiotics and prebiotics offer targeted approaches to modulate gut microbial composition and metabolite production for cardiovascular benefit. Probiotics, which are live beneficial bacteria, have the ability to increase the number of helpful microorganisms in the gut and therefore produce compounds that are favourable to health. Bifidobacterium and Lactobacillus strains, for example, lower inflammation and aid in the synthesis of SCFA, which may lower the risk of cardiovascular disease. However, prebiotics—non-digestible fibres that serve as food for good bacteria—promote the development of these microorganisms and increase the synthesis of SCFA. It has been demonstrated that probiotics and prebiotics can enhance lipid profiles, lower blood pressure, and lessen vascular inflammation, all of which can benefit cardiovascular health. Further research is needed to optimize probiotic and prebiotic formulations for targeted cardiovascular benefits, emphasizing the potential of microbiota-targeted interventions in cardiovascular disease management [15].

Faecal Microbiota Transplantation (FMT)

Faecal microbiota transplantation (FMT) represents a promising therapeutic approach aimed at restoring microbial balance and function in individuals with dysbiosis, potentially offering novel avenues for the management of cardiovascular diseases. Historically utilized primarily for the treatment of gastrointestinal disorders, FMT involves the transfer of faecal material from a healthy donor to a recipient, with the goal of introducing beneficial microbes and promoting microbial diversity in the recipient's gut.

The rationale behind using FMT for cardiovascular diseases lies in its ability to modify gut microbial metabolites, thereby influencing cardiovascular risk factors and disease progression. Dysbiosis-induced alterations in microbial composition and function can lead to dysregulation of microbial metabolites, including trimethylamine-N-oxide (TMAO) and short-chain fatty acids (SCFAs), which play key roles in cardiovascular health. By restoring microbial balance and diversity, FMT has the potential to mitigate dysbiosis-associated changes in metabolite profiles and improve cardiovascular outcomes.

One of the mechanisms through which FMT may exert its therapeutic effects on cardiovascular health is by reducing the formation of TMAO, a microbial metabolite implicated in atherosclerosis and cardiovascular risk. The microbial breakdown of dietary precursors such as choline, phosphatidylcholine, and carnitine produces TMAO, which has been linked to harmful cardiovascular effects. FMT has the potential to alter the gut microbiota composition in a way that reduces the abundance of TMAO-producing bacteria and promotes the growth of beneficial microbes that metabolize TMAO precursors differently, thereby lowering circulating TMAO levels and attenuating cardiovascular risk. Additionally, FMT may enhance the synthesis of SCFAs, which exert beneficial effects on cardiovascular health by modulating lipid metabolism, endothelial function, and inflammation. SCFAs, produced through the microbial fermentation of dietary fibers, have been shown to improve endothelial function, reduce inflammation, and lower blood pressure, all of which contribute to cardiovascular health. By establishing a healthy and diversified microbial population in the recipient's gut, FMT may promote the production of SCFAs and other beneficial metabolites, thereby conferring cardiovascular protective effects.

While the potential of FMT as a therapeutic strategy for cardiovascular diseases is promising, further investigation is needed to clarify its effectiveness and safety. Clinical trials evaluating the impact of FMT on cardiovascular outcomes, including changes in microbial composition, metabolite profiles, and disease progression, are warranted to establish its therapeutic potential and optimize treatment protocols. Moreover, long-term safety considerations, including the risk of microbial transmission and immune reactions, should be carefully evaluated to ensure the safety and efficacy of FMT in the management of cardiovascular diseases [16].

CLINICAL EVIDENCE AND STUDIES

The function of gut microbial metabolites in cardiovascular disorders must be clarified by clinical data and research. By means of thorough study, scientists want to comprehend the ways in which changes in the composition of the gut microbiota and the production of metabolites affect cardiovascular health. Through the use of diverse study designs and methodology, clinical research offers significant insights into the intricate relationships that exist between the gut microbiota, metabolites, and cardiovascular outcomes. These investigations aid in the creation of cutting-edge treatment strategies and interventions for the management and prevention of cardiovascular illnesses [17, 18].

Observational Studies

Observational studies provide crucial insights into the association between gut microbial metabolites and cardiovascular diseases. Large cohorts are used in this research to investigate relationships between metabolite profiles, gut microbiota makeup, and cardiovascular outcomes. Their findings clarify the processes connecting gut microbial metabolites to cardiovascular risk and pinpoint possible dysbiosis biomarkers. To better understand the intricate interactions between gut microbiota and cardiovascular health, observational studies are essential for formulating hypotheses and directing future investigation [19, 20].

Interventional Trials

Interventional trials investigate the therapeutic potential of modulating gut microbial metabolites for cardiovascular disease management. These studies modify the gut microbiota and its metabolites through a variety of treatments, including dietary changes, probiotics, prebiotics, and faecal microbiota transplantation (FMT). Interventional studies offer important evidence for the effectiveness and safety of gut microbiota-targeted therapeutics in the prevention and treatment of cardiovascular disease by evaluating changes in microbial composition, metabolite production, and cardiovascular outcomes pre- and post-intervention [21, 22].

Cardiovascular Outcomes

Clinical studies evaluate the impact of gut microbial metabolites on cardiovascular outcomes, including atherosclerosis, hypertension, myocardial infarction, and stroke. Through the analysis of cardiovascular health parameters such as blood pressure, endothelial function, lipid profile, and inflammation, these investigations clarify the processes that underlie the association between gut microbiota and cardiovascular disorders. Developing tailored therapies to reduce cardiovascular risk and enhance patient outcomes requires an understanding of how gut microbial metabolites affect cardiovascular outcomes [23, 24].

CHALLENGES AND FUTURE DIRECTIONS IN RESEARCH

The study of gut microbiota metabolites and cardiovascular illnesses continues to face a number of obstacles, even with notable progress. Determining the precise processes by which microbial metabolites affect cardiovascular health is a significant task. Though correlations between dysbiosis and cardiovascular outcomes have been noted, the specific mechanisms involved are still not fully understood. In order to overcome this challenge, further mechanistic studies are required to elucidate the impact of metabolites such as trimethylamine-N-oxide (TMAO), bile acids, and short-chain fatty acids (SCFAs) on cardiovascular disease and function [25, 26].

Unraveling Specific Metabolite Mechanisms

Though correlations between dysbiosis and cardiovascular outcomes have been noted, the specific mechanisms involved are still not fully understood. More mechanistic study is required to address this challenge and elucidate the impact of metabolites such trimethylamine-N-oxide (TMAO), bile acids, and short-chain fatty acids (SCFAs) on cardiovascular disease and function. In order to unravel these intricate pathways, cutting-edge molecular and cellular techniques—such as omics methods and animal models—will be crucial. Furthermore, novel imaging modalities and bioinformatics instruments can facilitate the integration of data from many biological levels, offering a thorough comprehension of the cardiovascular pathways regulated by metabolites [27, 28].

Personalized Approaches to Cardiovascular Care

Personalised cardiovascular care techniques based on individual gut bacteria profiles and chemical signatures provide a viable path for further research. With the use of machine learning algorithms and new developments in microbiome sequencing technology, physicians may now customise patient therapies to target certain dysbiosis patterns and metabolic abnormalities. Probiotic formulations, faecal microbiota transplantation techniques, and tailored dietary recommendations have the potential to improve cardiovascular outcomes by adjusting the gut microbial composition and metabolite synthesis to suit individual needs [29, 30].

Integration with Traditional Therapies

A potential approach to improving cardiovascular care is to include medicines that target gut bacteria metabolites with conventional medications. Combinatorial strategies may be more effective in controlling cardiovascular risk factors and delaying the advancement of the illness when they combine the synergistic effects of pharmaceutical therapies, lifestyle changes, and microbiota-targeted therapy. However, successful integration requires interdisciplinary collaboration between cardiologists, gastroenterologists, microbiologists, and other healthcare professionals to optimize treatment strategies and ensure patient safety and efficacy [31, 32].

CONCLUSION AND IMPLICATIONS FOR CARDIOVASCULAR HEALTH

In conclusion, research on cardiovascular diseases and gut microbial metabolites holds immense promise for revolutionizing cardiovascular care. Through the clarification of the complex interrelationships among gut microbiota, microbial metabolites, and cardiovascular health, scientists can discover new targets for therapeutic intervention, tailor treatments to individual needs, and enhance patient outcomes. However, the scientific community, healthcare professionals, legislators, and industry stakeholders will need to work together to solve the issues raised and integrate research findings into clinical practice. Ultimately, integrating microbiota-based approaches into routine cardiovascular care has the potential to usher in a new era of precision medicine, where tailored interventions based on individual microbial signatures optimize cardiovascular health and prevent disease burden.

CONSENT FOR PUBLICATIONS

We, the undersigned authors, hereby provide our consent for the publication of the book chapter titled **"Cardiovascular Diseases and Gut Microbial Metabolites"**. We certify that we made a substantial contribution to the idea, planning, and gathering of the data for the project that is detailed in the book chapter. Furthermore, we declare that the book chapter is entirely original material that has never been published before and is not presently being considered for publication anywhere.

CONFLICT OF INTEREST

We declare that we have no conflicts of interest that could influence the conduct or reporting of this work.

REFERENCES

[1] Kasahara K, Rey FE. The emerging role of gut microbial metabolism on cardiovascular disease. Curr Opin Microbiol 2019; 50: 64-70. [http://dx.doi.org/10.1016/j.mib.2019.09.007] [PMID: 31693963]

[2] Brial F, Le Lay A, Dumas ME, Gauguier D. Implication of gut microbiota metabolites in cardiovascular and metabolic diseases. Cell Mol Life Sci 2018; 75(21): 3977-90. [http://dx.doi.org/10.1007/s00018-018-2901-1] [PMID: 30101405]

[3] Jansen VLBI, Gerdes VEA, Middeldorp S, van Mens TE. Gut microbiota and their metabolites in cardiovascular disease. Best Pract Res Clin Endocrinol Metab 2021; 35(3): 101492. [http://dx.doi.org/10.1016/j.beem.2021.101492] [PMID: 33642219]

[4] Jin L, Shi X, Yang J, *et al.* Gut microbes in cardiovascular diseases and their potential therapeutic applications. Protein Cell 2021; 12(5): 346-59. [http://dx.doi.org/10.1007/s13238-020-00785-9] [PMID: 32989686]

[5] Shariff S, Kwan Su Huey A, Parag Soni N, *et al.* Unlocking the gut-heart axis: exploring the role of gut microbiota in cardiovascular health and disease. Ann Med Surg (Lond) 2024; 86(5): 2752-8. [http://dx.doi.org/10.1097/MS9.0000000000001744] [PMID: 38694298]

[6] Almeida C, Gonçalves-Nobre JG, Costa DA, Barata P. The potential links between human gut microbiota and cardiovascular health and disease-is there a gut-cardiovascular axis?. gut. 2023; 24: 25.

[7] Kasahara K, Rey FE. The emerging role of gut microbial metabolism on cardiovascular disease. Curr Opin Microbiol 2019; 50: 64-70. [http://dx.doi.org/10.1016/j.mib.2019.09.007] [PMID: 31693963]

[8] Chambers ES, Preston T, Frost G, Morrison DJ. Role of gut microbiota-generated short-chain fatty acids in metabolic and cardiovascular health. Curr Nutr Rep 2018; 7(4): 198-206.
[http://dx.doi.org/10.1007/s13668-018-0248-8] [PMID: 30264354]

[9] Carubelli V, Castrini AI, Lazzarini V, Gheorghiade M, Metra M, Lombardi C. Amino acids and derivatives, a new treatment of chronic heart failure? Heart Fail Rev 2015; 20(1): 39-51.
[http://dx.doi.org/10.1007/s10741-014-9436-9] [PMID: 24925377]

[10] Zhu Y, Shui X, Liang Z, *et al.* Gut microbiota metabolites as integral mediators in cardiovascular diseases (Review). Int J Mol Med 2020; 46(3): 936-48.
[http://dx.doi.org/10.3892/ijmm.2020.4674] [PMID: 32705240]

[11] Nesci A, Carnuccio C, Ruggieri V, *et al.* Gut Microbiota and Cardiovascular Disease: Evidence on the Metabolic and Inflammatory Background of a Complex Relationship. Int J Mol Sci 2023; 24(10): 9087.
[http://dx.doi.org/10.3390/ijms24109087] [PMID: 37240434]

[12] Wang H, Li Y, Wang R, Ji H, Lu C, Su X. Chinese Torreya grandis cv. Merrillii seed oil affects obesity through accumulation of sciadonic acid and altering the composition of gut microbiota. Food Sci Hum Wellness 2022; 11(1): 58-67.
[http://dx.doi.org/10.1016/j.fshw.2021.07.007]

[13] Ellis CJ, Legget ME, Edwards C, *et al.* High calcium scores in patients with a low Framingham risk of cardiovascular (CVS) disease: implications for more accurate CVS risk assessment in New Zealand. N Z Med J 2011; 124(1335): 13-26.
[PMID: 21946678]

[14] Khan SU, Khan MU, Riaz H, *et al.* Effects of nutritional supplements and dietary interventions on cardiovascular outcomes: an umbrella review and evidence map. Ann Intern Med 2019; 171(3): 190-8.
[http://dx.doi.org/10.7326/M19-0341] [PMID: 31284304]

[15] Azad MA, Sarker M, Li T, Yin J. Probiotic species in the modulation of gut microbiota: an overview. BioMed research international, 2018.
[http://dx.doi.org/10.1155/2018/9478630]

[16] Murphy K, O'Donovan AN, Caplice NM, Ross RP, Stanton C. Exploring the gut microbiota and cardiovascular disease. Metabolites 2021; 11(8): 493.
[http://dx.doi.org/10.3390/metabo11080493] [PMID: 34436434]

[17] Dzau VJ, Antman EM, Black HR, *et al.* The cardiovascular disease continuum validated: clinical evidence of improved patient outcomes: part I: Pathophysiology and clinical trial evidence (risk factors through stable coronary artery disease). Circulation 2006; 114(25): 2850-70.
[http://dx.doi.org/10.1161/CIRCULATIONAHA.106.655688] [PMID: 17179034]

[18] Zordoky BNM, Robertson IM, Dyck JRB. Preclinical and clinical evidence for the role of resveratrol in the treatment of cardiovascular diseases. Biochim Biophys Acta Mol Basis Dis 2015; 1852(6): 1155-77.
[http://dx.doi.org/10.1016/j.bbadis.2014.10.016] [PMID: 25451966]

[19] Rodríguez-Monforte M, Flores-Mateo G, Sánchez E. Dietary patterns and CVD: a systematic review and meta-analysis of observational studies. Br J Nutr 2015; 114(9): 1341-59.
[http://dx.doi.org/10.1017/S0007114515003177] [PMID: 26344504]

[20] Rosato V, Temple NJ, La Vecchia C, Castellan G, Tavani A, Guercio V. Mediterranean diet and cardiovascular disease: a systematic review and meta-analysis of observational studies. Eur J Nutr 2019; 58(1): 173-91.
[http://dx.doi.org/10.1007/s00394-017-1582-0] [PMID: 29177567]

[21] Evans RW, Shaten BJ, Hempel JD, Cutler JA, Kuller LH. Homocyst(e)ine and risk of cardiovascular disease in the Multiple Risk Factor Intervention Trial. Arterioscler Thromb Vasc Biol 1997; 17(10): 1947-53.

[http://dx.doi.org/10.1161/01.ATV.17.10.1947] [PMID: 9351358]

[22] Stamler J, Neaton JD, Cohen JD, *et al.* Multiple risk factor intervention trial revisited: a new perspective based on nonfatal and fatal composite endpoints, coronary and cardiovascular, during the trial. J Am Heart Assoc 2012; 1(5): e003640. [http://dx.doi.org/10.1161/JAHA.112.003640] [PMID: 23316301]

[23] Weiner DE, Tabatabai S, Tighiouart H, *et al.* Cardiovascular outcomes and all-cause mortality: exploring the interaction between CKD and cardiovascular disease. Am J Kidney Dis 2006; 48(3): 392-401. [http://dx.doi.org/10.1053/j.ajkd.2006.05.021] [PMID: 16931212]

[24] Schultz WM, Kelli HM, Lisko JC, *et al.* Socioeconomic status and cardiovascular outcomes: challenges and interventions. Circulation 2018; 137(20): 2166-78. [http://dx.doi.org/10.1161/CIRCULATIONAHA.117.029652] [PMID: 29760227]

[25] Hlatky MA, Douglas PS, Cook NL, *et al.* Future directions for cardiovascular disease comparative effectiveness research: report of a workshop sponsored by the National Heart, Lung, and Blood Institute. J Am Coll Cardiol 2012; 60(7): 569-80. [http://dx.doi.org/10.1016/j.jacc.2011.12.057] [PMID: 22796257]

[26] Stone EJ, Pearson TA, Fortmann SP, McKinlay JB. Community-based prevention trials: Challenges and directions for public health practice, policy, and research. Ann Epidemiol 1997; 7(7): S113-20. [http://dx.doi.org/10.1016/S1047-2797(97)80014-2]

[27] Basak T, Varshney S, Akhtar S, Sengupta S. Understanding different facets of cardiovascular diseases based on model systems to human studies: A proteomic and metabolomic perspective. J Proteomics 2015; 127(Pt A): 50-60. [http://dx.doi.org/10.1016/j.jprot.2015.04.027] [PMID: 25956427]

[28] Villette R, Kc P, Beliard S, *et al.* Unraveling host-gut microbiota dialogue and its impact on cholesterol levels. Front Pharmacol 2020; 11: 278. [http://dx.doi.org/10.3389/fphar.2020.00278] [PMID: 32308619]

[29] Smith N, de Vecchi A, McCormick M, *et al.* euHeart: personalized and integrated cardiac care using patient-specific cardiovascular modelling. Interface Focus 2011; 1(3): 349-64. [http://dx.doi.org/10.1098/rsfs.2010.0048] [PMID: 22670205]

[30] Blacher J, Femery V, Thorez F, *et al.* A novel personalized approach to cardiovascular prevention: The VIVOPTIM programme. Arch Cardiovasc Dis 2020; 113(10): 590-8. [http://dx.doi.org/10.1016/j.acvd.2020.02.005] [PMID: 33011157]

[31] Zou G, Wei X, Gong W, *et al.* Evaluation of a systematic cardiovascular disease risk reduction strategy in primary healthcare: an exploratory study from Zhejiang, China. J Public Health (Oxf) 2015; 37(2): 241-50. [http://dx.doi.org/10.1093/pubmed/fdu013] [PMID: 24696086]

[32] Zhao Y. Cardiovascular Disease Risk Assessment in Patients with Diabetes Mellitus. Los Angeles: University of California 2020.

CHAPTER 5

Gut Microbiota in Type 2 Diabetes

Atreyee Ganguly[1] and **Falguni Patra**[1,*]

[1] *Dr. B. C. Roy College of Pharmacy and Allied Health Sciences, Durgapur, West Bengal, India*

Abstract: Type 2 Diabetes mellitus (T2DM), a chronic metabolic disorder characterized by insulin resistance and relative insulin deficiency, has emerged as a significant public health challenge globally due to its rapidly increasing prevalence. Growing evidence, as demonstrated by various studies, show that there is a significant association between the development of T2DM and disturbance in the composition profile of gut microbiota, which has generated interest in establishing the roles played by various metabolites derived from the gut microbiota in the development of T2DM. New approaches to treat T2DM by regulating the gut microbiota using probiotics, prebiotics, synbiotics, and fecal microbiota transplantation have generated significant interest.

Keywords: Farnesoid X Receptor (FXR), Gut microbiota, Gut permeability, Gut microbial metabolites, Probiotics, Prebiotics, Type 2 diabetes mellitus.

INTRODUCTION

Type 2 Diabetes Mellitus (T2DM)

Type 2 diabetes mellitus (T2DM), which accounts for most of all diabetes (about 90%), is a chronic metabolic disorder characterized by insulin resistance and relative insulin deficiency. It has emerged as a significant public health concern globally due to its increasing prevalence, particularly in developed and developing countries.

In 2021, every tenth adult, or just above half a billion adults in the world (537 million) were reportedly suffering from diabetes. The prevalence has nearly tripled in the last two decades (from 2020) and if allowed to grow unchecked at the current rate, it is projected to reach an alarming level of more than three-quarters of a billion within the next two decades (783 million by 2045). A large

* **Corresponding author Falguni Patra:** Dr. B. C. Roy College of Pharmacy and Allied Health Sciences, Durgapur, West Bengal, India; E-mail: falgunipatra@gmail.com

proportion of that, about half of those adults suffering from diabetes (240 million), are not diagnosed and, therefore, unaware of their disease condition. Equally alarming is the estimate that a further half a billion adults (541 million) have impaired glucose tolerance which increases the risk of developing type 2 diabetes [1].

Gut Microbiota and Microbiomes

There is a complex ecosystem of microorganisms consisting of bacteria, archaea, fungi, viruses, and protozoa living inside and on the human body, and they are collectively called microbiota. The exact composition of the microbiota, both in number and type, changes from site to site like gut microbiota, oral microbiota, etc. The genomic information from this community of microorganisms including their microbial structural elements and metabolites is referred to as the Microbiome. The term ‘human microbiome’ was first defined by a Nobel Laureate Joshua Lederberg in 2002 as an “ecological community of commensal, symbiotic and pathogenic microorganisms that collectively share our body space” [2].

The gut microbiota, weighing about 1.5 kg in a healthy adult, is a collection of trillions of microorganisms (mostly bacteria, with a small minority of viruses, fungi, and eukaryotic) from more than a thousand species from 6 phyla namely *Firmicutes, Bacteroidetes, Actinobacteria, Proteobacteria, Fusobacteria,* and *Verrucomicrobi*. Of these, *Firmicutes* and *Bacteroidetes* make up the largest portions of the gut microbiota (64% and 23% respectively), followed by *Proteobacteria* (8%) and *Actinobacteria* (3%). Gut microbiota is well reported for a variety of symbiotic functions such as breakdown and absorption of complex carbohydrates, absorption of some electrolytes and minerals as well as effect on bowel movement, and synthesis of micronutrients. Additionally, the gut microbiota interacts with the immune system by sending signals that promote immune cell maturity and normal functions while preventing colonization by harmful bacteria [3].

EFFECT OF GUT MICROBIOTA ON TYPE 2 DIABETES AND ITS MECHANISM

A child at birth is introduced to the microbiota from the mother during birth and this plays a crucial role in developing the initial immunity of the child. After birth, breastfeeding also enriches the immune system of the by further contribution from the mother. Those born by Cesarean section are more prone to be colonized with microbiota of epidermal origin, while infants born naturally tend to have more microorganisms from the maternal vaginal flora (Table **1**). Formula-fed infants are known to show higher Proteobacteriaceae. This abundance leads to dysbiosis, which increases the probability of acquiring T2DM and obesity in the future [4 - 9].

Table 1. Gut microbiota acquisition during the first three years.

Influencing Factors	Species	References
MODE OF BIRTH	-	-
a. Normal Delivery	*Bifidobacteriaceae*, *Lactobacillus*, and *Prevotella spp.*	[4]
b. Cesarean	*Enterobacter hormaechei/ E. cancerogenus, Haemophilus parainfluenzae/ H. aegyptius/ H. influenzae/ H. haemolyticus, Staphylococcus saprophyticus/ S. lugdunensis/ S. aureus, Streptococcus australis, and Veillonella dispar/ V. parvula, Enterococcus and Klebsiella spp*	[5]
TYPE OF FEEDING	-	-
c. Breast milk	*L. gasseri, L. salivarius, Lactobacillus reuteri, L. fermentum, or Bifidobacterium breve*	[6]
d. Non-breastfed	*Prevotella*	[7]
e. Formula-fed	*Proteobacteriaceae*	[8]
f. Solid foods	*Fecal bacilli and Rosebacterium. R. intestinalis*	[9]

The adult gut is dominated by two phyla, namely *Firmicutes* and *Bacteroidaceae*. These phyla are involved in maintaining homeostasis in the gut and the host. Any change in their population and proportion may lead to a loss of that balance. A close correlation has been found between higher *Firmicutes* to *Bacteroidaceae* ratio and the development of T2DM [2, 3]. An investigation by Gurung *et al.* showed that administrating *Bacteroides uniformis* and *Bacteroides acidifaciens* in diabetic mice improved insulin resistance and glucose intolerance. This suggests that the *Bacteroides* play an advantageous role in glucose metabolism [10].

Bifidobacteriaceae is one of the most commonly reported genera negatively associated with T2DM [10 - 13]. Certain species, such as *Bifidobacterium adolescentis, Bifidobacterium dentium, Bifidobacterium pseudocatenulatum, Bifidobacterium bifidum* and *Bifidobacterium longum* are negatively associated with T2DM when metformin is administered [14 - 16]

Streptococcus mutans and *Eggerthela lenta* can trigger insulin resistance through mTORC1-p38γ by producing propionic acid imidazole [17].

Lactobacillus abundance in T2DM portrayed a positive association with fasting blood glucose and HbA1c [18]. Certain species, such as *Lactobacillus gasseri* [19], *Lactobacillus acidophilus* [20] and *Lactobacillus salivarius* [10] increased in T2DM patients. *Clostridium*, a genus belonging to phyla *Firmicutes*, is negatively associated with FBG, HbA1c, insulin, and plasma triglyceride and positively associated with HDL and adiponectin [21].

Faecalibacterium and *Roseburia* maintain gut permeability and prevent microbial translocation across the gut wall. In T2DM patients, these microbiotas are depleted. *Faecalibacterium prausnitzii* is an important butyrate-producing bacteria that is negatively associated with T2DM [22, 23].

Gut Microbial Metabolites and T2DM

Short Chain Fatty Acids (SCFAs)

Short-chain fatty acids, a gut microbiota (GM) derived metabolite, are produced by the anaerobic fermentation of dietary fibres. Chemically, SCFAs are organic compounds consisting of a carboxylic head attached to an aliphatic chain of 1 to 6 carbons [24, 25].

The three main types of SCFAs produced by the anaerobic colonic microbes are acetate (C2), propionate (C3), and butyrate (C4), in the molar ratio of 3:1:1 [26, 27]. The SCFA, once generated within the lumen of the colon, are absorbed into the colonocytes by various mechanisms such as SCFAs/HCO^{-3}, hydrogen coupled monocarboxylate transporter 1 (MCT1) and sodium monocarboxylate transporter 1(SMCT1) [26]. The two major phyla, *Firmicutes* and *Bacteroidetes*, ferment the dietary fibres and complex starches into SCFAs in the colon. *Firmicutes* are known to produce butyrate [28] and *Bacteroidetes* produce acetate and propionate [29]. GM utilizes Embden-Meyerhof-Parnas, Wood-Ljungdahl, acrylate, succinate, pentoses-phosphate, and propanediol pathways to produce SCFAs. *Bifidobacteria, Lactobacilli, Faecalibacterium prausnitzii*, and *Roseburia* act optimally at pH 5.5 to ferment fibres into SCFA and the accumulation of non-fermentable fibres in the distal colon, leading to a shift of the pH to 6.5 which obliterates almost entirely the butyrate-producing bacteria [30].

The colonocytes consist of receptors for SCFA signal transduction. These are G protein-coupled receptors (GPCR) namely free fatty acid receptor 2 (FFAR 2)/GPR43, free fatty acid receptor 3(FFAR 3)/GPR41, and GPR109a [26, 31]. The overall functions of SCFA are summarized in (Fig. **1**) and the same can be categorised under various heads.

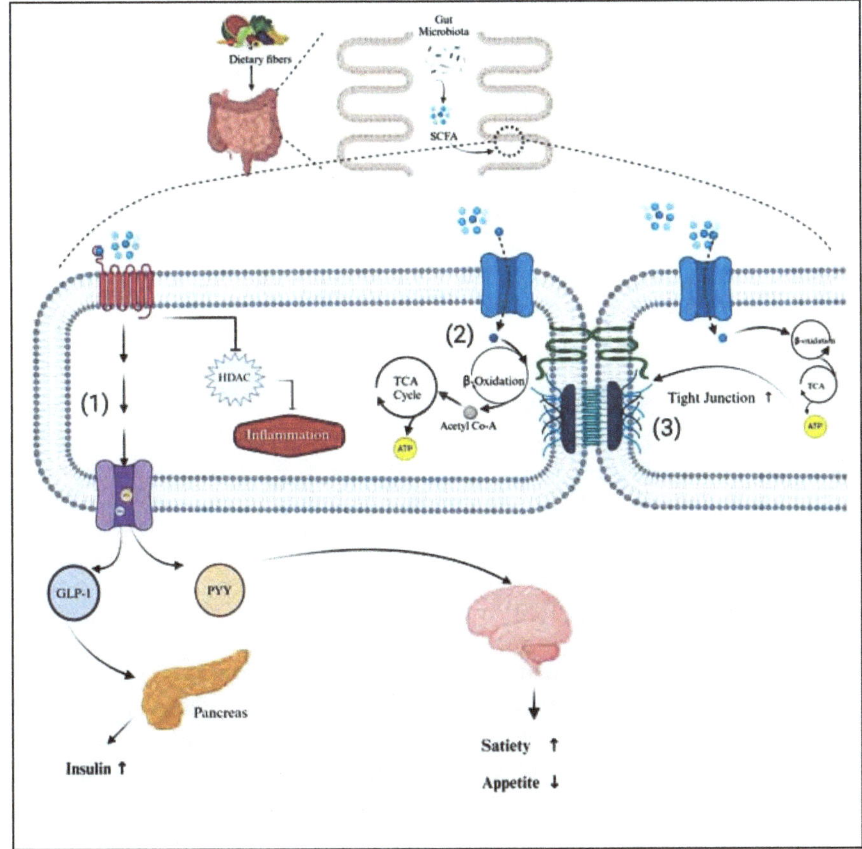

Fig. (1). Functions of Short-Chain Fatty Acids (SCFA).

Source of Energy

Acetate and butyrate undergo β-oxidation to produce acetyl CoA, whereas propionate produces propanyl CoA. These substances enter the TCA cycle to liberate ATP, which modulates the tight junction and regulates gut permeability [21].

Release of Metabolic Hormones

Intestinal L cells release two metabolic hormones glucagon-like peptide (GLP-1) and Peptide YY(PYY), upon activation of FFAR 2 and FFAR3. These hormones decrease gut motility, delay gastric emptying, increase insulin secretion, and decrease glucagon secretion [32]. In a study, propionate has been shown to enhance the GLP-1 and PYY expression in colonic cells, which leads to reduced weight and blood glucose levels [33].

HDAC Inhibition

SCFA inhibits the protease, which deacetylates the histone proteins. Butyrate is known to inhibit HDAC3, which represses the peroxisome proliferator-activated receptor (PPAR)-α expression, which enables the hepatic fibroblast growth factor 21 (Fgf21) transcription, resulting in triglyceride clearance and lipid oxidation. The beneficial effect of SCFA inhibition of HDAC in T2DM has been studied mainly in butyrate [34].

Gut Permeability Maintenance

T2DM patients' gut permeability is highly affected and damaged by mediators released from pro-inflammation. This results in the development of insulin resistance [21]. Butyrate, a GM metabolite, upregulates the expression of claudin 1 in the cell line model and assists in congregating the tight junction proteins. Propionate, another SCFA, enhances the expression of ZO-1 and occludins and improves paracellular transport [35].

Anti-inflammatory Mechanism

Chronic low-grade inflammation is a characteristic feature of T2DM patients. Butyrate is known to enhance the production of regulatory t cells (Treg), reducing inflammation, whereas propionate modulates the hematopoietic function of bone marrow cells in mice, which results in enhanced production of macrophages and dendritic cells [21]. GPR 109a regulates the AMP-activated protein kinase (AMPK), which stimulates Nrf2 nuclear import, leading to autophagy and thus possessing an anti-inflammatory effect [33].

Bile Acids

Chenodeoxycholic acids (CDCA) and cholic acids (CA) are two primary bile acids that have a significant role in digestion and a vital role in maintaining glucose homeostasis. These are synthesized by cholesterol within the hepatocytes [36]. Mitochondrial sterol 27-hydroxylase and sterol 12-hydroxylase (CYP8B1) catalyses the formation of CDCA and CA from corticosteroids [31]. Utilizing a bile salt export pump that couples with taurine or glycine, the bile acids are released into the digestive system. Within the digestive system, these bile acids are converted into secondary bile acids by the action of gut microbiota [37]. CA is converted into deoxycholic acid and CDCA is converted into lithocholic acid by the action of bile salt hydrolase (BSH) and 7α hydroxylase. BSH is produced by various microbes such as *Parasiticum, Staphylococcus, Enterococcus, Bifidobacterium, Clostridium perfringens*, and *Neococcus*, whereas *Clostridium perfringens* synthesizes 7α hydroxylase [31, 38, 39].

Bile acids modulate insulin susceptibility and thus regulate glucose homeostasis. These bile acids and secondary bile acids are the signalling molecules that show their effect in T2DM patients via activating farnesoid X receptor (FXR) and Takeda G protein-coupled receptor 5 (TGR5). The significance of bile acids in modulating insulin sensitivity and inflammation is summarized below by the activation of FXR and TGR5 [31].

Activation of FXR

FXRs are primarily present in the intestine and liver. The intestinal FXR, upon activation with endogenous ligand (CDCA), secretes fibroblast growth factor (FGF)15/19. This enters the liver via enterohepatic circulation and activates the FGFR 4/klotho complex, which inhibits bile acid synthesis by inhibiting the cholesterol 7-α hydroxylase (CYP7A1). Moreover, the activation of the FXR nuclear receptor in the liver elevates the transcriptional function of the small heterodimer (SHP), which inhibits the expression of CYP7A1 and decreases bile acid synthesis [40]. CYP7A1 attenuates all obesity-related disorders, such as insulin resistance, dyslipidemia, and glucose intolerance. Apart from this, hepatic FXR signalling impedes gluconeogenesis and advances glycogen synthesis. Enteroendocrinal FXR activation reduces GLP-1 production, whereas pancreatic β FXR activation leads to increased insulin secretion [41].

Activation of TGR5

Takeda receptor is a type of G protein-coupled receptor that is widely present in many cells within the body, such as enteroendocrine cells, pancreatic α, β cells, and brown adipose tissue. The secondary bile acids produced within the intestine by the action of gut microbiota activate the TGR5. Activation of TGR5 in enteroendocrine L cells promotes the secretion of GLP-1. TGR5 signalling in pancreatic β cells induces insulin secretion, and α cell activation of TGR5 leads to the production of GLP-1. Moreover, TGR5 signal transduction in brown adipose tissues enhances the deiodinase type 2(DIO2), which converts T4 into T3 and promotes energy expansion. Thus, the overall activation of TGR5 ameliorates glucose homeostasis and insulin production [40].

Toll-like receptor type 4 (TLR-4) expression on the macrophage or dendritic cells is induced by lipopolysaccharide, releasing inflammatory cytokines. In contrast, activation of Tgr5 inhibits the TLR4, reducing the inflammatory cytokines [42].

Branched Chain Amino Acids (BCAA)

BCAAs are not manufactured by the human body. Rather, they are taken from the diet. Leucine, isoleucine, and valine are BCAAs that are related to the pathogenesis of T2DM. Increased concentration of BCAAs is directly related to the precipitation of insulin resistance. An intermediate of dissimilation of BCAA is 3-Hydroxyisobutyrate, and T2DM patients have an elevated 3-Hydroxyisobutyrate in the plasma. This results in an increased breakdown of protein and leads to insulin insufficiency, which can be correlated with insulin deficiency [43].

Lipopolysaccharide (LPS)

The outer membrane of gram-negative bacterial cell walls comprises a characteristic structure known as LPS. Structurally, LPS consists of three domains: lipid A, core oligosaccharide, and terminal O-antigen [44]. LPS has the ability to bind with LPS-binding proteins (LBP) present in the macrophage, thus transmitting immune response through toll-like receptor 4 (TLR4). The LPS is drawn out from the cell wall of the gram-negative bacteria with the help of LBP and delivered to CD 14, which in turn transports it to TLR 4 [45]. Upon binding of LPS and recognizing it, the extracellular segment of TLR 4 dimerizes and recruits adaptor proteins such as Myd88, TRIAP, TRIF, and TRAM. Depending upon the type of the adaptor proteins, two different pathways are activated, resulting in the production of discrete inflammatory molecules. On recruitment of Myd88 and TRIAP to the intracytosolic toll/IL-1receptor (TIR) fragment of TLR 4 initiates Myd88 dependent pathway, whereas, the involvement of TRIF and TRAM triggers non-Myd88 dependent pathway producing pro-inflammatory cytokines and interferons, respectively [46].

On triggering the Myd88 pathway, mitogen-activated protein kinases (MAPK) and nuclear factor kappa B (NF-κ B) lead to the transcription of proinflammatory cytokine genes and releasing IL-1, IL-6, and TNF-α. This leads to inflammation and enhances insulin resistance [21, 45]. Alteration in the gut microbiota results in the accumulation of LPS-producing bacteria, leading to the generation of many inflammatory mediators [21]. This promotes chronic inflammation and pancreatic β cell apoptosis [43]. Hence, an adequate amount of insulin is not secreted, leading to insulin insufficiency and insulin resistance, contributing to the development of T2DM.

Trimethylamine N Oxide (TMAO)

TMAO is a gut microbial metabolite produced from dietary choline, betaine, and carnitine [47, 48]. Primarily, the later substances promote the formation of trimethylamine (TMA), a precursor for TMAO. The pathway of formation of TMAO is initiated by the conversion of choline, betaine, and carnitine to TMA by various bacterial enzymes such as choline lyase cleaving choline, carnitine monooxygenase catalysing the conversion of carnitine to TMA and betaine reductase acting on betaine. Thus, the TMA formed within the intestinal lumen can passively diffuse through the enterocytes and enter into the liver through enterohepatic circulation. Within the endoplasmic reticulum of hepatocytes, flavin-containing monooxygenase (FMO3) converts TMA to TMAO [49].

TMAO has the capability to produce insulin resistance by activating a cascade of reactions. Generally, TMAO causes activation of protein kinase R, like endoplasmic reticulum kinase (PERK) and FOXO1, contributing to ER stress, which plays a vital role in insulin resistance by expressing insulin receptor (INSR) [50]. T2DM patients are known to have a higher amount of TMAO in circulation as compared to prediabetics and normal individuals. Thus, reduced TMAO levels can be correlated with protection against T2DM. This can be achieved by modulating the TMA formation by gut microbiota. A study has shown that 3,3-dimethyl-1-butanol, a choline analogue, reduces TMAO levels in choline or carnitine-fed mice, which inhibits diet-induced atherosclerosis [49].

Tryptophan Metabolite

As an essential amino acid, tryptophan can be metabolized by the gut microbiota into different indole derivatives such as indole-3 propionic acid, indole-3 lactate, and indole-3 acetaldehyde. Certain bacterial genera are known to convert tryptophan into its metabolites, such as *Clostridium, Streptococcus,* and *Lactobacillus*. These metabolites are intricately associated with the pathogenesis of T2DM. Intestinal L cells are stimulated by indole to secrete GLP-1, which increases satiety, gastric motility, and insulin responsiveness. Aryl hydrocarbon receptor is the target receptor for indole-3 propionic acid, which shows its anti-inflammatory effect by activating these receptors [31].

Host Molecules that Induce Gut Microbiota Dysbiosis

The gut microbiota dysbiosis is one of the characteristic features of T2DM. Though the mechanism of such dysbiosis is still unclear, certain host molecules are known to maintain gut microbiota homeostasis. Abnormalities in these host molecules give rise to a dysbiotic GM environment and expedite T2DM. Here, we have explained the role of different host molecules in GM dysbiosis under two categories: a) Deletion of host molecules and b) overexpression of host molecules.

Deletion of Host Molecules

Sirtuin 1

Sirtuin 1 is known to have a protective effect against T2DM. Its protective effect was shown in a study where high-fat diet (HFD) fed mice were safeguarded against metabolic disorders by modulating the *Bacteriodetes* and *Firmicutes*. On the other hand, the absence of Sirtuin 1 in HFD-fed mice leads to hypertrophy of adipose tissue, resulting in hepatic steatosis and insulin resistance [51].

Intestinal FXR

In a study, db/db mice, when administered with fexaramine (FXR agonist), exhibited a drastic reduction in cholesterol and increased GLP-1 secretion, giving rise to glucose homeostasis. Fexaramine acts by stimulating the TGR5 receptor, promoting the secretion of GLP-1. This is achieved by modulating the lithocholic acid-secreting microbes such as *Bacteroides* and *Acetatifactor*. Hence, amelioration of overall glucose homeostasis is achieved [52].

Zinc Transporter 8 (ZnT8)

Zinc plays a crucial role in insulin secretion from the pancreatic β cells. Zinc ions can be transported by two categories of transporters namely: ZnT and Zip. In this chapter, we will focus only on the role of ZnT8 in the pathogenesis of T2DM and GM.

ZnT8 is expressed in the insulin granules and enables the movement of Zn^{2+} from the cytosol to the beta-cell insulin granules. The Zn^{2+} moves into the secretory granules, which hexamerizes with proinsulin. Lack of ZnT8 leads to glucose metabolism abnormality by modulating gut microbiota [53].

Tissue Inhibitor of Metalloproteinase 3 (Timp3)

According to Mavilio et al., a Timp3 knockout and high-fat diet-fed mouse has culminated in glucose intolerance and liver steatosis. These anomalies are contributed to the lack of timp3 that has caused GM dysbiosis. Furthermore, loss of timp3 triggers the activation of IL-6 receptors that, in turn, release the CD11c+, leading to metabolic inflammation. Thus, his findings concluded that timp3 has an important role in modulating GM, causing dysbiosis and leading to metabolic disorders [54].

Overexpression of Host Molecules

Mammalian Target of Rapamycin Complex 1 (mTorc 1)

mTorc1 is known to mediate insulin resistance and aggravate T2DM. Resveratrol, a stilbenoid, inhibits mTorc1, which ameliorates insulin resistance and glucose homeostasis. *Lactococcus, Clostridium XI*, *Hydrogenoanaerobacterium Flavonifractor* and *Oscillibacter* are reduced in high-fat diet-fed mice by resveratrol. These taxa are known to be related to fasting blood glucose levels.

Thus, it underlies the significance of mTorc1 causing a dysbiotic GM that is associated with diabetic phenotype [55].

Glucose Transporter 2 (GLUT2)

Schmitt et al, suggested that the deletion of GLUT 2 led to improved glucose homeostasis by modulating the gut microbiota composition [56].

Angiopoietin-like 4 (ANGPTL4)

In particular, in mice given diets high in fructose, cholesterol, and unsaturated fatty acids, the deletion of ANGPTL4 enhanced glucose tolerance and elevated insulin levels.

Additionally, Angptl4−/− mice's gut microbiota composition was different from wild-type mice's, exhibiting reduced levels of *Allobaculum* and greater levels of *Adlercreutzia and Lactobacillus*. This implies that ANGPTL4 may affect the gut flora in order to affect glucose metabolism. The study also discovered that in Angptl4−/− mice, suppressing the gut flora with antibiotics decreased glucose tolerance. This suggests that the advantageous effects of ANGPTL4 deletion on glucose metabolism may be dependent, at least in part, on the make-up and functionality of GM [57].

Monoglyceride lipase (MGLL)

The research conducted on mice lacking monoglyceride lipase (MGLL) provides insight into the possible function of MGLL in metabolic well-being and its association with the gut microbiota. Compared to wild-type mice, this study's HFD-fed MGLL knockout animals showed reduced adiposity and enhanced glucose tolerance. An interesting discovery was that, in contrast to wild-type mice, the gut microbiota of MGLL mutant mice reacted differently to a high-fat diet. To be more precise, HFD enhanced *Lactobacillus* abundance in wild-type mice but had no effect on MGLL knockout animals. This implies that MGLL may affect gut microbiota in order to affect metabolic health, at least somewhat. Potential explanations for the observed improvements could be the changed gut microbiota response in MGLL knockout mice to HFD diet [58].

Factors Affecting the GM

As of now, we have an idea about the composition of the gut microbiota and their capacity to modulate various physiological activities. This attribute of the GM contributes to their capacity to adjust to the changing environmental conditions. By intervening in various factors such as diet, physical activity, and antidiabetic drugs, GM benefits the host by modulating its composition and function. Thus, targeting GM with various external factors such as diet, physical exercise, and antidiabetic drugs can be an approach to the better management of T2DM.

Diet

Along with the use of antidiabetic drugs, a balanced diet and active lifestyle provide a benchmark strategy to manage T2DM well. Diet is a basic contributor to modifying the structure of GM. Thus, it is known to play a vital role in modulating and culminating a favourable role towards T2DM [59]. The gut microbiota inhabiting the human body is dominated by three enterotypes (types of microbiotas), namely: *Prevotella, Bacteroides*, and *Ruminococcus* [60]. A strong association has been drawn between each enterotype and diet. A Mediterranean diet high in fibres and unsaturated fatty acid is associated with *Prevotella,* which has been proven to be positively associated with T2DM, providing protection against metabolic syndrome and T2DM. This protective role of the Mediterranean diet can be explained by the high fibre content in the diet that gives rise to butyrate. Whereas *Bacteroides* levels are relatively reduced with an intake of a Western diet rich in saturated fatty acid. This directly influences the blood's LPS level, leading to endotoxemia and enhanced inflammation [30]. Moreover, according to a recent study, the amount of undigested food reaching the gut is estimated to be approximately 40g, 20g, and 10g for carbohydrates, proteins, and fats, respectively [61]. Thus, this amount of undigested food is liable to microbial metabolism producing diversified metabolites capable of modulating physiological actions.

Exercise

An active lifestyle is one of the most crucial aspects of T2DM management. Daily exercising affects blood sugar levels by enhancing insulin sensitivity, which leads to improved cell utilization of glucose. A study demonstrated the effect of regular exercising on the composition of GM of athletes, increasing *Akkermansia muciniphila* [62,63]. Regular physical activity also led to increased SCFA production that improved insulin resistance in skeletal muscles, thus contributing to the progressive management of T2DM [64]. Moreover, *Firmicutes* and *Proteobacteria* are greatly reduced, and *Bacteroidetes* are increased in a rodent model exposed to training. In a cohort study, Y. Liu *et al.* deduced that 12 weeks of physical activity modified the plethora of *Bacteroidetes, Proteobacteria*, and *Firmicutes* in humans [65].

Antidiabetic Drugs

The pharmacological intervention for T2DM is oral hypoglycaemic drugs (OHD). These drugs act by various mechanisms, such as increasing insulin sensitivity, decreasing hepatic glucose synthesis, stimulating β cells to release insulin, reducing glucose absorption, and converting polysaccharides to monosaccharides. Besides the above-mentioned mechanisms, all OHDs also act by modulating the GM. In this chapter, we will focus on the capacity of different OHDs to regulate the GM and bring about protective effects.

Metformin

Metformin, a biguanide, primarily increases insulin sensitivity and improves glucose metabolism [30]. But, our topic of discussion will be focussed on another mode of action of metformin i.e. modulation of GM.

The overall improved glucose metabolism by metformin can also be attributed to the enhanced species of *Bifidobacterium* and *Akkermansia muciniphila* [66]. These drugs also increase the production of SCFAs and thus improve insulin sensitivity, satiety, and gastric motility by the secretion of GLP-1 and PYY. Production of the SCFAs further reduces the inflammatory responses, improving insulin sensitivity. Further, metformin is also associated with managing weight in T2DM patients.

DPP-4 inhibitors

Dipeptidyl peptidase 4 enzyme degrades the incretin hormones such as GLP-1 and DPP-4 inhibitors inhibit the action of these enzymes. The first drug under this class was sitagliptin, which got approval in 2006 by the FDA [67]. A study showed a prominent effect of sitagliptin on a diabetic mouse that improved gut microbiota structure at a phylum level [68,69]. It escalates the *Bacteroidetes* and *Proteobacteria* and reduces *Firmicutes* [67]. Another preclinical study showed a reduction in *Blautia* and an increase in *Roseburia,* but no effect was found in the number of *Clostridium* in the sitagliptin-treated rat's faeces.

Zhang *et al.* deduced from their research that Vildagliptin strongly influences the various SCFAs-producing bacteria, and the treatment has shown an enhancement of the *Bacteroidetes* and reduced *Firmicutes* [70].

α glucosidase inhibitors

α-glucosidase inhibitors are complex oligosaccharides that are obtained by microbial fermentation. Thus, making it obvious to modulate the gut microbiota. Acarbose modifies the composition of GM by increasing the *Bifidobacterium* and *Lactobacillus,* whereas it reduces *Bacteroides* [71]. The effect on other SCFA-producing genera, such as Prevotella and Faecalibacterium, is also increased.

Firmicutes to *Bacteroidetes* ratio is decreased by another α-glucosidase inhibitor, Voglibose, in a high-fat diet-fed mice [72].

Glucagon-like peptide-1 receptor agonists

Glucagon-like peptide-1 (GLP-1) is an incretin hormone secreted by intestinal L cells. These hormones increase insulin and decrease glucagon secretion, thus reducing blood glucose levels. Liraglutide, a glucagon-like peptide-1 receptor agonist, emulates the GLP-1 and attenuates the hyperglycaemia [67].

Wang et al., in their preclinical study with mice, deduced that Liraglutide has a huge impact on gut microbiota. Various genera such as *Butyricimonas, Allobaculum, Blautia, Turicibacter, Desulfovibrio,* and *Lactobacillus* are increased. On the other hand, phyla such as *Bacteriodetes* (*Bacteriodales*) and *Firmicutes* (*Clostridales*) are reduced [73].

TREATMENT APPROACHES

Probiotics, prebiotics, synbiotics

Conventionally, management of T2DM involves a multifaceted approach aimed at controlling blood glucose levels, preventing complications, and improving overall quality of life. It includes a combination of therapeutic and behavioural approaches along with diet, physical activity, weight and stress management. With the development, as demonstrated by various studies, that there is a significant association between the development of T2DM and disturbance in the composition profile of gut microbiota, new approaches to regulate the gut microbiota using probiotics, prebiotics, and synbiotics have generated interest [74].

Probiotics are live microorganisms that are beneficial to our health when administered as dietary supplements whereas prebiotics are food components like indigestible polysaccharides or fibre that help the host by selectively benefiting the growth of the intended microorganisms [75]. Synbiotics are a combination of both probiotics with substrates promoting their selective growth [76,77].

Multiple studies based on the approach of including probiotics as adjuvant in T2DM management to improve insulin sensitivity have been reported. Probiotics rebalance the gut microbiota composition with minimal side effects and without affecting the efficacy of antidiabetic medication. They modulate the gut microbiota to improve glucose metabolism, inhibit α– glucosidase activity and lactic acid production, and strengthen the intestinal barrier, immune modulation, SCFAs production, and regulation of bile acid metabolism [78].

Probiotic treatment, especially with certain strains of *Lactobacillus* and *Bifidobacterium*, can enhance lipid profiles and decrease fasting blood sugar levels, insulin levels, and HbA1c levels. Additionally, the use of *Akkermansia muciniphila* has been suggested as an adjuvant to antidiabetic medication due to its capacity to restore the intestinal barrier, reduce inflammation, and enhance metabolic processes [79]. Several studies have reported that administering a combination of probiotics is more beneficial than administering individual strains to improve oxidative stress and fasting plasma glucose in people with diabetes [80].

For prebiotics, various complex carbohydrates and dietary fibers, polyphenols, and polyunsaturated fatty acids have been tested. Apart from helping in stool formation, they can also be fermented to SCFAs that help in strengthening the intestinal barrier, reducing inflammation. Oligo-fructose used as a prebiotic has demonstrated improvement in glucose metabolism, leptin sensitivity, GLP-1 production, and intestinal barrier integrity [81]. Similar supporting activity has been reported with the use of berberine, capsaicin, resveratrol, betacyanin, alliin, and cranberry proanthocyanins [78]. With growing evidence of the ability of probiotics and prebiotics to improve antidiabetic drug therapy, combining drug therapy with both prebiotics and probiotics as synbiotics could potentially further improve glycaemic control in T2DM. Probiotics of *Bacteroides* (especially enterotypes) taken with capsaicin as a prebiotic have shown positive effects in controlling obesity, and cardiovascular diseases, and with arabinoxylan, and hemicellulose,an improvement in weight gain was observed [82].

Fecal Microbiota Transplantation

Fecal microbiota transplantation (FMT), also known as stool transplantation, has been investigated as a supporting strategy for antidiabetic therapy through the modulation of microbiota. It involves transferring fecal material from a healthy donor to a recipient to modulate the recipient's intestinal microbiota [83]. Various reports have consistently shown that FMT helps to improve insulin sensitivity in T2DM and also positively modulates autoimmunity [84,85]. Although promising, FMT suffers from the risk of infection from pathogens in the donor flora as well as uncertain clinical results of such studies warrant more investigation.

CONCLUSION

Type 2 diabetes mellitus (T2DM) is a chronic metabolic disorder characterized by peripheral insulin resistance, impaired regulation of hepatic glucose production, and declining β-cell function, eventually leading to β -cell failure. Management of T2DM involves a combination of therapeutic and behavioural approaches along with diet, physical activity, weight, and stress management. Our Gut microbiota is a complex ecosystem of microorganisms consisting of bacteria, archaea, fungi, viruses, and protozoa involved in maintaining homeostasis in the gut and the host. There is a significant association between the development of T2DM and disturbance in the composition profile of gut microbiota. Targeting the gut microbiota and its metabolites is currently gaining traction as a possible treatment strategy for type 2 diabetes. Strategies such as the use of FMT, probiotics, prebiotics, and synbiotics are being investigated by various researchers. The lack of detailed understanding of the complex interplay between the gut microbiota, its metabolites, and the physiological processes of the host in normal and diseased conditions pose a significant challenge in harnessing the power of gut microbiota in the treatment of T2DM.

REFERENCES

[1] International Diabetes Federation. IDF Diabetes Atlas, 10th edn. Brussels, Belgium: 2021. Available from: https://www.diabetesatlas.org

[2] Lederberg J, McCray A. Ome sweet omics—a genealogical treasury of words. Scientist 2001; 15(7): 8.

[3] Liu BN, Liu XT, Liang ZH, Wang JH. Gut microbiota in obesity. World J Gastroenterol 2021; 27(25): 3837-50.
[http://dx.doi.org/10.3748/wjg.v27.i25.3837] [PMID: 34321848]

[4] Dominguez-Bello MG, Costello EK, Contreras M, *et al.* Delivery mode shapes the acquisition and structure of the initial microbiota across multiple body habitats in newborns. Proc Natl Acad Sci USA 2010; 107(26): 11971-5.
[http://dx.doi.org/10.1073/pnas.1002601107] [PMID: 20566857]

[5] Bäckhed F, Roswall J, Peng Y, *et al.* Dynamics and Stabilization of the Human Gut Microbiome during the First Year of Life. Cell Host Microbe 2015; 17(6): 852.
[http://dx.doi.org/10.1016/j.chom.2015.05.012] [PMID: 26308884]

[6] Bokulich NA, Chung J, Battaglia T, *et al.* Antibiotics, birth mode, and diet shape microbiome maturation during early life. Sci Transl Med 2016; 8(343): 343ra82.
[http://dx.doi.org/10.1126/scitranslmed.aad7121] [PMID: 27306664]

[7] Fernández L, Langa S, Martín V, *et al.* The human milk microbiota: Origin and potential roles in health and disease. Pharmacol Res 2013; 69(1): 1-10.
[http://dx.doi.org/10.1016/j.phrs.2012.09.001] [PMID: 22974824]

[8] Ding T, Schloss PD. Dynamics and associations of microbial community types across the human body. Nature 2014; 509(7500): 357-60.
[http://dx.doi.org/10.1038/nature13178] [PMID: 24739969]

[9] Torow N, Hornef MW. The Neonatal Window of Opportunity: Setting the Stage for Life-Long Host-Microbial Interaction and Immune Homeostasis. J Immunol 2017; 198(2): 557-63.
[http://dx.doi.org/10.4049/jimmunol.1601253] [PMID: 28069750]

[10] Gurung M, Li Z, You H, *et al.* Role of gut microbiota in type 2 diabetes pathophysiology. EBioMedicine 2020; 51: 102590.
[http://dx.doi.org/10.1016/j.ebiom.2019.11.051] [PMID: 31901868]

[11] Gao R, Zhu C, Li H, *et al.* Dysbiosis Signatures of Gut Microbiota Along the Sequence from Healthy, Young Patients to Those with Overweight and Obesity. Obesity (Silver Spring) 2018; 26(2): 351-61.
[http://dx.doi.org/10.1002/oby.22088] [PMID: 29280312]

[12] Sedighi M, Razavi S, Navab-Moghadam F, *et al.* Comparison of gut microbiota in adult patients with

type 2 diabetes and healthy individuals. Microb Pathog 2017; 111: 362-9.
[http://dx.doi.org/10.1016/j.micpath.2017.08.038] [PMID: 28912092]

[13] Wu X, Ma C, Han L, *et al.* Molecular characterisation of the faecal microbiota in patients with type II diabetes. Curr Microbiol 2010; 61(1): 69-78.
[http://dx.doi.org/10.1007/s00284-010-9582-9] [PMID: 20087741]

[14] Murphy R, Tsai P, Jüllig M, Liu A, Plank L, Booth M. Differential Changes in Gut Microbiota After Gastric Bypass and Sleeve Gastrectomy Bariatric Surgery Vary According to Diabetes Remission. Obes Surg 2017; 27(4): 917-25.
[http://dx.doi.org/10.1007/s11695-016-2399-2] [PMID: 27738970]

[15] Barengolts E, Green SJ, Eisenberg Y, *et al.* Gut microbiota varies by opioid use, circulating leptin and oxytocin in African American men with diabetes and high burden of chronic disease. PLoS One 2018; 13(3): e0194171.
[http://dx.doi.org/10.1371/journal.pone.0194171] [PMID: 29596446]

[16] Wu H, Esteve E, Tremaroli V, *et al.* Metformin alters the gut microbiome of individuals with treatment-naive type 2 diabetes, contributing to the therapeutic effects of the drug. Nat Med 2017; 23(7): 850-8.
[http://dx.doi.org/10.1038/nm.4345] [PMID: 28530702]

[17] Koh A, Molinaro A, Ståhlman M, *et al.* Microbially Produced Imidazole Propionate Impairs Insulin Signaling through mTORC1. Cell 2018; 175(4): 947-961.e17.
[http://dx.doi.org/10.1016/j.cell.2018.09.055] [PMID: 30401435]

[18] Chen PC, Chien YW, Yang SC. The alteration of gut microbiota in newly diagnosed type 2 diabetic patients. Nutrition 2019; 63-64: 51-6.
[http://dx.doi.org/10.1016/j.nut.2018.11.019] [PMID: 30933725]

[19] Yun SI, Park HO, Kang JH. Effect of *Lactobacillus gasseri* BNR17 on blood glucose levels and body weight in a mouse model of type 2 diabetes. J Appl Microbiol 2009; 107(5): 1681-6.
[http://dx.doi.org/10.1111/j.1365-2672.2009.04350.x] [PMID: 19457033]

[20] Moroti C, Souza Magri LF, de Rezende Costa M, Cavallini DCU, Sivieri K. Effect of the consumption of a new symbiotic shake on glycemia and cholesterol levels in elderly people with type 2 diabetes mellitus. Lipids Health Dis 2012; 11(1): 29.
[http://dx.doi.org/10.1186/1476-511X-11-29] [PMID: 22356933]

[21] Zhang L, Chu J, Hao W, *et al.* Gut Microbiota and Type 2 Diabetes Mellitus: Association, Mechanism, and Translational Applications. Mediators Inflamm 2021; 2021: 1-12.
[http://dx.doi.org/10.1155/2021/5110276] [PMID: 34447287]

[22] Di Vincenzo F, Del Gaudio A, Petito V, Lopetuso LR, Scaldaferri F. Gut microbiota, intestinal permeability, and systemic inflammation: a narrative review. Intern Emerg Med 2024; 19(2): 275-93.
[http://dx.doi.org/10.1007/s11739-023-03374-w] [PMID: 37505311]

[23] Nie K, Ma K, Luo W, *et al. Roseburia intestinalis*: A Beneficial Gut Organism From the Discoveries in Genus and Species. Front Cell Infect Microbiol 2021; 11: 757718.
[http://dx.doi.org/10.3389/fcimb.2021.757718] [PMID: 34881193]

[24] McMurdie PJ, Stoeva MK, Justice N, *et al.* Increased circulating butyrate and ursodeoxycholate during probiotic intervention in humans with type 2 diabetes. BMC Microbiol 2022; 22(1): 19.
[http://dx.doi.org/10.1186/s12866-021-02415-8] [PMID: 34996347]

[25] Hoving LR, Heijink M, van Harmelen V, van Dijk KW, Giera M. GC-MS Analysis of Short-Chain Fatty Acids in Feces, Cecum Content, and Blood Samples. In: Giera M, Ed. Clinical Metabolomics: Methods and Protocols. New York, NY: Springer New York 2018; pp. 247-56.
[http://dx.doi.org/10.1007/978-1-4939-7592-1_17]

[26] Anachad O, Taouil A, Taha W, Bennis F, Chegdani F. The Implication of Short-Chain Fatty Acids in Obesity and Diabetes. Microbiol Insights 2023; 16: 11786361231162720.

[http://dx.doi.org/10.1177/11786361231162720] [PMID: 36994236]

[27] Sun S. The Impacts of SCFAs on Intestinal Homeostasis, and Glucose-Lipid metabolism. 2022; Vol. 2022.

[28] Zhu LB, Zhang YC, Huang HH, Lin J. Prospects for clinical applications of butyrate-producing bacteria. World J Clin Pediatr 2021; 10(5): 84-92.
[http://dx.doi.org/10.5409/wjcp.v10.i5.84] [PMID: 34616650]

[29] Nkosi BVZ, Padayachee T, Gront D, Nelson DR, Syed K. Contrasting Health Effects of *Bacteroidetes* and *Firmicutes* Lies in Their Genomes: Analysis of P450s, Ferredoxins, and Secondary Metabolite Clusters. Int J Mol Sci 2022; 23(9): 5057.
[http://dx.doi.org/10.3390/ijms23095057] [PMID: 35563448]

[30] Martínez-López YE, Esquivel-Hernández DA, Sánchez-Castañeda JP, Neri-Rosario D, Guardado-Mendoza R, Resendis-Antonio O. Type 2 diabetes, gut microbiome, and systems biology: A novel perspective for a new era. Gut Microbes 2022; 14(1): 2111952.
[http://dx.doi.org/10.1080/19490976.2022.2111952] [PMID: 36004400]

[31] Wu J, Yang K, Fan H, Wei M, Xiong Q. Targeting the gut microbiota and its metabolites for type 2 diabetes mellitus. Front Endocrinol (Lausanne) 2023; 14: 1114424.
[http://dx.doi.org/10.3389/fendo.2023.1114424] [PMID: 37229456]

[32] F. Moraes AC, De Almeida-Pittito B, Ferreira SRG. The Gut Microbiome in Vegetarians. Microbiome and Metabolome in Diagnosis, Therapy, and other Strategic Applications, Elsevier; 2019, p. 393–400.
[http://dx.doi.org/10.1016/B978-0-12-815249-2.00041-5]

[33] Zhang Y, Li X, Huang G, *et al.* Propionate stimulates the secretion of satiety hormones and reduces acute appetite in a cecal fistula pig model. Anim Nutr 2022; 10: 390-8.
[http://dx.doi.org/10.1016/j.aninu.2022.06.003] [PMID: 35949198]

[34] Tang R, Li L. Modulation of Short-Chain Fatty Acids as Potential Therapy Method for Type 2 Diabetes Mellitus. Can J Infect Dis Med Microbiol 2021; 2021: 1-13.
[http://dx.doi.org/10.1155/2021/6632266] [PMID: 33488888]

[35] Wang HB, Wang PY, Wang X, Wan YL, Liu YC. Butyrate enhances intestinal epithelial barrier function via up-regulation of tight junction protein Claudin-1 transcription. Dig Dis Sci 2012; 57(12): 3126-35.
[http://dx.doi.org/10.1007/s10620-012-2259-4] [PMID: 22684624]

[36] Hofmann AF. The continuing importance of bile acids in liver and intestinal disease. Arch Intern Med 1999; 159(22): 2647-58.
[http://dx.doi.org/10.1001/archinte.159.22.2647] [PMID: 10597755]

[37] Larabi AB, Masson HLP, Bäumler AJ. Bile acids as modulators of gut microbiota composition and function. Gut Microbes 2023; 15(1): 2172671.
[http://dx.doi.org/10.1080/19490976.2023.2172671] [PMID: 36740850]

[38] Huang F, Zheng X, Ma X, *et al.* Theabrownin from Pu-erh tea attenuates hypercholesterolemia via modulation of gut microbiota and bile acid metabolism. Nat Commun 2019; 10(1): 4971.
[http://dx.doi.org/10.1038/s41467-019-12896-x] [PMID: 31672964]

[39] Kiriyama Y, Nochi H. Physiological Role of Bile Acids Modified by the Gut Microbiome. Microorganisms 2021; 10(1): 68.
[http://dx.doi.org/10.3390/microorganisms10010068] [PMID: 35056517]

[40] Feng X, Deng M, Zhang L, Pan Q. Impact of gut microbiota and associated mechanisms on postprandial glucose levels in patients with diabetes. J Transl Int Med 2023; 11(4): 363-71.
[http://dx.doi.org/10.2478/jtim-2023-0116] [PMID: 38130636]

[41] Liu H, Pathak P, Boehme S, Chiang JL. Cholesterol 7α-hydroxylase protects the liver from inflammation and fibrosis by maintaining cholesterol homeostasis. J Lipid Res 2016; 57(10): 1831-44.
[http://dx.doi.org/10.1194/jlr.M069807] [PMID: 27534992]

[42] Lun W, Yan Q, Guo X, *et al.* Mechanism of action of the bile acid receptor TGR5 in obesity. Acta Pharm Sin B 2024; 14(2): 468-91.
[http://dx.doi.org/10.1016/j.apsb.2023.11.011] [PMID: 38322325]

[43] Fu Y, Li S, Xiao Y, Liu G, Fang J. A Metabolite Perspective on the Involvement of the Gut Microbiota in Type 2 Diabetes. Int J Mol Sci 2023; 24(19): 14991.
[http://dx.doi.org/10.3390/ijms241914991] [PMID: 37834439]

[44] Farhana A, Khan YS. Biochemistry. Lipopolysaccharide 2024.

[45] Soares JB, Pimentel-Nunes P, Roncon-Albuquerque R Jr, Leite-Moreira A. The role of lipopolysaccharide/toll-like receptor 4 signaling in chronic liver diseases. Hepatol Int 2010; 4(4): 659-72.
[http://dx.doi.org/10.1007/s12072-010-9219-x] [PMID: 21286336]

[46] Lannoy V, Côté-Biron A, Asselin C, Rivard N. TIRAP, TRAM, and Toll-Like Receptors: The Untold Story. Mediators Inflamm 2023; 2023: 1-13.
[http://dx.doi.org/10.1155/2023/2899271] [PMID: 36926280]

[47] Cho CE, Taesuwan S, Malysheva OV, *et al.* Trimethylamine□ *N* □oxide (TMAO) response to animal source foods varies among healthy young men and is influenced by their gut microbiota composition: A randomized controlled trial. Mol Nutr Food Res 2017; 61(1): 1600324.
[http://dx.doi.org/10.1002/mnfr.201600324] [PMID: 27377678]

[48] Zhu C, Sawrey-Kubicek L, Bardagjy AS, *et al.* Whole egg consumption increases plasma choline and betaine without affecting TMAO levels or gut microbiome in overweight postmenopausal women. Nutr Res 2020; 78: 36-41.
[http://dx.doi.org/10.1016/j.nutres.2020.04.002] [PMID: 32464420]

[49] Constantino-Jonapa LA, Espinoza-Palacios Y, Escalona-Montaño AR, *et al.* Contribution of Trimethylamine N-Oxide (TMAO) to Chronic Inflammatory and Degenerative Diseases. Biomedicines 2023; 11(2): 431.
[http://dx.doi.org/10.3390/biomedicines11020431] [PMID: 36830968]

[50] Chen S, Henderson A, Petriello MC, *et al.* Trimethylamine N-Oxide Binds and Activates PERK to Promote Metabolic Dysfunction. Cell Metab 2019; 30(6): 1141-1151.e5.
[http://dx.doi.org/10.1016/j.cmet.2019.08.021] [PMID: 31543404]

[51] Caron AZ, He X, Mottawea W, *et al.* The SIRT1 deacetylase protects mice against the symptoms of metabolic syndrome. FASEB J 2014; 28(3): 1306-16.
[http://dx.doi.org/10.1096/fj.13-243568] [PMID: 24297700]

[52] Pathak P, Xie C, Nichols RG, *et al.* Intestine farnesoid X receptor agonist and the gut microbiota activate G-protein bile acid receptor-1 signaling to improve metabolism. Hepatology 2018; 68(4): 1574-88.
[http://dx.doi.org/10.1002/hep.29857] [PMID: 29486523]

[53] Zhou Z, Sun B, Yu D, Zhu C. Gut Microbiota: An Important Player in Type 2 Diabetes Mellitus. Front Cell Infect Microbiol 2022; 12: 834485.
[http://dx.doi.org/10.3389/fcimb.2022.834485] [PMID: 35242721]

[54] Mavilio M, Marchetti V, Fabrizi M, *et al.* A Role for Timp3 in Microbiota-Driven Hepatic Steatosis and Metabolic Dysfunction. Cell Rep 2016; 16(3): 731-43.
[http://dx.doi.org/10.1016/j.celrep.2016.06.027] [PMID: 27373162]

[55] Jung MJ, Lee J, Shin NR, *et al.* Chronic Repression of mTOR Complex 2 Induces Changes in the Gut Microbiota of Diet-induced Obese Mice. Sci Rep 2016; 6(1): 30887.
[http://dx.doi.org/10.1038/srep30887] [PMID: 27471110]

[56] Schmitt CC, Aranias T, Viel T, *et al.* Intestinal invalidation of the glucose transporter GLUT2 delays tissue distribution of glucose and reveals an unexpected role in gut homeostasis. Mol Metab 2017; 6(1): 61-72.

[http://dx.doi.org/10.1016/j.molmet.2016.10.008] [PMID: 28123938]

[57] Janssen AWF, Katiraei S, Bartosinska B, Eberhard D, Willems van Dijk K, Kersten S. Loss of angiopoietin-like 4 (ANGPTL4) in mice with diet-induced obesity uncouples visceral obesity from glucose intolerance partly via the gut microbiota. Diabetologia 2018; 61(6): 1447-58. [http://dx.doi.org/10.1007/s00125-018-4583-5] [PMID: 29502266]

[58] Dione N, Lacroix S, Taschler U, *et al. Mgll* Knockout Mouse Resistance to Diet-Induced Dysmetabolism Is Associated with Altered Gut Microbiota. Cells 2020; 9(12): 2705. [http://dx.doi.org/10.3390/cells9122705] [PMID: 33348740]

[59] Makki K, Deehan EC, Walter J, Bäckhed F. The Impact of Dietary Fiber on Gut Microbiota in Host Health and Disease. Cell Host Microbe 2018; 23(6): 705-15. [http://dx.doi.org/10.1016/j.chom.2018.05.012] [PMID: 29902436]

[60] Ubags NDJ, Marsland BJ. Obesity and the microbiome: Big changes on a small scale? Mechanisms and Manifestations of Obesity in Lung Disease. Elsevier 2019; pp. 281-300. [http://dx.doi.org/10.1016/B978-0-12-813553-2.00012-9]

[61] Shortt C, Hasselwander O, Meynier A, *et al.* Systematic review of the effects of the intestinal microbiota on selected nutrients and non-nutrients. Eur J Nutr 2018; 57(1): 25-49. [http://dx.doi.org/10.1007/s00394-017-1546-4] [PMID: 29086061]

[62] Clarke SF, Murphy EF, O'Sullivan O, *et al.* Exercise and associated dietary extremes impact on gut microbial diversity. Gut 2014; 63(12): 1913-20. [http://dx.doi.org/10.1136/gutjnl-2013-306541] [PMID: 25021423]

[63] Reddy V, Avtanski D. Environmental and Lifestyle Factors Influencing Inflammation and Type 2 Diabetes. Obesity, Diabetes and Inflammation: Molecular Mechanisms and Clinical Management. Cham: Springer International Publishing 2023; pp. 165-83. [http://dx.doi.org/10.1007/978-3-031-39721-9_8]

[64] Yang L, Lin H, Lin W, Xu X. Exercise Ameliorates Insulin Resistance of Type 2 Diabetes through Motivating Short-Chain Fatty Acid-Mediated Skeletal Muscle Cell Autophagy. Biology (Basel) 2020; 9(8): 203. [http://dx.doi.org/10.3390/biology9080203] [PMID: 32756447]

[65] Liu Y, Wang Y, Ni Y, *et al.* Gut Microbiome Fermentation Determines the Efficacy of Exercise for Diabetes Prevention. Cell Metab 2020; 31(1): 77-91.e5. [http://dx.doi.org/10.1016/j.cmet.2019.11.001] [PMID: 31786155]

[66] Shin NR, Lee JC, Lee HY, *et al.* An increase in the *Akkermansia* spp. population induced by metformin treatment improves glucose homeostasis in diet-induced obese mice. Gut 2014; 63(5): 727-35. [http://dx.doi.org/10.1136/gutjnl-2012-303839] [PMID: 23804561]

[67] Chaithanya V, Kumar J, Leela KV, Angelin M, Satheesan A, Murugesan R. Metabolic consequences of alterations in gut microbiota induced by antidiabetic medications. Diabetes Epidemiology and Management 2024; 13: 100180. [http://dx.doi.org/10.1016/j.deman.2023.100180]

[68] Yan X, Feng B, Li P, Tang Z, Wang L. Microflora Disturbance during Progression of Glucose Intolerance and Effect of Sitagliptin: An Animal Study. J Diabetes Res 2016; 2016: 1-10. [http://dx.doi.org/10.1155/2016/2093171] [PMID: 27631013]

[69] Olivares M, Hernández-Calderón P, Cárdenas-Brito S, Liébana-García R, Sanz Y, Benítez-Páez A. Gut microbiota DPP4-like enzymes are increased in type-2 diabetes and contribute to incretin inactivation. Genome Biol 2024; 25(1): 174. [http://dx.doi.org/10.1186/s13059-024-03325-4] [PMID: 38961511]

[70] Zhang Q, Xiao X, Li M, *et al.* Vildagliptin increases butyrate-producing bacteria in the gut of diabetic rats. PLoS One 2017; 12(10): e0184735.

[http://dx.doi.org/10.1371/journal.pone.0184735] [PMID: 29036231]

[71] Su B, Liu H, Li J, *et al.* Acarbose treatment affects the serum levels of inflammatory cytokines and the gut content of bifidobacteria in C hinese patients with type 2 diabetes mellitus. J Diabetes 2015; 7(5): 729-39.
[http://dx.doi.org/10.1111/1753-0407.12232] [PMID: 25327485]

[72] Do HJ, Lee YS, Ha MJ, *et al.* Beneficial effects of voglibose administration on body weight and lipid metabolism <i>via</i> gastrointestinal bile acid modification. Endocr J 2016; 63(8): 691-702.
[http://dx.doi.org/10.1507/endocrj.EJ15-0747] [PMID: 27349182]

[73] Wang L, Li P, Tang Z, Yan X, Feng B. Structural modulation of the gut microbiota and the relationship with body weight: compared evaluation of liraglutide and saxagliptin treatment. Sci Rep 2016; 6(1): 33251.
[http://dx.doi.org/10.1038/srep33251] [PMID: 27633081]

[74] Cunningham AL, Stephens JW, Harris DA. Gut microbiota influence in type 2 diabetes mellitus (T2DM). Gut Pathog 2021; 13(1): 50.
[http://dx.doi.org/10.1186/s13099-021-00446-0] [PMID: 34362432]

[75] Wang X, Zhang P, Zhang X. Probiotics Regulate Gut Microbiota: An Effective Method to Improve Immunity. Molecules 2021; 26(19): 6076.
[http://dx.doi.org/10.3390/molecules26196076] [PMID: 34641619]

[76] Schrezenmeir J, de Vrese M. Probiotics, prebiotics, and synbiotics—approaching a definition. Am J Clin Nutr 2001; 73(2) (Suppl.): 361s-4s.
[http://dx.doi.org/10.1093/ajcn/73.2.361s] [PMID: 11157342]

[77] Lee S, Choi SP, Choi HJ, Jeong H, Park YS. A comprehensive review of synbiotics: an emerging paradigm in health promotion and disease management. World J Microbiol Biotechnol 2024; 40(9): 280.
[http://dx.doi.org/10.1007/s11274-024-04085-w] [PMID: 39060821]

[78] Adeshirlarijaney A, Gewirtz AT. Considering gut microbiota in treatment of type 2 diabetes mellitus. Gut Microbes 2020; 11(3): 253-64.
[http://dx.doi.org/10.1080/19490976.2020.1717719] [PMID: 32005089]

[79] Cani PD, de Vos WM. Next-Generation Beneficial Microbes: The Case of *Akkermansia muciniphila.* Front Microbiol 2017; 8: 1765.
[http://dx.doi.org/10.3389/fmicb.2017.01765] [PMID: 29018410]

[80] Raygan F, Rezavandi Z, Bahmani F, *et al.* The effects of probiotic supplementation on metabolic status in type 2 diabetic patients with coronary heart disease. Diabetol Metab Syndr 2018; 10(1): 51.
[http://dx.doi.org/10.1186/s13098-018-0353-2] [PMID: 29946368]

[81] Paone P, Suriano F, Jian C, *et al.* Prebiotic oligofructose protects against high-fat diet-induced obesity by changing the gut microbiota, intestinal mucus production, glycosylation and secretion. Gut Microbes 2022; 14(1): 2152307.
[http://dx.doi.org/10.1080/19490976.2022.2152307] [PMID: 36448728]

[82] Christensen L, Sørensen CV, Wøhlk FU, *et al.* Microbial enterotypes beyond genus level: *Bacteroides* species as a predictive biomarker for weight change upon controlled intervention with arabinoxylan oligosaccharides in overweight subjects. Gut Microbes 2020; 12(1): 1847627.
[http://dx.doi.org/10.1080/19490976.2020.1847627] [PMID: 33319645]

[83] Gupta A, Khanna S. Fecal Microbiota Transplantation. JAMA 2017; 318(1): 102.
[http://dx.doi.org/10.1001/jama.2017.6466] [PMID: 28672320]

[84] Murri M, Leiva I, Gomez-Zumaquero JM, *et al.* Gut microbiota in children with type 1 diabetes differs from that in healthy children: a case-control study. BMC Med 2013; 11(1): 46.
[http://dx.doi.org/10.1186/1741-7015-11-46] [PMID: 23433344]

[85] Yang Y, Yan J, Li S, *et al.* Efficacy of fecal microbiota transplantation in type 2 diabetes mellitus: a systematic review and meta-analysis. Endocrine 2023; 84(1): 48-62. [http://dx.doi.org/10.1007/s12020-023-03606-1] [PMID: 38001323]

CHAPTER 6

The Role of Gut Microbiota in Ocular Diseases

Tapas Kumar Roy[1], **Arnab Roy**[2], **Swati Bairagya**[3] and **Sanjay Dey**[4,*]

[1] *Department of Ocular Pharmacology and Pharmacy Division, Dr. R.P.Centre, AIIMS, New Delhi, India*

[2] *Department of Biological Sciences (Pharmacology and Toxicology), National Institute of Pharmaceutical Education and Research (NIPER), Hyderabad, Telangana, India*

[3] *Department of Pharmacology/Biotechnology, Delhi Pharmaceutical Sciences and Research University, New Delhi, India*

[4] *Department of Pharmaceutical Technology, School of Health and Medical Sciences, Adamas University, Barasat-Barrackpore Road, Kolkata – 700126, West Bengal, India*

Abstract: The adaptive environment that is crucial to the host's health is the microbiome. Several research works have revealed that dysbiosis, or changes in the gut microbiota of humans can have an involvement in the etiology of a number of prevalent ailments, including diabetes, cancer, and neuropsychiatric disorders. Nonetheless, recent findings indicate the potential for a gut-eye axis, in which gut dysbiosis suggests a crucial role in the progression and development of an array of ocular conditions, that include uveitis, diabetic retinopathy, glaucoma and age-related macular degeneration. Current therapeutic strategies include probiotic and prebiotic supplementation, which seems to be the most economical and practical way to avoid ocular diseases and return the gut microbiome to a healthy state. In this chapter, we discuss the present understanding of gut dysbiosis linked with the pathophysiology of common eye disorders along with potential therapeutic implications for future translational studies in this research area.

Keywords: Age-related macular degeneration, Bacteriophage Therapy, Diabetic Retinopathy, Dysbiosis, Fecal transplant, Glaucoma, Gut-Eye Axis, Keratitis, Microbial-derived metabolites, Ocular disease, Retinal artery occlusion.

INTRODUCTION

The gut microbiome (GM), producing numerous small molecules, and shaping mammalian physiology profoundly in health and disease [1], stands out as the largest, with a predominance of bacteria whose quantity (3.8×10^{13}) closely matches the count of cells in the human body (3.0×10^{13}) [2]. The gut microbiome

[*] **Corresponding author Sanjay Dey:** Department of Pharmaceutical Technology, School of Health and Medical Sciences, Adamas University, Barasat-Barrackpore Road, Kolkata – 700126, West Bengal, India;
E-mail: sanju1980dey@gmail.com

Sandipan Dasgupta & Moitreyee Chattopadhyay (Eds.)

contributes to digestion, short-chain fatty acids (SCFA) synthesis, vitamin production, and immune system development, while SCFAs from microbes like *Bacteroides* regulate Treg and Th17 cells systemically [3]. The dynamic interplay between the host's immune system and the GM is crucial for preserving intestinal balance and suppressing inflammatory responses. Numerous studies have found a connection between changes in gut bacteria and eye diseases. A precise understanding of the gut microbiome is critically important for maintaining host health and managing disease. The eye is equipped with unique anatomic structures to maintain a highly regulated and confined environment for its function. There are mainly two blood-ocular barriers present in the human eye *i.e.* blood-aqueous barrier (BAB) and blood-retinal barrier (BRB) [4]. The endothelial cells lining the blood vessels in the iris, along with the non-pigmented cell layer of the ciliary epithelium, collectively constitute the BAB. Additionally, tight junctions between the non-pigmented epithelial cells further limit drug movement from the ciliary processes into the posterior chamber. Compared to immunocompetent tissue, privileged sites like the eye are particularly susceptible to inflammatory diseases resulting from changes in the gut microbiome. As people age, changes in the microbiome occur, potentially contributing to degenerative diseases like age-related macular degeneration (AMD) through altered ratios of Bacteroidetes to Firmicutes, as noted by Mariat *et al.* [5, 6]. In this manuscript, we summarized the association between gut microbiota and common eye diseases, including autoimmune uveitis, diabetic retinopathy, AMD, keratitis, glaucoma, and retinal artery occlusion, sheds light on the microbial involvement in ocular disease pathogenesis.

GUT MICROBIOME FUNCTIONS

The gut microbiome is beneficial for human health in numerous ways. Complex carbohydrates, fibres, and other indigestible substances that the human body is unable to handle on its own are broken down by gut bacteria. Furthermore, gut bacteria produce enzymes that help the body absorb nutrients like vitamins, minerals, and short-chain fatty acids. Theinteraction between the gut microbiota and the immune system helps regulate the functions of the immune system. It aids in the formation and upkeep of a well-balanced immune response, which is necessary to protect the body from infections while preventing detrimental inflammation or autoimmune reactions.

GUT MICROBIOME AND ITS AGE-DEPENDENT FEATURES

The microbiome in infancy undergoes significant changes influenced by various factors including the method of birth (cesarean section or vaginal delivery), feeding practices (breastfeeding or formula feeding, and introduction to solid foods), family lifestyle, location, genetic factors, and antibiotic usage [7]. Between approximately 3 to 4 years of age, the microbiome undergoes dynamic alterations, eventually transitioning to a more stable adult state [8]. As individuals age, the microbiome composition shifts due to senescence, with some degenerative diseases being linked to these changes in the aging microbiome. Research conducted by Mariat *et al.* revealed a modified ratio of Bacteroidetes to Firmicutes in older age groups, characterized by a higher proportion of Bacteroidetes among the elderly [5]. This ratio has demonstrated implications for various diseases, including AMD, which affects eye health [6]. Hence, to uphold a high quality of life and mitigate age-related ailments, it becomes imperative to comprehend the dynamics of the gut microbiome in older individuals. A recent study demonstrated that individuals aged 65 years and above (n = 145) differed from those below 65 years (n = 133) in both taxonomic and functional aspects of their gut microbiome [9]. These modifications could have a considerable impact on overall health, an elevated presence of *Proteobacteria* may serve as a potential indicator of an unstable gut microbiome and heightened susceptibility to diseases [10]. These discoveries carry significance for preventative strategies against age-related degenerative ailments and conditions such as AMD and retinal artery blockages. Utilizing interventions that target the microbiome, such as antibiotic or probiotic treatments, may offer promising avenues for preventive strategies.

INTERDEPENDENT REGULATION OF THE HOST IMMUNE SYSTEM AND GUT MICROBIOME

The interplay between the host immune system and gut microbiome has an important role in preserving intestinal balance and preventing inflammation. Acting as a barrier, the epithelial layer of the gut forms a biochemical and physiological shield that separates the host from commensal microbes, food antigens, pathogens, and toxins. Overlaying this epithelial barrier is a mucin layer composed of heavily glycosylated mucins, forming a gel-like substance, and containing various molecules like immunoglobulin A and antimicrobial agents such as lactoferrin [11]. Furthermore, another barrier to microbial invasion is the immunological defense system composed of specialized lymphoid structures known as Peyer's patches and lymphoid follicles. These follicles house a diverse array of immune cells like neutrophils, T cells, B cells, and dendritic cells. Goblet cells, predominantly found in the small intestine, facilitate the presentation of acquired luminal antigens to CD103+ dendritic cells, forming goblet cell-associated antigen passages [12]. The gut microbiota generates a multitude of metabolites, known as gut microbiota-derived metabolites, including short-chain fatty acids (SCFAs) and lipopolysaccharides (LPS), which facilitate communication between immune cells and gut epithelium, further playing a crucial role in inflammatory signalling. SCFAs have a direct binding affinity for

G-coupled receptors (like GPR43), also referred to as the free fatty acid receptor, exerting numerous crucial functions depending on the cell and tissue type. Apart from regulating the function of the intestinal barrier and safeguarding against invasion from pathogens, SCFAs demonstrate anti-inflammatory actions on immune cells by diminishing pro-inflammatory mediator levels and increasing the levels of anti-inflammatory cytokines [13]. When LPS binds to the TLR4, it initiates inflammatory processes, causing inflammation locally and allowing immune cells to travel to remote areas like the retina. Conversely, immune cells have receptors specialized in recognizing microbial metabolites, such as toll-like receptors [14]. This interaction is required for the immune system to manage the presence of microbes effectively—tolerating their existence while remaining vigilant against potential threats—thus maintaining the host's overall balance. The interplay between the immune system and microbiome hinges on their capacity to differentiate between non-pathogenic (commensal or mutualistic) and pathogenic symbionts. Commensals derive benefits from the host without causing harm or providing direct advantages, while mutualistic symbionts are involved in mutually benefitting relationships. Conversely, symbionts that are pathogenic form harmful associations with the host, leading to disease [15]. Nevertheless, following translocation across the mucosa or under circumstances like immunodeficiency, commensals have the potential to transition into pathogens (referred to as commensal-to-pathogen transition) [16]. If there is a shift in the balanced composition of the gut microbiota, characterized by a decrease in mutualistic symbionts and/or an increase in pathogens and their associated metabolites, this condition, known as dysbiosis, could play a role in the onset of various immune-mediated diseases [17].

GUT MICROBIOME AND DYSBIOSIS

The trillions of bacteria that reside in the gastrointestinal tract and make up the gut microbiome are essential for immune system function, metabolism, and digestion. However, when the balance of this complex ecosystem is disrupted, a condition known as dysbiosis occurs. Dysbiosis refers to an imbalance in the composition and function of the gut microbiome, characterized by a decrease in beneficial microorganisms (such as probiotics) and/or an increase in harmful or pathogenic bacteria [18]. This imbalance can result from various factors, including diet, lifestyle, antibiotic usage, stress, and underlying medical conditions. The consequences of dysbiosis can be far-reaching, impacting not only gastrointestinal health but also contributing to the development of numerous systemic disorders. Studies have connected dysbiosis to disorders like obesity, metabolic syndrome, autoimmune diseases, irritable bowel syndrome (IBS), inflammatory bowel disease (IBD), and even neurological ailments like anxiety and depression [19]. Dysbiosis can manifest in different ways, including alterations in microbial diversity, changes in the abundance of specific bacterial taxa, and disruptions in microbial metabolite production. These alterations may weaken the intestinal barrier's integrity, resulting in a leaky gut and increased intestinal permeability. They may also cause dangerous bacteria and microbiological products to enter the circulation, which can cause immunological dysregulation and systemic inflammation [20]. Addressing dysbiosis often involves interventions aimed at restoring microbial balance and promoting gut health. Strategies may include dietary modifications (such as increasing fibre intake and consuming fermented foods), probiotic supplementation, prebiotic fibres to support beneficial bacteria, lifestyle changes to reduce stress, and targeted antimicrobial therapies [21]. Personalized approaches tailored to individual microbial profiles and health conditions are increasingly being explored to optimize treatment outcomes. The gut microbiome plays a vital role in maintaining overall health, and dysbiosis can have significant implications for health and disease. Understanding the complex interactions within the gut ecosystem and implementing strategies to restore microbial balance are key steps in managing dysbiosis and promoting gastrointestinal and systemic well-being.

EVIDENCE THAT BACTERIA IN THE GUT MICROBIOME ARE ASSOCIATED WITH OCULAR DISEASE

There may be a direct gut-retina axis role and potential influence of the gut microbiome for several retinal disorders including diabetic retinopathy, retinitis pigmentosa, and AMD. The multifactorial nature of AMD is caused by a complicated interplay between environmental and genetic factors. Given the significance of microbiome integrity in host control and immune response generation, intestinal microbiota may serve as a potential mediator of the interaction between genetic susceptibility and environmental variables that contribute to AMD [22]. Dysbiosis in the gut microbiome may lead to increased intestinal permeability, allowing gut-derived metabolites to modulate immune cells specific to the retina. Additionally, chronic inflammation triggered by substances like LPS has been observed to hasten neurodegeneration in dystrophic retinas. Zinkernagel and colleagues investigated the gut microbiomes of AMD patients and found associations between certain bacterial genera and species and neovascular AMD [6]. These microbial variations may impact retinal health by affecting pathways related to neurotransmission and retinal degeneration. Conversely, the presence of *Bacteroides eggerthii* in healthy individuals might provide protective effects against the disease through the production of SCFAs, which help regulate inflammation [6]. Dietary factors could also play a role in the gut-retina connection, as shown by studies linking dietary glycemic index to changes in gut microbiome composition and subsequent effects on AMD features [23]. Furthermore, alterations in gastrointestinal metabolite production due to dysbiosis may contribute to inflammatory states and metabolic disturbances, exacerbating retinal inflammation and vascular damage in conditions like DR [24]. In mouse models, RP has been associated with changes in gut microbiome composition, with diseased animals exhibiting higher levels of certain bacteria compared to healthy controls. These findings suggest a potential interplay between gut microbiota changes and retinal degeneration [24]. Grasping the concept of the gut-retina axis and its relevance to retinal disorders could lead to the development of focused therapeutic approaches aimed at adjusting the gut microbiome to enhance ocular well-being.

GUT-EYE AXIS

To maintain the human body in homeostasis, the microbiome must be in good health. Systemic inflammation is caused by changes in the gut microbiota and its metabolites, which further leads to stimulation of the innate and adaptive immune responses. Various studies on both humans and animals have suggested that this inflammation can go on to damage tissues throughout the body, which can result in the emergence of numerous diseases, including those that affect the eyes [25]. Even in the absence of infection, the eye is susceptible to developing inflammatory disorders, which may be influenced by gut microbiome dysbiosis. Ocular disorders and inflammatory intestinal diseases have a relevant correlation. In fact, 10% of patients with inflammatory bowel disease are associated with eye conditions like uveitis, conjunctivitis, or episcleritis [26]. Numerous studies have demonstrated the presence of a gut-eye axis, in which immunity in distant locations, such as the eye, can be influenced by gut bacteria [27]. Furthermore, other research has demonstrated that the microbiome of the intestines and its metabolic products, particularly the SCFA, can affect the epigenome of various cell types in a direct or indirect way, which in turn can influence important immune cell activities [28]. An immune system reaction that threatens vision and damages the eye is a hallmark of inflammatory diseases affecting the eyes. Gut microbiome alterations have been linked with AMD, uveitis, glaucoma, infectious keratitis, diabetic retinopathy, and Sjogren's disease associated with eye dryness [29]. However, the data validating these connections are still in preliminary stages.

IMPLICATIONS OF DYSBIOSIS ON EYE DISEASES

Maintaining intestinal homeostasis and preventing inflammatory processes require the gut microbiome and immune system of the host to cooperate dynamically. Dysregulation of immune responses can occur due to gut dysbiosis by causing mucosal barrier malfunction and allowing pathogenic microbes to translocate across the epithelial barrier. Several disorders, including those affecting the eyes, may begin because of inflammation and progress to tissue death. Bacteria and their metabolites are translocated to extraintestinal organs in a surplus of immune cells like the eye by mesenteric lymphatics or the bloodstream. The blood-aqueous and blood-retina barriers, along with the tolerogenic response of the immune system, shield the retina from internal and external assaults. This makes the retina an immune-favoured tissue. Blood-retina barrier is made up of an interior and an exterior barrier. Alterations in these blood-retina barriers have the potential to attract inflammatory cells and subsequently cause ocular inflammation, which could result in the occurrence of retinal diseases including uveitis. The retina is also shielded to preserve retinal homeostasis by the complement system and microglia that make up its very own innate immune system. When a stimulus occurs, microglia cells move to the affected area, release reactive oxygen species (ROS) and pro-inflammatory cytokines to counteract the damage, and phagocyte the cell debris to hinder waste materials accumulation. There are three distinct pathways for triggering the complement system, which is made up of more than 30 proteins. Although these pathways require distinct molecules to initiate, they eventually come together to produce a common set of effector chemicals that aid in pathogen opsonization, death, and inflammatory cell recruitment [30]. Antigen-antibody complexes initiate the traditional pathway. Mannan-binding lectin, a serum component, initiates the mannose-binding lectin pathway and pathogen surfaces directly initiate the alternative pathway. Immune responses often serve as a homeostatic mechanism, limiting the ability for processes of regeneration and repair while maintaining tissue processes and minimizing detrimental immune responses by regulating the development and appearance of intraocular inflammatory conditions. The eye and other immune-favoured tissues are therefore more vulnerable than immune-competent tissue to developing inflammatory conditions brought on by gut microbiome changes. The translocation of bacteria by the gut-eye axis constitutes a potential pathway for the same. Nevertheless, while numerous researches have demonstrated that gut microbiome has a role in the pathophysiology of specific illnesses, it remains unclear if mucosal inflammation causes or results from dysbiosis. Yet, microbiome-modifying tactics could be helpful in preserving gut-barrier integrity and homeostasis, which would further support avoiding systemic inflammation. The gut microbiome dysbiosis causes different ocular diseases, which are given in Fig. (**1**).

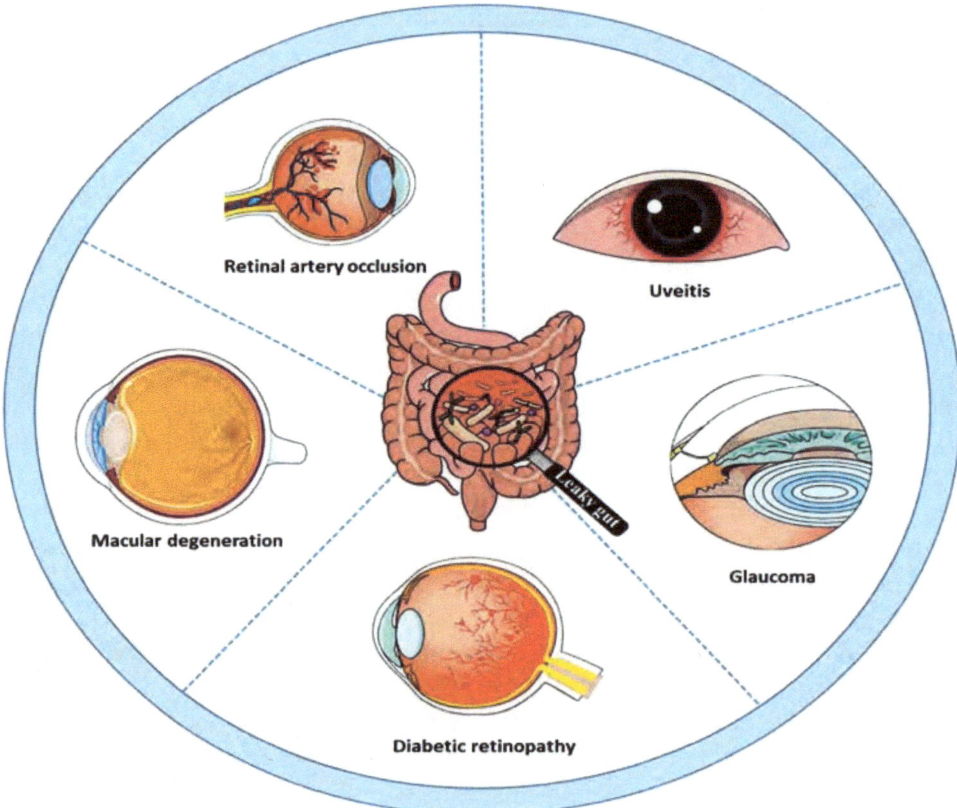

Fig. (1). Gut microbiome dysbiosis and ocular diseases.

GUT MICROBIOME DYSBIOSIS AND OCULAR DISEASES

Gut Microbiome Dysbiosis and Uveitis

Uveitis refers to inflammation in the vascular uveal tract of the eye, encompassing the iris, ciliary body, and choroid. However, it can also affect nearby structures like the retina, optic nerve, vitreous, and sclera [31]. Uveitis contributes to approximately 5 to 20% of blindness in both the United States and Europe [32], while about 25% of blindness in India and other developing countries is attributed to uveitis [33]. The International Uveitis Study Group (IUSG) categorized uveitis into four anatomical types: anterior uveitis, intermediate uveitis, posterior uveitis, and panuveitis [34]. In 2019, WHO estimated at least 2.2 billion people globally, who were suffering from vision impairment or blindness [35]. Uveitis can stem from various causes, including infections, inflammatory conditions, trauma, and cases of unknown origin (idiopathic) [36]. Systemic microbial infections, such as those resulting from dysbiosis in the GM, may play a significant role in driving uveitis [37]. Depending on its underlying cause, uveitis can be categorized as either infectious or noninfectious. Noninfectious uveitis, often termed autoimmune uveitis, is predominantly associated with autoimmunity, potentially sight-threatening inflammation within the eye that impacts the neuroretina [38]. Its pathogenesis might be linked to the abnormal activation of T helper cells (Th cells), particularly an imbalance between inflammatory Th1/Th17 cells and regulatory T cells (Treg cells) [31]. Recently, emerging evidence suggests that the gut microbiota may play a crucial role in the development of uveitis. Kalyana *et al.* have demonstrated dysbiosis in the gut bacterial communities of patients with uveitis compared to healthy individuals from a South Indian population [39]. It has been shown that depleting the gut microbiota reduces the severity of autoimmune uveitis in mouse models [40]. Retina-specific T cells receive an activation signal in the gut from antigens derived from commensal microbiota, which may lead to the initiation of autoimmune uveitis [41]. 16S sequencing of gastrointestinal contents suggests the presence of both protective and potentially uveitogenic gut microbiota [42]. Dysbiosis leads to autoimmune uveitis through a variety of interconnected mechanisms. See Fig. (**2**).

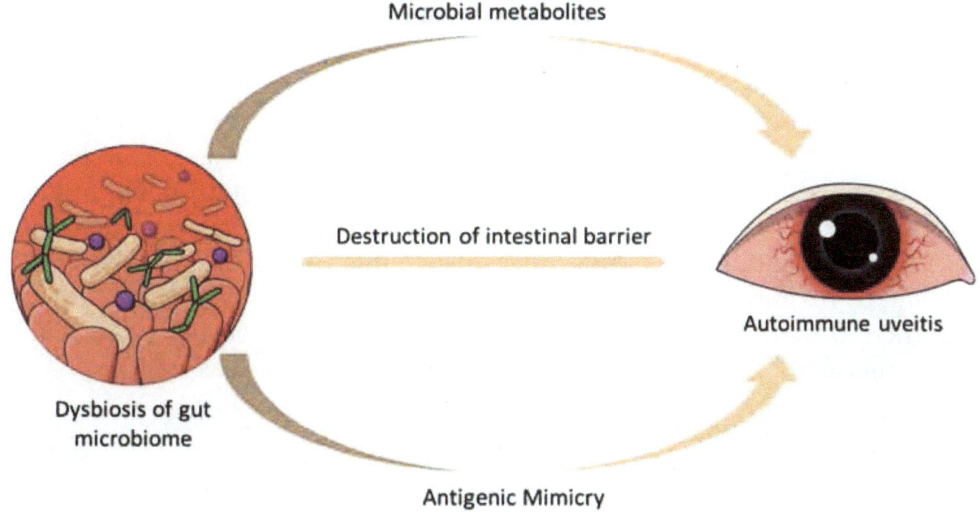

Fig. (2). Mechanisms of autoimmune uveitis caused by the gut microbiome.

The Role of Microbial Metabolites

Gut microorganisms can generate thousands of metabolites, with SCFAs such as acetic acid, propionic acid, and butyric acid being the most prevalent. SCFAs are believed to alleviate uveitis by promoting the proliferation of Tregs in the colon and cervical lymph nodes. Additionally, they may reduce the migration of effector

T cells between the intestine and spleen during uveitis [43]. In patients with acute anterior uveitis (AAU), the expression of seven fecal metabolites, including 6-deoxy-D-glucose and palmitoleic acid, was found to be elevated compared to the control group [44]. Microbial metabolites like LPS or other endotoxins are known to potentially trigger uveitis [45].

The Role of the Gut Microbiome in Antigenic Mimicry

Antigenic mimicry, also known as molecular mimicry, refers to the mechanism by which autoreactive T cells are produced due to the cross-reactivity between peptides derived from gut microbes and self-antigens [46]. The commensal gut flora, even without pathogenic agents, plays a crucial role in initiating immune responses that result in a relapsing-remitting autoimmune disease driven by myelin-specific CD4+ T cells [47]. Caspi *et al.* demonstrated that T cell activation in the gut is associated with spontaneous uveitis in R161H mice. The elimination of gut microbiota lessens disease severity and decreases T cell activation in the gut [48].

Destruction of the Intestinal Barrier: Increased Intestinal Permeability

Dysbiosis of the gut microbiome has the potential to disrupt the intestinal barrier, alter intestinal permeability, and lead to intestinal leakage [49]. In individuals with ankylosing spondylitis, dysfunction in the gut vascular barrier was observed, which showed a correlation with increased serum levels of LPS-binding protein (LPS-BP), intestinal fatty acid-binding protein (iFABP), and zonulin [50]. Intestinal dysbiosis is often associated with a disturbance in intestinal homeostasis in autoimmune uveitis. However, it is worth noting that adjuvant-killed mycobacterial antigen (MTB) alone can also induce intestinal disruption [51]. Human leukocyte antigen (HLA)-B27-dependent dysbiosis, changes in intestinal permeability, and molecular mimicry can all affect the composition and function of the gut microbiota, potentially mediating acute anterior uveitis AAU [52].

Gut Microbiome Dysbiosis and Glaucoma

Glaucoma, characterized by the progressive degeneration of retinal ganglion cells (RGCs), constitutes a group of optic neuropathies and is the primary cause of irreversible blindness in developed countries [53]. Glaucoma involves an elevation in intraocular pressure (IOP) and changes in the drainage of aqueous humor. Globally, it is projected that the number of individuals with glaucoma will increase to approximately 110 million by the year 2040 [54]. Potential alterations in the cellular immune system in patients with glaucoma were identified by measuring levels of T lymphocyte subsets, cytokine IL-2, and the soluble IL-2 receptor in peripheral blood [55]. There have been limited studies exploring the potential association between gut microbiota and glaucoma. For the first time in 2000, Kountouras *et al.* demonstrated the link between *Helicobacter pylori* (H. pylori) infection and glaucoma [56]. In patients with primary open-angle glaucoma (POAG), *Prevotellaceae*, unidentified *Enterobacteriaceae*, and *Escherichia coli* showed the most significant increases compared to controls. Conversely, *Megamonas* and *Bacteroides plebeius* exhibited significant decreases in POAG patients [57]. This conclusion suggests that patients with POAG have distinct gut microbiota and serum metabolites compared to healthy individuals. The results of the Mendelian randomization (MR) analysis indicated that the family *Oxalobacteraceae* and the genus *Eggerthella* had a detrimental impact on glaucoma. Conversely, the genus *Bilophila* and *Ruminiclostridium* had a beneficial effect on glaucoma [58]. Elevated IOP triggers T-cell infiltration in mice, leading to sustained retinal damage. Heat shock proteins are identified as targets of T-cell responses in glaucoma [59]. Skrzypecki *et al.* demonstrated that trimethylamine (TMA) levels are elevated in the aqueous humor of patients with glaucoma [60]. This same group also found that Butyrate, a metabolite produced by gut bacteria, reduces IOP in normotensive rats but not in hypertensive rats [61].

Gut Microbiome Dysbiosis and Age-Related Macular Degeneration (AMD)

Age-related macular degeneration (AMD) stands as one of the most prevalent ophthalmic conditions among the elderly in industrialized countries. It targets the macula, resulting in irreversible loss of central vision and, eventually, legal blindness [62]. It is estimated that approximately 196 million people worldwide are affected by AMD [63]. AMD is a condition influenced by multiple genes and environmental factors. It presents in two main types: dry and wet (neovascular) AMD. Dry AMD may advance to wet AMD. In dry AMD, there is a build-up of drusen and cellular debris underneath the retinal pigment epithelium (RPE) and Bruch's membrane [64]. Regulated immune activation in AMD involves the recruitment of microglia, macrophages, mast cell activation, and immune activation of RPE [65]. *Lactobacillus paracasei* KW3110 has been shown to activate macrophages and suppress inflammation in both mice and humans. The consumption of*L. paracasei* KW3110 has been found to alleviate age-related chronic inflammation by modulating the composition of gut microbiota and immune system functions in aged mice. Additionally, it has been observed to reduce age-related loss of retinal ganglion cells (RGCs) [66]. Zhang *et al.* showed that the downregulation of the peroxisome proliferator-activated receptor-gamma coactivator 1-alpha (PGC-1α) gene, when combined with a high-fat diet, can lead to the development of AMD-like characteristics in mice [67]. Toll-like receptors (TLRs) recognize microbe-specific molecules in the gastrointestinal tract, mediating immune communication with gut microbiota. Neovascular AMD is associated with higher *Firmicutes* prevalence, while *Bacteroides* species may offer protection, linked to the genetic risk factor like complement factor H (CFH) [68]. These findings indicate that alterations in the intestinal microbiome are linked to AMD.

Gut Microbiome Dysbiosis and Diabetic Retinopathy

Diabetic retinopathy (DR), is a major illness related to type 2 diabetes mellitus resulting in visual impairment in working age population [69]. By 2030, there are estimated to be approximately 191 million cases of this condition [70, 71]. Its occurrence is linked to numerous kinds of mechanisms, including cellular degradation and inflammation, which cause endothelial and neurological damage [70]. The gut microbiota is a complex system and it regulates the microenvironment of the human body. DR is closely associated with dysbiosis [72]. Recent studies indicate that the onset and progression of diabetic retinopathy are intricate processes influenced by various factors, including the management of blood pressure, blood sugar levels, and the duration of a patient's diabetes [73]. DR can occur as a result of these conditions because they might cause vascular dysfunction and damage the activity of cells that maintain retinal structures [74]. In general, the mechanism associated with microangiopathy triggered by elevated glucose levels involves oxidative stress and dysfunction of the endothelium mediated by glucose. Earlier research suggested that ROS could disrupt the body's antioxidant defense mechanisms and impact abnormalities in retinal metabolism. Additionally, the apoptosis and inflammation observed in retinal pigment epithelial cells, connected with heightened blood sugar levels, are fundamental aspects contributing to the progression of DR [75]. Various microorganisms have been detected in the intestines of individuals with diabetes mellitus (DM), with some in accretive proportion and others showing a negative correlation. Many studies have utilized the abundance of these bacteria as a key metric [76]. The top two prevalent microorganisms are *Firmicutes* and *Bacteroidetes* [77]. The microbial community residing on the surface of the eye is mainly made up of *Proteobacteria and Actinobacteria* [78]. Diabetes and obesity are closely linked with an imbalance in gut microbiota. Certainly, a change in the balance of gut bacteria can initiate mild, ongoing inflammation and oxidative stress, potentially influencing the development and advancement of diabetic retinopathy. Research suggests that an imbalance in gut microbes contributes to persistent inflammation and weakened immune responses over time [79]. Interestingly, DR patients showed a significant enrichment of families such as *Acidaminococcaceae, Oscillospiraceae, Christensenellaceae,* and *Anaerovoracaceae* compared to those with DM [80, 81]. Remarkably, the *Enterococcus* and *Cloacibacillus* genera were exclusively found in DR. However, a separate investigation revealed heightened levels of the *Faecalibacterium, Roseburia, Lachnospira, and Romboutsia genera,* while the *Akkermansia muciniphila* species was reduced in DR. Relative to individuals with DM, those with DR showed higher levels of genera *Agathobacteria, Prevotella, Faecalibacterium, Subdoligranulum,* and *Olsenella*, and decreased levels of genera *Bacillus, Veillonella,* and *Pantoea* [82]. A connection between the gut and the retina is recognized, and altering the gut microbiome through dietary changes, probiotics, or antibiotics can influence the onset of retinal diseases. Understanding this gut-retina axis could provide valuable insights into conditions such as retinopathy of prematurity, where an underdeveloped gut microbiome and prolonged antibiotic use might play a role [83]. Research demonstrated that HFD have the ability to directly influence the retinal transcriptome without being influenced by the gut microbiome. It is universally observed in all studies that dysbacteriosis is a shared characteristic of DR [84].

Gut Microbiome Dysbiosis and Bacterial Keratitis (BK)

Keratitis is an inflammatory eye condition in which the cornea becomes inflamed, leading to redness, pain, itching, and substantial vision impairment [85]. Bacterial keratitis, the most prevalent type of keratitis, poses serious threats to vision, such as corneal scarring, endophthalmitis, perforation, and potential blindness [86]. Bacterial keratitis remains a primary reason for visual impairment and global blindness, with major risk factors including injury, the health of the eye's surface, and the wearing of contact lenses. In the Indian population, the yearly occurrence rate of bacterial keratitis is 2.79 cases per 10,000 individuals [87]. A research study demonstrated that an imbalanced gut microbiome in mice made them more susceptible to ocular pathogens that can lead to keratitis [88]. Over the past 25 years, the types of microorganisms causing Bacterial Keratitis have shown a consistent pattern, with *Staphylococci (S. aureus, S. epidermidis)* and *Streptococci (S. pneumoniae)* being the predominant gram-positive organisms frequently encountered and documented globally [89]. *Pseudomonas aeruginosa (P. aeruginosa)* ranks among the most commonly found gram-negative bacteria in patients diagnosed with bacterial keratitis [86]. However, numerous other bacteria have been identified in cases of BK. The research indicated a continual rise in the prevalence of pathogenic bacteria and imbalanced alterations in the bacterial microbiome of the conjunctiva and cornea among bacterial keratitis patients in comparison to healthy controls. This could potentially contribute to the initiation or aggravation of inflammation on the surface of the eye [90]. Healthy individuals exhibited elevated levels of beneficial bacteria and fungi possessing anti-inflammatory, antibacterial, and probiotic properties, while individuals with BK disease showed reduced levels of these microorganisms. The decline in beneficial bacteria and the rise in pro-inflammatory and pathogenic bacteria among BK subjects may play an important role in the disease phenotype [91].

Gut Microbiome Dysbiosis and Fungal Keratitis

Fungal keratitis (FK) is recognized as one of the most acute forms of microbial keratitis, characterized by a poor visual prognosis and the risk of eventual blindness [92]. Fungal keratitis is known to be a more prolonged and severe disease than bacterial keratitis [87]. Also, according to the findings of the Asia Cornea Society Infectious Keratitis Study (ACS IKS), fungal keratitis is a prevalent form of microbial keratitis (MK), coming after BK with a ratio of 33% for fungal keratitis compared to 38% for bacterial keratitis [93, 94]. FK typically presents substantial difficulties in diagnosis and treatment. It is predominantly observed in tropical/subtropical countries and areas with significant agricultural activity, constituting between 23% and 63% of all infectious keratitis cases in such regions [95, 96]. Aspergillus is a pathogen that affects humans and is one of the usual suspects in cases of fungal Keratitis [97]. Climate is also a significant factor in determining pathogens. For instance, within the temperate climate of Denmark, 52% of patients with fungal keratitis were found to be infected with *Candida*, 20% with *Fusarium*, 16% with *Aspergillus*, and 12% with a combination of filamentous fungi [98]. The research has found that Fungal keratitis results in decreased diversity and changes in the ocular surface microbiome in both affected and unaffected eyes. *Corynebacterium* and *Staphylococcus* are less prevalent, while *Pseudomonas* and *Cryophilus* are more common [99]. A recent study conducted within an Indian cohort demonstrated that individuals diagnosed with FK closely resembled healthy controls in terms of the composition of their fungal gut microbiomes. In contrast, there was a significant decrease in the richness and diversity of gut bacteria in FK patients, indicating an imbalance in their gut microbiomes compared to healthy controls [100]. Studies indicate that the lower levels of beneficial bacteria and higher levels of inflammatory and pathogenic bacteria in FK subjects could be a factor in the clinical symptoms observed in FK [92].

Gut Microbiome and Retinal Artery Occlusion

Retinal artery occlusion (RAO) poses a significant threat to vision and often arises as a complication of cardiovascular disease. It commonly occurs as a result of underlying atherosclerosis [101]. RAO is characterized by the blockage of blood flow to the retina due to a blood clot or fat deposit in one of the small arteries supplying blood to the retina. Bacteria from the gut may be associated with disease markers of atherosclerosis [102]. In patients with RAO, there was a decrease in the relative abundance of Bacteroidetes compared to controls. Conversely, the phylum Proteobacteria showed an increase in relative abundance in patients with RAO compared to controls [101]. The gut microbiota metabolizes choline, phosphatidylcholine, L-carnitine, and betaine into trimethylamine

(TMA), which is further oxidized into trimethylamine-N-oxide (TMAO) by hepatic flavin monooxygenases (FMO3) [103]. TMAO was significantly higher in patients with RAO compared to controls [101].

MODULATION OF THE GUT MICROBIOME AS A THERAPY/ FUTURE THERAPEUTIC APPROACHES: MICROBIAL THERAPEUTICS

Throughout the evolutionary timeline, humans have co-evolved alongside a wide array of microbial species in their environment, fostering symbiotic relationships [2]. The human microbiome comprises the entirety of microorganisms along with their metabolites and products that have been detected within and on the human body [104]. Variations in hygiene, social habits, genetics, and dietary choices contribute diversity of microbiota at specific anatomical sites among individuals [105]. Yet, when there is a disruption in this microbial balance, it can lead to various disorders [106]. Given the significant involvement of microbes in maintaining human health, there's immense promise in utilizing them as therapeutic agents for treating diseases. Modulation of gut microbiome as therapy holds immense potential for treating severe diseases and represents a promising avenue for achieving personalized therapy objectives, addressing challenges such as individual variation and environmental stability [107] (Fig. **3**). For the majority of contemporary medical history, germ theory depicted microbes as foes; however, it is now widely acknowledged that they can function as therapeutic agents [108]. For managing IBD, strategies involve triggering the body's natural defenses through synthetic microbial byproducts or engineered bacterial strains, employing bacteriophages to combat harmful microbes, and hindering bacterial adhesion and blocking bacterial receptors. Additionally, efforts aim to enhance the oxygen-deprived environment to support the growth of beneficial anaerobic bacteria [109, 110]. Microbes possess the capacity to mitigate the onset of diseases by engaging with the host, thereby serving as valuable assets in the development of microbiome-based therapeutics [111]. *Christensenella* sp. is recognized for its ability to decrease symptoms of depression and anxiety [112]. *Bifidobacterium longum* mitigates the severity of Crohn's disease [113]. The expanding knowledge about the capabilities of gut microbes has led to a new realm of possibilities in therapeutics, offering fresh optimism for disease diagnosis, testing techniques, and innovative methods of data collection and analysis [112].

Probiotics and Relative Metabolites

Probiotics are live microorganisms that provide particular benefits to hosts when ingested in sufficient amounts [114]. Probiotics can speed up digestion, and shield against harmful pathogens. They also function as immune boosters and aid in growth promotion. Additionally, probiotics reduce the occurrence of infections caused by bacterial pathogens [115, 116]. Recent progress in synthetic biology has opened up the potential for precise cell therapies by engineering probiotics to target particular cells, tissues, or pathways [117]. *Lactobacilli, Bifidobacteria,* and *E. coli* have been utilized as probiotics with success in the treatment of a variety of diseases [118, 119]. Probiotics function by engaging in competition with pathogens through actions such as producing bacteriocins, competing for attachment sites and nutrients, modifying pathogen functions, and enhancing the host's immune response and nutritional status [120]. Probiotics have proven effective in treating various conditions like ulcerative colitis, IBD, diarrhea, Crohn's disease (CD), and cancer [112].

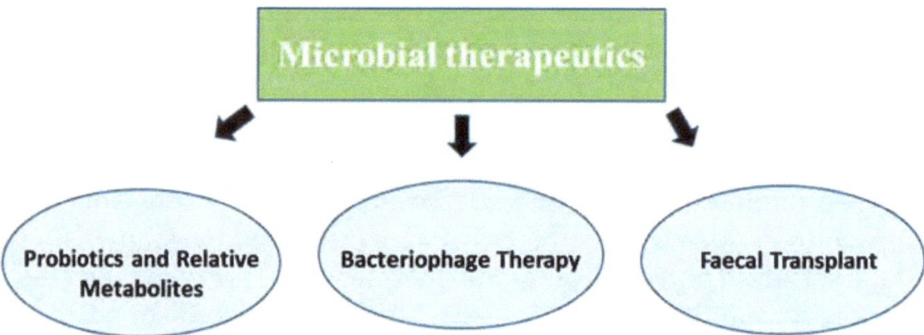

Fig. (3). Modulation of the gut microbiome as a therapy.

Bacteriophage Therapy

Bacteriophages are viruses that target a particular type of bacteria. Since bacteriophages insert their genetic material into their particular bacteria and lead to the breakdown of bacterial membranes, they are employed to combat antibiotic-resistant pathogens [121]. Phages and their derivatives are utilized in the treatment of various diseases caused by microbial pathogens that are resistant to antibiotics. Bacteriophage treatment effectively eliminated methicillin-resistant Staphylococcus aureus causing osteomyelitis [122]. Staphylococcus bacteriophage sb-1 was applied in the treatment of foot ulcers for healing [123]. The bacteriophages MR299-2 and NH-4 have demonstrated effectiveness in treating lung infections caused by Pseudomonas, while the bacteriophage targeting *Propionibacterium* acnes has been proven successful in treating acne [124, 125]. Engineered bacteriophages offer an intriguing and promising approach to modulating the gut microbiota. However, ongoing clinical trials predominantly utilize phages for antimicrobial purposes or diagnostic testing, with little exploration of their potential in gut microbiota modulation [126].

Fecal Transplant

Fecal Microbiota Transplantation (FMT) involves introducing a solution containing fecal material from a donor into the recipient's gastrointestinal tract. This procedure can be carried out using different forms, such as enema, colonoscopy, or capsules. A fecal transplant has the potential to directly alter the composition of the gut microbiota. Prior research has demonstrated the effectiveness of FMT in addressing conditions related to microbial imbalance, notably recurrent *Clostridoides* difficile infection and ulcerative colitis [127, 128]. The current recommendations for FMT in clinical settings suggest a structured four-step selection procedure, which includes a clinical assessment, blood and stool analysis, additional questionnaires, and direct molecular stool testing on the day of donation [129]. Currently and over time, FMT has become recognized as a dependable therapeutic option for recurrent *Clostridioides* difficile infection (CDI), serving as an effective alternative to vancomycin and fidaxomicin [130, 131]. In recent years, there has been a rise in the number of studies examining how FMT could be used to treat noncommunicable chronic conditions, spanning from IBD and IBS to psychiatric disorders, metabolic disorders, liver disease, autoimmune disorders, and cancer [132].

CONCLUSION

The emerging evidence linking the gut microbiome to eye diseases underscores the intricate relationship between gut health and eye health. Numerous retinal disorders, such as AMD, diabetic retinopathy, and retinitis pigmentosa have been linked to dysbiosis in the gut microbiome. The gut-retina axis plays a crucial role in the pathogenesis of these diseases, with dysbiosis contributing to systemic inflammation, metabolic disturbances, and immune dysregulation that ultimately impact retinal health. Unravelling the processes by which ocular disorders are influenced by the gut microbiome opens exciting opportunities for the development of novel therapeutic strategies. Targeted interventions aimed at modulating the gut microbiome, such as dietary modifications, probiotic supplementation, and fecal microbiota transplantation, hold promise for mitigating the progression of retinal diseases and improving patient outcomes. Further research is needed to elucidate the intricate interactions between the gut microbiome and ocular healthfully. By unravelling the complexities of the gut-retina axis, we can pave the way for innovative approaches to prevent, diagnose, and treat ocular diseases, ultimately enhancing the quality of life for individuals affected by these conditions.

CONSENT FOR PUBLICATION

All authors have consented to publish the book chapter "The role of gut microbiota in ocular diseases" in this book.

REFERENCES

[1] Koppel N, Maini Rekdal V, Balskus EP. Chemical transformation of xenobiotics by the human gut microbiota. Science (80-). 2017; 356(6344): eaag2770.
[http://dx.doi.org/10.1126/science.aag2770]

[2] Sender R, Fuchs S, Milo R. Are we really vastly outnumbered? Revisiting the ratio of bacterial to host cells in humans. Cell 2016; 164(3): 337-40.
[http://dx.doi.org/10.1016/j.cell.2016.01.013] [PMID: 26824647]

[3] Zeng H, Chi H. Metabolic control of regulatory T cell development and function. Trends Immunol 2015; 36(1): 3-12.
[http://dx.doi.org/10.1016/j.it.2014.08.003] [PMID: 25248463]

[4] Cunha-Vaz J. The blood-retinal barrier in the management of retinal disease: EURETINA award lecture. Ophthalmologica 2017; 237(1): 1-10.
[http://dx.doi.org/10.1159/000455809] [PMID: 28152535]

[5] Mariat D, Firmesse O, Levenez F, *et al.* The Firmicutes/Bacteroidetes ratio of the human microbiota changes with age. BMC Microbiol 2009; 9(1): 123.
[http://dx.doi.org/10.1186/1471-2180-9-123] [PMID: 19508720]

[6] Zinkernagel MS, Zysset-Burri DC, Keller I, *et al.* Association of the Intestinal Microbiome with the Development of Neovascular Age-Related Macular Degeneration. Sci Rep 2017; 7(1): 40826.
[http://dx.doi.org/10.1038/srep40826] [PMID: 28094305]

[7] Zhuang L, Chen H, Zhang S, Zhuang J, Li Q, Feng Z. Intestinal Microbiota in Early Life and Its Implications on Childhood Health. Genomics Proteomics Bioinformatics 2019; 17(1): 13-25.
[http://dx.doi.org/10.1016/j.gpb.2018.10.002] [PMID: 30986482]

[8] Kumbhare SV, Patangia DV, Patil RH, Shouche YS, Patil NP. Factors influencing the gut microbiome in children: from infancy to childhood. J Biosci 2019; 44(2): 49.
[http://dx.doi.org/10.1007/s12038-019-9860-z] [PMID: 31180062]

[9] Herzog EL, Wäfler M, Keller I, Wolf S, Zinkernagel MS, Zysset-Burri DC. The importance of age in compositional and functional profiling of the human intestinal microbiome. PLoS One 2021; 16(10): e0258505.
[http://dx.doi.org/10.1371/journal.pone.0258505] [PMID: 34662347]

[10] Rizzatti G, Lopetuso LR, Gibiino G, Binda C, Gasbarrini A. Proteobacteria: A common factor in human diseases. 2017.
[http://dx.doi.org/10.1155/2017/9351507]

[11] Singh PK, Parsek MR, Greenberg EP, Welsh MJ. A component of innate immunity prevents bacterial biofilm development. Nature 2002; 417(6888): 552-5.
[http://dx.doi.org/10.1038/417552a] [PMID: 12037568]

[12] Howe SE, Lickteig DJ, Plunkett KN, Ryerse JS, Konjufca V. The uptake of soluble and particulate antigens by epithelial cells in the mouse small intestine. PLoS One 2014; 9(1): e86656.
[http://dx.doi.org/10.1371/journal.pone.0086656] [PMID: 24475164]

[13] Yoo J, Groer M, Dutra S, Sarkar A, McSkimming D. Gut microbiota and immune system interactions. Vol. 8. Microorganisms 2020; 8(10): 1587.
[http://dx.doi.org/10.3390/microorganisms8101587]

[14] Hajjar AM, Ernst RK, Tsai JH, Wilson CB, Miller SI. Human Toll-like receptor 4 recognizes host-

specific LPS modifications. Nat Immunol 2002; 3(4): 354-9.
[http://dx.doi.org/10.1038/ni777] [PMID: 11912497]

[15] Tipton L, Darcy JL, Hynson NA. A developing symbiosis: Enabling cross-talk between ecologists and microbiome scientists. Front Microbiol 2019; 10(FEB): 292.
[http://dx.doi.org/10.3389/fmicb.2019.00292] [PMID: 30842763]

[16] Tlaskalová-Hogenová H, Štěpánková R, Kozáková H, *et al.* The role of gut microbiota (commensal bacteria) and the mucosal barrier in the pathogenesis of inflammatory and autoimmune diseases and cancer: contribution of germ-free and gnotobiotic animal models of human diseases. Cell Mol Immunol 2011; 8(2): 110-20.
[http://dx.doi.org/10.1038/cmi.2010.67] [PMID: 21278760]

[17] Lin P. Altering the intestinal microbiota for therapeutic benefit in uveitis. Ann Eye Sci 2020; 5(September): 26. Available from: https://aes.amegroups.org/article/view/5585
[http://dx.doi.org/10.21037/aes-19-114]

[18] Carding S, Verbeke K, Vipond DT, Corfe BM, Owen LJ. Dysbiosis of the gut microbiota in disease. Microb Ecol Health Dis 2015; 26(1): 26191.
[http://dx.doi.org/10.3402/mehd.v26.26191] [PMID: 25651997]

[19] Davies C, Bergman J, Eshraghi AA, Mittal R, Eshraghi RS. The Gut Microbiome: Potential Clinical Applications in Disease Management. In: Gut?Brain Connection, Myth or Reality?. ; : p. (). 2020; : p.
[http://dx.doi.org/10.1142/9789811221156_0009]

[20] Hollander D, Kaunitz JD. The "Leaky Gut": Tight Junctions but Loose Associations? Dig Dis Sci 2020; 65(5): 1277-87.
[http://dx.doi.org/10.1007/s10620-019-05777-2] [PMID: 31471860]

[21] Shah BR, Li B, Al Sabbah H, Xu W, Mráz J. Effects of prebiotic dietary fibers and probiotics on human health: With special focus on recent advancement in their encapsulated formulations. Trends Food Sci Technol 2020; 102: 178-92.
[http://dx.doi.org/10.1016/j.tifs.2020.06.010] [PMID: 32834500]

[22] Lin P. Importance of the intestinal microbiota in ocular inflammatory diseases: A review. Clin Exp Ophthalmol 2019; 47(3): 418-22.
[http://dx.doi.org/10.1111/ceo.13493] [PMID: 30834680]

[23] Rowan S, Jiang S, Korem T, *et al.* Involvement of a gut–retina axis in protection against dietary glycemia-induced age-related macular degeneration. Proc Natl Acad Sci USA 2017; 114(22): E4472-81.
[http://dx.doi.org/10.1073/pnas.1702302114] [PMID: 28507131]

[24] Kutsyr O, Maestre-Carballa L, Lluesma-Gomez M, Martinez-Garcia M, Cuenca N, Lax P. Retinitis pigmentosa is associated with shifts in the gut microbiome. Sci Rep 2021; 11(1): 6692.
[http://dx.doi.org/10.1038/s41598-021-86052-1] [PMID: 33758301]

[25] Floyd JL, Grant MB. The Gut–Eye Axis: Lessons Learned from Murine Models. Ophthalmol Ther 2020; 9(3): 499-513.
[http://dx.doi.org/10.1007/s40123-020-00278-2] [PMID: 32617914]

[26] Vavricka SR, Schoepfer A, Scharl M, Lakatos PL, Navarini A, Rogler G. Extraintestinal Manifestations of Inflammatory Bowel Disease. Inflamm Bowel Dis 2015; 21(8): 1982-92.
[http://dx.doi.org/10.1097/MIB.0000000000000392] [PMID: 26154136]

[27] Kugadas A, Wright Q, Geddes-McAlister J, Gadjeva M. Role of Microbiota in Strengthening Ocular Mucosal Barrier Function Through Secretory IgA. Invest Ophthalmol Vis Sci 2017; 58(11): 4593-600.
[http://dx.doi.org/10.1167/iovs.17-22119] [PMID: 28892827]

[28] Woo V, Alenghat T. Host–microbiota interactions: epigenomic regulation. Curr Opin Immunol 2017; 44: 52-60. Available from: https://www.sciencedirect.com/science/article/pii/S0952791516301558
[http://dx.doi.org/10.1016/j.coi.2016.12.001] [PMID: 28103497]

[29] Cavuoto KM, Banerjee S, Galor A. Relationship between the microbiome and ocular health. Ocul Surf 2019; 17(3): 384-92. Available from: https://www.sciencedirect.com/science/article/pii/S154201241930028X
[http://dx.doi.org/10.1016/j.jtos.2019.05.006] [PMID: 31125783]

[30] Akhtar-Schäfer I, Wang L, Krohne TU, Xu H, Langmann T. Modulation of three key innate immune pathways for the most common retinal degenerative diseases. EMBO Mol Med 2018; 10(10): e8259.
[http://dx.doi.org/10.15252/emmm.201708259] [PMID: 30224384]

[31] Lee RW, Nicholson LB, Sen HN, Chan C-C, Wei L, Nussenblatt RB, *et al.* Autoimmune and autoinflammatory mechanisms in uveitis. Seminars in immunopathology. Springer 2014; pp. 581-94.

[32] Bodaghi B, Cassoux N, Wechsler B, *et al.* Chronic severe uveitis: etiology and visual outcome in 927 patients from a single center. Medicine (Baltimore) 2001; 80(4): 263-70.
[http://dx.doi.org/10.1097/00005792-200107000-00005] [PMID: 11470987]

[33] Rao N. Uveitis in developing countries. Indian J Ophthalmol 2013; 61(6): 253-4.
[http://dx.doi.org/10.4103/0301-4738.114090] [PMID: 23803475]

[34] Deschenes J, Murray PI, Rao NA, Nussenblatt RB. International Uveitis Study Group (IUSG): clinical classification of uveitis. Ocul Immunol Inflamm 2008; 16(1-2): 1-2.
[http://dx.doi.org/10.1080/09273940801899822] [PMID: 18379933]

[35] Kumari R. Blindness and Visual Impairment. Health Science Journal. 2023; 17(12): 1-4.

[36] Tsirouki T, Dastiridou A, Symeonidis C, Tounakaki O, Brazitikou I, Kalogeropoulos C, Androudi S. A focus on the epidemiology of uveitis. Ocular immunology and inflammation. 2018 Jan 2; 26(1): 2-16.

[37] Ye Z, Wu C, Zhang N, *et al.* Altered gut microbiome composition in patients with Vogt-Koyanag--Harada disease. Gut Microbes 2020; 11(3): 539-55.
[http://dx.doi.org/10.1080/19490976.2019.1700754] [PMID: 31928124]

[38] Forrester JV, Kuffova L, Dick AD. Autoimmunity, autoinflammation, and infection in uveitis. Am J Ophthalmol 2018; 189: 77-85.
[http://dx.doi.org/10.1016/j.ajo.2018.02.019] [PMID: 29505775]

[39] Kalyana Chakravarthy S, Jayasudha R, Sai Prashanthi G, *et al.* Dysbiosis in the gut bacterial microbiome of patients with uveitis, an inflammatory disease of the eye. Indian J Microbiol 2018; 58(4): 457-69.
[http://dx.doi.org/10.1007/s12088-018-0746-9] [PMID: 30262956]

[40] Heissigerova J, Seidler Stangova P, Klimova A, Svozilkova P, Hrncir T, Stepankova R, *et al.* The microbiota determines susceptibility to experimental autoimmune uveoretinitis. J Immunol Res. 2016; 2016.

[41] Horai R, Zárate-Bladés CR, Dillenburg-Pilla P, *et al.* Microbiota-dependent activation of an autoreactive T cell receptor provokes autoimmunity in an immunologically privileged site. Immunity 2015; 43(2): 343-53.
[http://dx.doi.org/10.1016/j.immuni.2015.07.014] [PMID: 26287682]

[42] Nakamura YK, Metea C, Karstens L, *et al.* Gut microbial alterations associated with protection from autoimmune uveitis. Invest Ophthalmol Vis Sci 2016; 57(8): 3747-58.
[http://dx.doi.org/10.1167/iovs.16-19733] [PMID: 27415793]

[43] Nakamura YK, Janowitz C, Metea C, *et al.* Short chain fatty acids ameliorate immune-mediated uveitis partially by altering migration of lymphocytes from the intestine. Sci Rep 2017; 7(1): 11745.
[http://dx.doi.org/10.1038/s41598-017-12163-3] [PMID: 28924192]

[44] Huang X, Ye Z, Cao Q, *et al.* Gut microbiota composition and fecal metabolic phenotype in patients with acute anterior uveitis. Invest Ophthalmol Vis Sci 2018; 59(3): 1523-31.
[http://dx.doi.org/10.1167/iovs.17-22677] [PMID: 29625474]

[45] Yoshino S, Sasatomi E, Ohsawa M. Bacterial lipopolysaccharide acts as an adjuvant to induce autoimmune arthritisin mice. Immunology 2000; 99(4): 607-14.
[http://dx.doi.org/10.1046/j.1365-2567.2000.00015.x] [PMID: 10792509]

[46] Rojas M, Restrepo-Jiménez P, Monsalve DM, *et al.* Molecular mimicry and autoimmunity. J Autoimmun 2018; 95: 100-23.
[http://dx.doi.org/10.1016/j.jaut.2018.10.012] [PMID: 30509385]

[47] Berer K, Mues M, Koutrolos M, *et al.* Commensal microbiota and myelin autoantigen cooperate to trigger autoimmune demyelination. Nature 2011; 479(7374): 538-41.
[http://dx.doi.org/10.1038/nature10554] [PMID: 22031325]

[48] Horai R, Za CR, Dillenburg-pilla P, Rachel R. Microbiota-Dependent Activation of an Autoreactive T Cell Receptor Provokes Autoimmunity in an Immunologically Privileged Site Article Microbiota-Dependent Activation of an Autoreactive T Cell Receptor Provokes Autoimmunity in an Immunologically Privilege. 2015; 343–53.

[49] Fu X, Chen D. Role of Gut Microbiome in Autoimmune Uveitis 2021; 610041: 168-77.

[50] Ciccia F, Guggino G, Rizzo A, *et al.* Dysbiosis and zonulin upregulation alter gut epithelial and vascular barriers in patients with ankylosing spondylitis. Ann Rheum Dis 2017; 76(6): 1123-32.
[http://dx.doi.org/10.1136/annrheumdis-2016-210000] [PMID: 28069576]

[51] Janowitz C, Nakamura YK, Metea C, *et al.* Disruption of intestinal homeostasis and intestinal microbiota during experimental autoimmune uveitis. Invest Ophthalmol Vis Sci 2019; 60(1): 420-9.
[http://dx.doi.org/10.1167/iovs.18-24813] [PMID: 30695094]

[52] Parthasarathy R, Santiago F, McCluskey P, Kaakoush NO, Tedla N, Wakefield D. The microbiome in HLA-B27-associated disease: implications for acute anterior uveitis and recommendations for future studies. Trends Microbiol 2023; 31(2): 142-58.
[http://dx.doi.org/10.1016/j.tim.2022.08.008] [PMID: 36058784]

[53] Jayaram H, Kolko M, Friedman DS, Gazzard G. Glaucoma: now and beyond. Lancet 2023; 402(10414): 1788-801.
[http://dx.doi.org/10.1016/S0140-6736(23)01289-8] [PMID: 37742700]

[54] Allison K, Patel D, Alabi O. Epidemiology of glaucoma: the past, present, and predictions for the future. Cureus 2020; 12(11): e11686.
[http://dx.doi.org/10.7759/cureus.11686] [PMID: 33391921]

[55] Yang J, Patil RV, Yu H, Gordon M, Wax MB. T cell subsets and sIL-2R/IL-2 levels in patients with glaucoma. Am J Ophthalmol 2001; 131(4): 421-6.
[http://dx.doi.org/10.1016/S0002-9394(00)00862-X] [PMID: 11292402]

[56] Kountouras J, Mylopoulos N, Boura P, *et al.* Relationship between Helicobacter pylori infection and glaucoma11The authors have no commercial interests in the products or devices mention herein. Ophthalmology 2001; 108(3): 599-604.
[http://dx.doi.org/10.1016/S0161-6420(00)00598-4] [PMID: 11237916]

[57] Gong H, Zhang S, Li Q, *et al.* Gut microbiota compositional profile and serum metabolic phenotype in patients with primary open-angle glaucoma. Exp Eye Res 2020; 191: 107921.
[http://dx.doi.org/10.1016/j.exer.2020.107921] [PMID: 31917963]

[58] Wu Y, Shi R, Chen H, *et al.* Effect of the gut microbiome in glaucoma risk from the causal perspective. BMJ Open Ophthalmol 2024; 9(1): e001547.
[http://dx.doi.org/10.1136/bmjophth-2023-001547] [PMID: 38286567]

[59] Chen H, Cho KS, Vu THK, *et al.* Commensal microflora-induced T cell responses mediate progressive neurodegeneration in glaucoma. Nat Commun 2018; 9(1): 3209.
[http://dx.doi.org/10.1038/s41467-018-05681-9] [PMID: 30097565]

[60] Skrzypecki J, Izdebska J, Kamińska A, *et al.* Glaucoma patients have an increased level of

trimethylamine, a toxic product of gut bacteria, in the aqueous humor: a pilot study. Int Ophthalmol 2021; 41(1): 341-7.
[http://dx.doi.org/10.1007/s10792-020-01587-y] [PMID: 32914277]

[61] Skrzypecki J, Żera T, Ufnal M. Butyrate, a gut bacterial metabolite, lowers intraocular pressure in normotensive but not in hypertensive rats. J Glaucoma 2018; 27(9): 823-7.
[http://dx.doi.org/10.1097/IJG.0000000000001025] [PMID: 30001267]

[62] Zysset-burri DC, Morandi S, Herzog EL, Berger LE, Zinkernagel MS. Progress in Retinal and Eye Research The role of the gut microbiome in eye diseases. Prog Retin Eye Res. 2023; 92(September 2022): 101117.

[63] Wong WL, Su X, Li X, *et al.* Global prevalence of age-related macular degeneration and disease burden projection for 2020 and 2040: a systematic review and meta-analysis. Lancet Glob Health 2014; 2(2): e106-16.
[http://dx.doi.org/10.1016/S2214-109X(13)70145-1] [PMID: 25104651]

[64] Ambati J, Fowler BJ. Mechanisms of age-related macular degeneration. Neuron 2012; 75(1): 26-39.
[http://dx.doi.org/10.1016/j.neuron.2012.06.018] [PMID: 22794258]

[65] Handa JT, Bowes Rickman C, Dick AD, *et al.* A systems biology approach towards understanding and treating non-neovascular age-related macular degeneration. Nat Commun 2019; 10(1): 3347.
[http://dx.doi.org/10.1038/s41467-019-11262-1] [PMID: 31350409]

[66] Morita Y, Jounai K, Sakamoto A, *et al.* Long-term intake of *Lactobacillus paracasei* KW3110 prevents age-related chronic inflammation and retinal cell loss in physiologically aged mice. Aging (Albany NY) 2018; 10(10): 2723-40.
[http://dx.doi.org/10.18632/aging.101583] [PMID: 30341255]

[67] Zhang M, Chu Y, Mowery J, Konkel B, Galli S, Theos AC. Pgc-1 α repression and high-fat diet induce age-related macular degeneration-like phenotypes in mice. 2018;1–10.

[68] Zysset-burri DC, Zinkernagel MS, Keller I, Berger LE, Largiadèr CR, Wittwer M, *et al.* Associations of the intestinal microbiome with the complement system in neovascular age-related macular degeneration. npj. Genomic Med 3: 1-11.

[69] Zhou H, Peng C, Huang DS, Liu L, Guan P. microRNA expression profiling based on microarray approach in human diabetic retinopathy: a systematic review and meta-analysis. DNA Cell Biol 2020; 39(3): 441-50.
[http://dx.doi.org/10.1089/dna.2019.4942] [PMID: 32101049]

[70] Sharma A. Emerging simplified retinal imaging. Manag Diabet Retin. 2017; 60: 56–62.

[71] Sharma A. Emerging simplified retinal imaging. Dev Ophthalmol 2017; 60: 56-62.
[http://dx.doi.org/10.1159/000459690] [PMID: 28427065]

[72] Cai Y, Kang Y. Gut microbiota and metabolites in diabetic retinopathy: insights into pathogenesis for novel therapeutic strategies. Biomed Pharmacother. 2023; 164: 114994.
[http://dx.doi.org/10.1016/j.biopha.2023.114994]

[73] Grauslund J. Long-term mortality and retinopathy in type 1 diabetes. Acta Ophthalmol. 2010; 88(thesis1): 1–14.

[74] Srivastava B, Ramya B, Prathiba V, Mohan V. Systemic factors affecting diabetic retinopathy. Journal of Diabetology 2018; 9(3): 73-7.
[http://dx.doi.org/10.4103/jod.jod_35_17]

[75] Jiao J, Yu H, Yao L, Li L, Yang X, Liu L. Recent insights into the role of gut microbiota in diabetic retinopathy. J Inflamm Res 2021; 14: 6929-38.
[http://dx.doi.org/10.2147/JIR.S336148] [PMID: 34938095]

[76] Gurung M, Li Z, You H, *et al.* Role of gut microbiota in type 2 diabetes pathophysiology. EBioMedicine 2020; 51: 102590.

[http://dx.doi.org/10.1016/j.ebiom.2019.11.051] [PMID: 31901868]

[77] Eckburg PB, Bik EM, Bernstein CN, Purdom E, Dethlefsen L, Sargent M, *et al.* Diversity of the human intestinal microbial flora. Science (80-). 2005; 308(5728): 1635–8. [http://dx.doi.org/10.1126/science.1110591]

[78] Huang Y, Yang B, Li W. Defining the normal core microbiome of conjunctival microbial communities. Clin Microbiol Infect 2016; 22(7): 643.e7-643.e12. [http://dx.doi.org/10.1016/j.cmi.2016.04.008] [PMID: 27102141]

[79] Fernandes R, Viana SD, Nunes S, Reis F. Diabetic gut microbiota dysbiosis as an inflammaging and immunosenescence condition that fosters progression of retinopathy and nephropathy. Biochim Biophys Acta Mol Basis Dis 2019; 1865(7): 1876-97. [http://dx.doi.org/10.1016/j.bbadis.2018.09.032] [PMID: 30287404]

[80] Huang Y, Wang Z, Ma H, *et al.* Dysbiosis and implication of the gut microbiota in diabetic retinopathy. Front Cell Infect Microbiol 2021; 11: 646348. [http://dx.doi.org/10.3389/fcimb.2021.646348] [PMID: 33816351]

[81] Das T, Jayasudha R, Chakravarthy S, *et al.* Alterations in the gut bacterial microbiome in people with type 2 diabetes mellitus and diabetic retinopathy. Sci Rep 2021; 11(1): 2738. [http://dx.doi.org/10.1038/s41598-021-82538-0] [PMID: 33531650]

[82] Zhou Z, Zheng Z, Xiong X, *et al.* Gut microbiota composition and fecal metabolic profiling in patients with diabetic retinopathy. Front Cell Dev Biol 2021; 9: 732204. [http://dx.doi.org/10.3389/fcell.2021.732204] [PMID: 34722512]

[83] Rowan S, Taylor A. The role of microbiota in retinal disease. Retin Degener Dis Mech Exp Ther 2018; pp. 429-35. [http://dx.doi.org/10.1007/978-3-319-75402-4_53]

[84] Dao D, Xie B, Nadeem U, *et al.* High-fat diet alters the retinal transcriptome in the absence of gut microbiota. Cells 2021; 10(8): 2119. [http://dx.doi.org/10.3390/cells10082119] [PMID: 34440888]

[85] Pascolini D, Mariotti SP. Global estimates of visual impairment: 2010. Br J Ophthalmol 2012; 96(5): 614-8. [http://dx.doi.org/10.1136/bjophthalmol-2011-300539] [PMID: 22133988]

[86] Al-Mujaini A, Al-Kharusi N, Thakral A, Wali UK. Bacterial keratitis: perspective on epidemiology, clinico-pathogenesis, diagnosis and treatment. Sultan Qaboos Univ Med J 2009; 9(2): 184-95. [PMID: 21509299]

[87] Prajna V, Prajna L, Muthiah S. Fungal keratitis: The Aravind experience. Indian J Ophthalmol 2017; 65(10): 912-9. [http://dx.doi.org/10.4103/ijo.IJO_821_17] [PMID: 29044053]

[88] Kugadas A, Christiansen SH, Sankaranarayanan S, *et al.* Impact of microbiota on resistance to ocular Pseudomonas aeruginosa-induced keratitis. PLoS Pathog 2016; 12(9): e1005855. [http://dx.doi.org/10.1371/journal.ppat.1005855] [PMID: 27658245]

[89] Miller D, Cavuoto KM, Alfonso EC. Bacterial keratitis. Infect Cornea Conjunctiva 2021; pp. 85-104.

[90] Shivaji S, Jayasudha R, Chakravarthy SK, *et al.* Alterations in the conjunctival surface bacterial microbiome in bacterial keratitis patients. Exp Eye Res 2021; 203: 108418. [http://dx.doi.org/10.1016/j.exer.2020.108418] [PMID: 33359511]

[91] Jayasudha R, Kalyana Chakravarthy S, Sai Prashanthi G, *et al.* Alterations in gut bacterial and fungal microbiomes are associated with bacterial Keratitis, an inflammatory disease of the human eye. J Biosci 2018; 43(5): 835-56. [http://dx.doi.org/10.1007/s12038-018-9798-6] [PMID: 30541945]

[92] Kuo MT, Chen JL, Hsu SL, Chen A, You HL. An omics approach to diagnosing or investigating

fungal keratitis. Int J Mol Sci 2019; 20(15): 3631.
[http://dx.doi.org/10.3390/ijms20153631] [PMID: 31349542]

[93] Kuo MT, Hsu SL, You HL, *et al.* Diagnosing Fungal Keratitis and Simultaneously Identifying *Fusarium* and *Aspergillus* Keratitis with a Dot Hybridization Array. J Fungi (Basel) 2022; 8(1): 64.
[http://dx.doi.org/10.3390/jof8010064] [PMID: 35050004]

[94] Khor WB, Prajna VN, Garg P, *et al.* The Asia Cornea Society Infectious Keratitis Study: a prospective multicenter study of infectious keratitis in Asia. Am J Ophthalmol 2018; 195: 161-70.
[http://dx.doi.org/10.1016/j.ajo.2018.07.040] [PMID: 30098351]

[95] Ting DSJ, Ho CS, Deshmukh R, Said DG, Dua HS. Infectious keratitis: an update on epidemiology, causative microorganisms, risk factors, and antimicrobial resistance. Eye (Lond) 2021; 35(4): 1084-101.
[http://dx.doi.org/10.1038/s41433-020-01339-3] [PMID: 33414529]

[96] Ting DSJ, Galal M, Kulkarni B, *et al.* Clinical characteristics and outcomes of fungal keratitis in the United Kingdom 2011–2020: a 10-year study. J Fungi (Basel) 2021; 7(11): 966.
[http://dx.doi.org/10.3390/jof7110966] [PMID: 34829253]

[97] Thomas PA, Kaliamurthy J. Mycotic keratitis: epidemiology, diagnosis and management. Clin Microbiol Infect 2013; 19(3): 210-20.
[http://dx.doi.org/10.1111/1469-0691.12126] [PMID: 23398543]

[98] Nielsen SE, Nielsen E, Julian HO, *et al.* Incidence and clinical characteristics of fungal keratitis in a D anish population from 2000 to 2013. Acta Ophthalmol 2015; 93(1): 54-8.
[http://dx.doi.org/10.1111/aos.12440] [PMID: 24836583]

[99] Zhou Y, Holland MJ, Makalo P, *et al.* The conjunctival microbiome in health and trachomatous disease: a case control study. Genome Med 2014; 6(11): 99.
[http://dx.doi.org/10.1186/s13073-014-0099-x] [PMID: 25484919]

[100] Kalyana Chakravarthy S, Jayasudha R, Ranjith K, *et al.* Alterations in the gut bacterial microbiome in fungal Keratitis patients. PLoS One 2018; 13(6): e0199640.
[http://dx.doi.org/10.1371/journal.pone.0199640] [PMID: 29933394]

[101] Zysset-Burri DC, Keller I, Berger LE, *et al.* Retinal artery occlusion is associated with compositional and functional shifts in the gut microbiome and altered trimethylamine-N-oxide levels. Sci Rep 2019; 9(1): 15303.
[http://dx.doi.org/10.1038/s41598-019-51698-5] [PMID: 31653902]

[102] Koren O, Spor A, Felin J, *et al.* Human oral, gut, and plaque microbiota in patients with atherosclerosis. Proc Natl Acad Sci USA 2011; 108(Suppl 1) (Suppl. 1): 4592-8.
[http://dx.doi.org/10.1073/pnas.1011383107] [PMID: 20937873]

[103] Vourakis M, Mayer G, Rousseau G. The role of gut microbiota on cholesterol metabolism in atherosclerosis. Int J Mol Sci 2021; 22(15): 8074.
[http://dx.doi.org/10.3390/ijms22158074] [PMID: 34360839]

[104] Walter J, Ley R. The human gut microbiome: ecology and recent evolutionary changes. Annu Rev Microbiol 2011; 65(1): 411-29.
[http://dx.doi.org/10.1146/annurev-micro-090110-102830] [PMID: 21682646]

[105] Flint HJ. The impact of nutrition on the human microbiome. Nutr Rev. 2012; 70(1): S10--S13.
[http://dx.doi.org/10.1111/j.1753-4887.2012.00499.x]

[106] Gupta A, Saha S, Khanna S. Therapies to modulate gut microbiota: Past, present and future. World J Gastroenterol 2020; 26(8): 777-88.
[http://dx.doi.org/10.3748/wjg.v26.i8.777] [PMID: 32148376]

[107] Kashyap PC, Chia N, Nelson H, Segal E, Elinav E. Microbiome at the frontier of personalized medicine. Mayo Clinic Proceedings. Elsevier 2017; pp. 1855-64.
[http://dx.doi.org/10.1016/j.mayocp.2017.10.004]

[108] Jimenez M, Langer R, Traverso G. Microbial therapeutics: New opportunities for drug delivery. J Exp Med 2019; 216(5): 1005-9.
[http://dx.doi.org/10.1084/jem.20190609] [PMID: 31028093]

[109] Byndloss MX, Olsan EE, Rivera-Chávez F, Tiffany CR, Cevallos SA, Lokken KL, *et al.* Microbiota-activated PPAR-γ signaling inhibits dysbiotic Enterobacteriaceae expansion. Science (80-). 2017; 357(6351): 570–5.

[110] Litvak Y, Byndloss MX, Tsolis RM, Bäumler AJ. Dysbiotic Proteobacteria expansion: a microbial signature of epithelial dysfunction. Curr Opin Microbiol 2017; 39: 1-6.
[http://dx.doi.org/10.1016/j.mib.2017.07.003] [PMID: 28783509]

[111] Thaiss CA, Elinav E. The remedy within: will the microbiome fulfill its therapeutic promise? J Mol Med (Berl) 2017; 95(10): 1021-7.
[http://dx.doi.org/10.1007/s00109-017-1563-z] [PMID: 28656322]

[112] Yadav M, Chauhan NS. Microbiome therapeutics: exploring the present scenario and challenges. Gastroenterol Rep (Oxf) 2022; 10: goab046.
[http://dx.doi.org/10.1093/gastro/goab046] [PMID: 35382166]

[113] Joossens M, De Preter V, Ballet V, Verbeke K, Rutgeerts P, Vermeire S. Effect of oligofructose-enriched inulin (OF-IN) on bacterial composition and disease activity of patients with Crohn's disease: results from a double-blinded randomised controlled trial: Table 1. Gut 2012; 61(6): 958.
[http://dx.doi.org/10.1136/gutjnl-2011-300413] [PMID: 21749983]

[114] Van Doan H, Hoseinifar SH, Ringø E, Ángeles Esteban M, Dadar M, Dawood MAO, *et al.* Host-associated probiotics: a key factor in sustainable aquaculture. Rev Fish Sci Aquac. 2020; 28(1): 16–42.
[http://dx.doi.org/10.1080/23308249.2019.1643288]

[115] Wang C, Chuprom J, Wang Y, Fu L. Beneficial bacteria for aquaculture: nutrition, bacteriostasis and immunoregulation. J Appl Microbiol 2020; 128(1): 28-40.
[http://dx.doi.org/10.1111/jam.14383] [PMID: 31306569]

[116] Pérez-Sánchez T, Ruiz-Zarzuela I, de Blas I, Balcázar JL. Probiotics in aquaculture: a current assessment. Rev Aquacult 2014; 6(3): 133-46.
[http://dx.doi.org/10.1111/raq.12033]

[117] Charbonneau MR, Isabella VM, Li N, Kurtz CB. Developing a new class of engineered live bacterial therapeutics to treat human diseases. Nat Commun 2020; 11(1): 1738.
[http://dx.doi.org/10.1038/s41467-020-15508-1] [PMID: 32269218]

[118] Cuello-Garcia CA, Brożek JL, Fiocchi A, *et al.* Probiotics for the prevention of allergy: A systematic review and meta-analysis of randomized controlled trials. J Allergy Clin Immunol 2015; 136(4): 952-61.
[http://dx.doi.org/10.1016/j.jaci.2015.04.031] [PMID: 26044853]

[119] Fujiya M, Ueno N, Kohgo Y. Probiotic treatments for induction and maintenance of remission in inflammatory bowel diseases: a meta-analysis of randomized controlled trials. Clin J Gastroenterol 2014; 7(1): 1-13.
[http://dx.doi.org/10.1007/s12328-013-0440-8] [PMID: 26183502]

[120] Kesarcodi-Watson A, Kaspar H, Lategan MJ, Gibson L. Probiotics in aquaculture: The need, principles and mechanisms of action and screening processes. Aquaculture 2008; 274(1): 1-14.
[http://dx.doi.org/10.1016/j.aquaculture.2007.11.019]

[121] Weynberg KD, Jaschke PR. Building better bacteriophage with biofoundries to combat antibiotic-resistant bacteria. Phage (New Rochelle) 2020; 1(1): 23-6.
[http://dx.doi.org/10.1089/phage.2019.0005] [PMID: 36147618]

[122] Drilling AJ, Ooi ML, Miljkovic D, *et al.* Long-term safety of topical bacteriophage application to the frontal sinus region. Front Cell Infect Microbiol 2017; 7: 49.
[http://dx.doi.org/10.3389/fcimb.2017.00049] [PMID: 28286740]

[123] Fish R, Kutter E, Wheat G, Blasdel B, Kutateladze M, Kuhl S. Compassionate use of bacteriophage therapy for foot ulcer treatment as an effective step for moving toward clinical trials. Bacteriophage Ther from lab to Clin Pract. 2018; 159–70.
[http://dx.doi.org/10.1007/978-1-4939-7395-8_14]

[124] Alemayehu D, Casey PG, McAuliffe O, *et al.* Bacteriophages φMR299-2 and φNH-4 can eliminate Pseudomonas aeruginosa in the murine lung and on cystic fibrosis lung airway cells. MBio 2012; 3(2): e00029-12.
[http://dx.doi.org/10.1128/mBio.00029-12] [PMID: 22396480]

[125] Brown TL, Petrovski S, Dyson ZA, Seviour R, Tucci J. The formulation of bacteriophage in a semi solid preparation for control of Propionibacterium acnes growth. PLoS One 2016; 11(3): e0151184.
[http://dx.doi.org/10.1371/journal.pone.0151184] [PMID: 26964063]

[126] Voorhees PJ, Cruz-Teran C, Edelstein J, Lai SK. Challenges & opportunities for phage-based in situ microbiome engineering in the gut. J Control Release 2020; 326: 106-19.
[http://dx.doi.org/10.1016/j.jconrel.2020.06.016] [PMID: 32569705]

[127] Brandt LJ. Fecal transplantation for the treatment of Clostridium difficile infection. Gastroenterol Hepatol. 2012; 8(3): 191.

[128] Borody TJ, Clancy A. Fecal microbiota transplantation for ulcerative colitis—where to from here? Transl Gastroenterol Hepatol 2019; 4: 48.
[http://dx.doi.org/10.21037/tgh.2019.06.04] [PMID: 31304425]

[129] Ianiro G, Porcari S, Bibbò S, *et al.* Donor program for fecal microbiota transplantation: A 3-year experience of a large-volume Italian stool bank. Dig Liver Dis 2021; 53(11): 1428-32.
[http://dx.doi.org/10.1016/j.dld.2021.04.009] [PMID: 34030988]

[130] Baunwall SMD, Lee MM, Eriksen MK, *et al.* Faecal microbiota transplantation for recurrent *Clostridioides difficile* infection: An updated systematic review and meta-analysis. EClinicalMedicine 2020; 29-30: 100642.
[http://dx.doi.org/10.1016/j.eclinm.2020.100642] [PMID: 33437951]

[131] Cammarota G, Masucci L, Ianiro G, Bibbò S, Dinoi G, Costamagna G, *et al.* Randomised clinical trial: faecal microbiota transplantation by colonoscopy vs. vancomycin for the treatment of recurrent Clostridium difficile infection. Aliment Pharmacol Ther. 2015; 41(9): 835–43.

[132] Airola C, Severino A, Porcari S, *et al.* Future modulation of gut microbiota: from eubiotics to FMT, engineered bacteria, and phage therapy. Antibiotics (Basel) 2023; 12(5): 868.
[http://dx.doi.org/10.3390/antibiotics12050868] [PMID: 37237771]

CHAPTER 7

Neurological Disorders and the Gut-Brain Axis

Moitreyee Chattopadhyay[1,*], **Ansar Laskar**[1], **Sk Safiur Rahaman**[1] and **Ananya Chanda**[2]

[1] *Department of Pharmaceutical Technology, Maulana Abul Kalam Azad University of Technology W.B. Haringhata Nadia-741249, West Bengal, India*

[2] *Adamas University, Barasat-Barrackpore Road, Barbaria, Jagannathpur, 24 Parganas (North), Kolkata-700126, West Bengal, India*

Abstract: The term "gut microbiota" refers to the group of microbes that reside in the GI tract, which extends from the mouth to the rectum. The term "microbiome," which refers to the substance of these microbes, is also used to describe this collection of microorganisms. A complex and reciprocal relationship between the stomach and the central nervous system (CNS), the gut-brain axis influences both health and disease. The hypothalamic-pituitary-adrenal (HPA) axis, sympatho-adrenal axis, autonomic nervous system (ANS), enteric nervous system (ENS), and descending monoaminergic pathways are the routes that are engaged in this communication. Mesenteric lymphoid tissues can become translocated with compounds produced by gut bacteria and molecular patterns associated with microbes due to dysbiosis in the gut and a weakened gut barrier. The complex immunological interaction between the gut bacteria and host cells allows for their mutually beneficial existence. When commensal bacteria are present, the gut's immune system must gently maintain equilibrium in order to continue performing its essential defensive role. Our goal is to understand how gut microbes relate to neurological conditions, particularly anxiety, depression, Parkinson's disease, autism spectrum disorders, and Alzheimer's disease. Further nutritional therapies can be utilized to improve overall gut health, induce eubiosis, and alter the composition of the gut microbiota and associated metabolites in addition to current medicinal approaches.

Keywords: Autism spectrum disorders, Alzheimer's disease, Anxiety, Depression, Eubiosis, Gut microbiota, Homeostasis, HPA axis, Immunological interaction, Microbiome, Metabolites, Nutritional, Parkinson's disease.

INTRODUCTION

The collection of microorganisms that live in the GI tract, from the mouth to the rectum is known as the gut microbiota. This group of microorganisms is also refe-

* **Corresponding author Moitreyee Chattopadhyay:** Department of Pharmaceutical Technology, Maulana Abul Kalam Azad University of Technology W.B. Haringhata Nadia-741249, West Bengal, India;
E-mail: pharmacol2015@gmail.com

Sandipan Dasgupta & Moitreyee Chattopadhyay (Eds.)

rred to as the microbiome, which represents the material of these microbes [1]. The makeup of the microbes, in the system varies in parts like the stomach, small intestine, and colon. These microbes and bacteria have a relationship with the host. While archaea, yeast, and fungi are also present in the GI tract, our knowledge about them is still limited. Previously thought to start after birth, it now appears that the establishment of gut microbiota begins during development [2]. The gut microbiota's composition is influenced by a range of factors, including antibiotic use, age, obesity, gastrointestinal disorders, and environment and nutrition. The bacteria, viruses, eukaryotic organisms, and archaea that make up the human body's enormous microbial ecosystem are between 10 and 100 trillion in number, individually [3]. Numerous environmental elements, including pH and oxygen content, are present in the body's habitat and have an impact on the ability of different bacteria to colonize. As a result, the exact anatomical site of colonization greatly influences the composition of the microbiota. In the human gut, microorganisms belonging to the families Firmicutes and Bacteroidetes predominate. Actinobacteria, Proteobacteria, Verrucomicrobia, Fusobacteria, Cyanobacteria, and Tenericutes are also present, albeit in fewer amounts [4].

The complex interactions that gut microorganisms have with each other and the host are a result of their direct and indirect interactions. The dynamics of the gut microbiome are closely related to the health of the gastrointestinal tract and other organ systems, including the brain [5]. Dietary materials such as fiber are used by gut microorganisms in greater quantities than the host can absorb. These microorganisms produce a wide range of compounds that have recently been dubbed "postbiotics." These include lactic acid, ammonia, volatile fatty acids (VFAs, sometimes called short-chain fatty acids), and gases like hydrogen, carbon dioxide, and methane [6].

The gut microbiome is essential for promoting adult development and preserving bodily equilibrium. Its influence on human metabolic processes is one of its primary functions since it breaks down complex polysaccharides included in meals. Furthermore, these microorganisms help regulate gut motility, the gut barrier, and the body's fat distribution. By controlling the growth of gut-associated lymphoid tissue and halting the colonization of dangerous pathogens, they also contribute to immune function. They may also have an impact on the host's mitochondrial and energy metabolism [7]. Comprehending the variety of gut microbes and their functions in physiology has been the focus of recent research. By changing these bacteria' makeup, this understanding may someday help prevent and cure illnesses. Certain gut floras, for example, have been found in trials to improve the efficacy of conventional chemotherapy medications [8]. Diet and age have a big impact on the makeup of the gut microbiota. Various studies, involving both humans and animals, have demonstrated that dietary practices can cause substantial changes in the microbiome. For example, due to their different diets, people in rural Africa and Europe have quite different gut bacterial compositions [9]. Wu *et al.* found that a diet high in animal fats and proteins was linked to greater levels of Bacteroides, whereas a diet high in carbohydrates was linked to higher levels of Prevotella after analyzing stool samples from 98 people [10]. Disease and infection can also upset the balance of the gut flora, potentially leading to adverse effects on the host. The human body and bacteria cohabit symbiotically to produce a complex micro-ecological system. Variations in the number and kind of gut microbes can affect how well the gut barrier functions, secrete more toxic compounds and less helpful ones, and perhaps cause several gastrointestinal and systemic illnesses [11]. Three basic approaches are usually used to identify gut microorganisms: high-throughput sequencing technologies, conventional molecular biology methods that do not require culture and bacterial culture. In contrast, the latter two techniques, on the other hand, extract bacterial DNA for quick identification from stool samples and provide a more thorough understanding of the types of bacteria present [12].

Emotional dysregulation, dementia, developmental disorders, and other immune-related neurological illnesses are linked to changes in the gut microbiota and the creation of microbial metabolites as described in Fig. (**1**). The brain is made up of several neuronal and non-neuronal cell types that are connected by complex structural networks [13]. The brain is the organ that controls all behavior. More than 98% of the bacteria in the body reside in the gastrointestinal (GI) tract; these bacteria are referred to as gut microbiota [14]. The rise of omics approaches has allowed us to better understand the role of the gut microbiota in regulating gut-brain connections. Research on both human and animal gut microbiota has shown that the microbiota may affect immune responses, metabolites, hormone synthesis, and brain behavior and development [15, 16]. This implies that improving or maybe treating brain disorders could be possible by altering the gut flora. Additionally, through intricate neurohumoral networks, messages from the brain can affect the sensory and secretory processes of the stomach [17]. Similarly, signals from the gastrointestinal tract that are visceral afferents can influence brain activity. As a significant factor in controlling normal brain function and contributing to the development of neuropathological illnesses, recent research has brought attention to the gut-brain axis [18]. The processes relating gut microbiota to brain diseases still require comprehensive confirmation. There are new technologies that can go beyond correlation to find biological pathways that could lead to effective treatments. As a significant factor in controlling normal brain function and contributing to the development of neuropathological illnesses, recent research has brought attention to the gut-brain axis [19]. The processes relating gut microbiota to brain diseases still require comprehensive confirmation, though. There are new technologies that can go beyond correlation to find biological pathways that could lead to effective treatments [20]. Scientists explore the function of microbiota in neurological illnesses, including schizophrenia, ASD, anxiety, depression, Parkinson's disease, Alzheimer's disease, and multiple sclerosis, as well as the interactions and signalling networks between the gut and the brain [21].

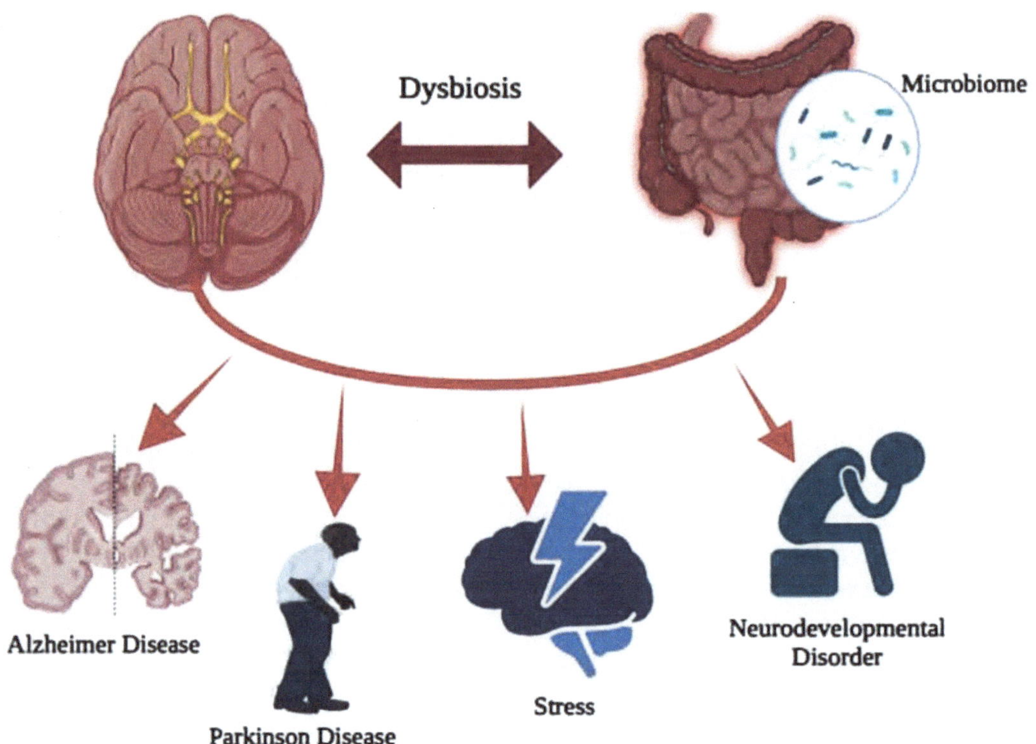

Fig. (1). Different neuronal complications due to gut microbiota

GUT-BRAIN AXIS

Gut and Nervous System Interaction

The gut-brain axis is a complex, reciprocal link between the gut and the central nervous system (CNS) that affects both health and disease. This relationship enables the vagus nerve to send visceral signals from the gut that impact CNS processes, such as mood and reflexes. On the other hand, by sending signals to the stomach, the CNS can control other activities including the physiology of the gut. The pathways that are involved in this communication include the autonomic nervous system (ANS), enteric nervous system (ENS), hypothalamic-pituitar--adrenal (HPA) axis, sympatho-adrenal axis, and descending monoaminergic pathways. Afferent neurons are responsible for carrying signals in, while efferent neurons are responsible for carrying signals out [22, 23]. These pathways and systems are highly linked and subject to different regulatory mechanisms. Innervating gut motility (peristalsis), secretion, and absorption are all greatly influenced by the ENS, an intricate network of neurons. These functions are controlled by the myenteric and submucosal plexuses, two ganglionated plexuses that make up this structure. Through intestinofugal neurons, the enteric nervous system (ENS) connects to the sympathetic nervous system (SNS) ganglia and communicates with the central nervous system (CNS) [24]. In gut-brain signaling, sensory data is sent by primary afferent neurons *via* vagal afferent pathways. A neural relay network made up of sympathetic (splanchnic) and parasympathetic (vagal-sacral) nerves is known as the autonomic nervous system (ANS). The ANS controls respiration, heart rate, and CNS-mediated alterations in gastrointestinal processes like motility, permeability, and digestion in addition to neuronal and neuroendocrine transmission [25]. Bile secretion, glucose levels, mucosal mechanical deformation, luminal osmolality, mucus synthesis, and mucosal immunological responses are among the other functions it regulates. Through CNS-mediated reactions, the ANS directly affects gut physiology [26]. Through their metabolites, which are detected by host cells and interact with ANS gut synapses, the gut microbiota can communicate with one another. Furthermore, the ANS can adjust the processes of the gut epithelium, which can either directly or indirectly activate the immune system by changing how gut immune cells respond to microorganisms.

Gut-Brain Axis and the Microbiota

Recent studies suggest that the gut microbiota plays a crucial role in the gut-brain axis. This reciprocal link emphasizes the important influence of gut bacteria on neurological functioning and is commonly known as the microbiota/gut-brain axis as in Table **1**. Disruption in the makeup of gut bacteria can affect neurological functions and vice versa [27]. According to studies, pattern recognition receptors including Toll-like receptors 2 and 4 are activated by the gut microbiota, which can then impact the central nervous system (CNS) and enteric nervous system (ENS). Dysbiosis in the gut, along with a compromised gut barrier, can cause chemicals produced by gut bacteria and molecular patterns linked to microbes to be translocated into mesenteric lymphoid tissues [28]. Research on animals has demonstrated that variations in the makeup of the gut microbiota or the lack of enteric bacteria can impact the number of myenteric neurons and the function of the bowel muscles. In addition, compared to regular control mice, germ-free animals display aberrant hormone signaling, decreased brain-derived neurotrophic factor (BDNF) production, and variations in neurotransmission and amino acid metabolism. Furthermore, studies using Drosophila have demonstrated that gut bacteria can modulate locomotor activity by increasing more metabolites [29].

Table 1. Bacterial components of microbiota influencing the gut-brain axis [32].

Bacteria	Role
Bifidobacter infantis	Reverses stress response in germ-free mice; Normalizes HPA axis following perinatal stress.
Trichuris muris	Elevates pro-inflammatory cytokines and induces anxiety.
Lactobacillus rhamnosus, Bifidibacterium longum	Probiotics decrease anxiety and serum cortisol level.
Bifidibacterium breve	Elevates fatty acid concentration in the brain.
Escherichia coli	After a perinatal stress event, detrimental effects on the HPA axis occur.
Bifidobacter infantis 35624	Raises the pain threshold and diminishes pain behavior after colorectal distension.
Lactobacillus acidophilus	Reduces visceral hypersensitivity.
Lactobacillus paracasei	Reversed colorectal hypersensitivity and distension.
Helicobacter pylori	Associated with peptic ulcer disease.

The frontal cortex, striatum, and hippocampus of GF mice showed decreased expressions of occluding and claudin-5 and increased blood-brain barrier (BBB) [30]. By upregulating the expression of tight-junction proteins, colonization with *B. thetaiotaomicron* and *C. tyrobutyricum* in GF mice decreased paracellular permeability. Remarkable abnormalities were observed in the GF mice's ENS; however, these anomalies vanished following colonization with altered Schaedler flora (ASF), underscoring the significance of particular bacterial flora in the establishment of the ENS. Intrinsic sensory signaling deficiencies, which are critical for central nervous system communication, were noted in GF mice, but these deficits were corrected in animals colonized with microbiota from certain pathogen-free (SPF) donor mice [31]. The terminologies in the gut-brain axis are mentioned in Table **2**.

Table 2. Glossary of terms related to the gut-brain axis [57].

Term	Definition
Gut-brain axis	The complex network integrates the central nervous system, neuroendocrine and neuroimmune systems, the gastrointestinal tract, and components of the enteric and autonomic nervous system.
Microbiota	The collection of microbes (bacteria, fungi, and viruses) that prevails at a particular site.
Microbiome	The total microbial genus belonging to a particular site.
Host	The organism that harbours a specific microbial population.

(Table 2) cont.....

Term	Definition
Commensal microorganisms	The intrinsic microorganisms dwelling within the host.
Prebiotic	Non-digestible foods with beneficial effects on hosts' microbiome.
Probiotic	Living organisms that contribute positively to the health of the host when consumed in adequate quantities.
Germ-free	A host lacking a microbiome is commonly observed in mice and rats born and raised in a sterile environment to prevent the microbiome.

Microbial Metabolites and Cellular Components on CNS and ENS

Recent studies have shown the molecular mechanisms through which the gut microbiota influences the central nervous system (CNS) and enteric nervous system (ENS). The significance of metabolites and cellular constituents originating from the gut microbiota in preserving brain homeostasis and impacting the emergence of neuropsychological diseases is highlighted by these discoveries [33]. *Via* the production of several metabolites and neurotransmitters with neuromodulator qualities, the gut microbiota can interact with the central nervous system and the encephalon. Branched-chain amino acids (BCAAs), glutamine, histamine, gamma-aminobutyric acid (GABA), lipopolysaccharides (LPS), short-chain fatty acids (SCFAs), bile acids, 5-hydroxytryptamine (5-HT), and catecholamines are among those that are important in regulating vital processes like neurogenesis, glial cell function, myelination, synaptic pruning, and blood-brain barrier function [34].

Under these conditions, changes in the gut microbiota may affect the development of the central nervous system and the ENS [35]. Microbes and the host create GABA, the main inhibitory neurotransmitter in the host nervous system, by converting the amino acid glutamate. It has been shown that some probiotic bacteria, including *Lactobacillus* and *Escherichia* spp., may manufacture GABA both in vitro and in vivo. It has been demonstrated that human intestinal isolates like *Lactobacillus* and *Bifidobacterium* raise GABA levels in the ENS, where its receptors are widely dispersed [36]. GABA receptor mRNA levels were discovered to be modulated in an animal study by administering L. *rhamnosus* [JB-1], which relieved anxiety-like symptoms in mice through the vagus nerve. The specific roles of GABA in the gut-brain communication are yet unknown. In the central nervous system (CNS) and epilepsy, glutamate is also a neurotransmitter. It is known that the bidirectional manipulation of glutamatergic receptors affects physiological responses in the stomach and brain [37]. Both dietary sources and microbes can create glutamate. Glutamate, which is absorbed by colonocytes and moved from the lumen to the portal circulation, is produced by bacterial strains such as *Corynebacterium glutamicum*, *Brevibacterium* spp., L. *plantarum*, and L. *lactis* [38]. Neurons in the central nervous system (CNS) can create glutamine by the deamination of glutamine by glutaminase enzyme or by employing α-ketoglutarate from the tricarboxylic acid cycle. Glutamate is stored in the cytoplasm of astrocytes, released into the extracellular fluid, taken up by neurons, and changed by deaminase into glutamate, which affects neuronal excitability [39]. Primary afferent neurons contain glutamate, which may play a function in enteric neurons as a sensory transmitter that carries messages from the mucosal layer to the enteric nervous system (ENS). The primary cause of the rising glutamatergic neurotoxicity is the difference in the activation of extrasynaptic and synaptic N-methyl-D-aspartate (NMDA) receptors. This suggests that glutamate has a role in the gut-brain crosstalk as a neurotransmitter [40].

TPH1, or tryptophan hydroxylase 1, is an enzyme that the gut microbiota uses to help generate 5-hydroxytryptamine (5-HT), a neurotransmitter. Comparing TPH-1 faulty GF mice with gut bacteria to GF and conventional THP1 transgenic mice, studies have revealed a decrease in the number of enteric neurons [41]. In addition, the enteric nervous system (ENS) architecture and intestinal transit rates of GF mice that were given microorganisms from conventional mice were changed. These alterations were linked to an increase in enteric neural progenitor proliferation and neuronal and mucosal 5-HT production [42]. While treatment of GF mice with 5-HT receptors preserved normal gut physiology, the presence of a 5-HT receptor antagonist had differing effects on the functioning of the ENS. This suggests that changes in intestinal transit rates in vivo are caused by the microbiota's 5-HT-dependent action on the ENS. Another enzyme that limits the synthesis of 5-HT is TPH2. In comparison to control mice, TPH2-mutant animals displayed aberrant ENS formation and ENS-mediated gastrointestinal functions [43]. Additionally, animals with TPH2 mutations showed decreased 5-HT levels in enteric neurons, gut transit rates, and colon motility. There appears to be a connection between depression and neuronal 5-HT synthesis because the administration of slow-release 5-HTP (5-HTP-SR) restored 5-HT levels in enteric neurons, total intestinal transit, and colonic motility [44]. It has been demonstrated that *Clostridium perfringens*, a component of the gut microbiota of humans and rodents, increases colonic and blood 5-HT synthesis in mice *via* way of TPH1 [45]. Furthermore, the metabolites of gut microorganisms (SCFAs) have an impact on colonic 5-HT synthesis in vivo.

Derived from the gut's fermentation of food fibers, short-chain fatty acids (SCFAs) are essential metabolites for gut microbes. Butyrate, propionate, and acetate are the main compounds produced by *Firmicutes* and *Bacteroidetes* [46]. After they are created, the brain and other peripheral tissues are swiftly reached by these SCFAs as they are taken up by the portal circulation. There, through their interactions with Olfactory receptor 78 (Olfr78), GRP41 and GRP43, also known as free fatty acid receptors or FFAR3 and FFAR2, and GRP109A, and by inhibiting histone deacetylases or HDACs, they play a crucial role in regulating neurological activities [47]. Microglial cell immaturity and altered cell shape have been demonstrated to be reversed in germ-free mice treated with SCFAs. SCFAs may affect immunological, vagal, endocrine, and humoral pathways in the brain. They increase the production of gut-derived peptides and regulatory cytokines by immunological, endocrine, and vagal neuronal cells, which in turn alter brain functioning. Additionally, it has been observed that SCFA treatment enhances the neurochemical phenotype of the enteric nervous system (ENS) and increases the percentage of myenteric neurons in rats that are immunoreactive to choline acetyltransferase (ChAT) [48]. A function for SCFAs in ENS homeostasis and physiology is suggested by the fact that butyrate-induced increase in ChAT-immunoreactive myenteric neurons in vivo may be prevented by silencing monocarboxylate transporter 2, which is crucial for the synthesis of enteric neurons. Mice treated with SCFAs have been demonstrated to have reduced psychosocial stress-induced changes as well as increased gut permeability and stress response. Nevertheless, SCFA therapy did not alter the composition of the microbiota, body weight gain, fecal SCFAs, colonic gene expression, or SCFA receptors in mice, suggesting that SCFAs have an in vivo role in mitigating diseases brought on by psychosocial stress. Studies on humans and animals have demonstrated a reduction in intestinal and fecal SCFA levels in alcoholic liver disease (ALD) and Parkinson's disease (PD) [49]. Acute oral butyrate treatment reduced the activity of neurons in the nucleus tractus solitaries (NTS), dorsal vagal complex, and hypothalamus of mice, indicating a dynamic control of butyrate on the gut-brain neural circuitry. Butyrate stimulation lowered the lipopolysaccharide (LPS)-induced inflammatory response in vitro in rat microglial and hippocampus cells, but it increased inflammation in mouse microglial cells [50].

Dysfunction of the Gut-Brain Axis

The gut microbiota can coexist happily with the host's cells thanks to an intricate immunological interplay depicted in Fig. (**2**). With commensal bacteria present, the immune system of the gut must remain delicately in balance to maintain its vital defensive function. Illnesses could result from a variety of pathological reasons upsetting this complex and sensitive interaction. A key component in many disorders is the makeup of the gut microbiota. An imbalance in the gut microbiota known as dysbiosis has been connected to problems in other organs and systems in addition to gastrointestinal illnesses. T-cell activation is one way that dysbiosis can affect the immune system; it is associated with autoimmune uveitis and may also affect other autoimmune illnesses [52]. Additionally, commensal gut bacteria may have a role in several illnesses by influencing the systemic levels of pro-inflammatory cytokines. Allergies have also been connected to modifications in the composition of the gut microbiome. Dysbiosis may be associated with several disorders *via* increasing intestinal permeability, sometimes known as "leaky gut." Local pathogenic processes frequently cause this state, which may allow gut bacteria and their metabolites to enter the circulatory system of the host and, if they can pass the blood-brain barrier, even reach the brain [53]. The regular operation of remote structures may be interfered with by this intrusion. Research conducted on mice has demonstrated that a decrease in the presence of pathogen-free gut microbiota can reduce the permeability of the blood-brain barrier, which is linked to the lack of normal gut microbiota [54]. As individuals with hepatic encephalopathy have shown, illnesses may arise in numerous circumstances that require both gut dysbiosis and a leaky gut [55]. In such cases, the elevated amounts of cytokines and bacterial endotoxins in the circulation, which ultimately cause cognitive dysfunction, are caused by the increased permeability of the gut wall, which is frequently secondary to hepatic dysfunction. *Alcaligenaceae* and *Porphyromonadaceae* overrepresentation in affected patients, which has been connected to cognitive impairment, highlights the significance of gut dysbiosis in these settings [56].

EFFECT OF GUT MICROBIOTA ON NEUROLOGICAL DISORDER AND ITS MECHANISM

There is a link between modifications in the gut microbiota and neurological and neuropsychiatric diseases [58]. These disorders have an impact on the peripheral and central nervous systems, which may lead to damage to the brain, spinal cord, nerves, and neuromuscular junctions, among various physiological components. Several diseases, problems of the developing neurological system, injuries to the spinal cord or brain, brain tumors, and vascular diseases are among the circumstances that can result in brain hemorrhage. Various neurological conditions have been linked to dysbiosis of the human gut microbiome [59]. Comparing the microbiota compositions of patients with various disorders to those of healthy individuals indicates significant variations. Permanent communication between the gut microbiota and the brain has been linked to behavioral disorders such as anxiety and depression, neurodegenerative diseases like Parkinson's and Alzheimer's, and neurodevelopmental disorders like autism spectrum disorder (ASD). Changes in microbial diversity may have an impact on the central nervous system (CNS) and be associated with unfavorable health outcomes, including anxiety, depression, and autism spectrum disorders (ASD) [60]. These results are supported by recent association studies conducted on humans and animals. Numerous other researchers have also documented associations between these neurological and mental illnesses and the composition of the microbiome. Accordingly, changes in the microbiota's makeup could have an impact on how the brain works [61]. Examining the relationship between gut microbiota and neurological disorders, this perspective looks at recent developments in neuromicrobiology. We aim to comprehend the role of gut microorganisms in neurological illnesses, specifically ASD, AD, PD, depression, and anxiety disorders.

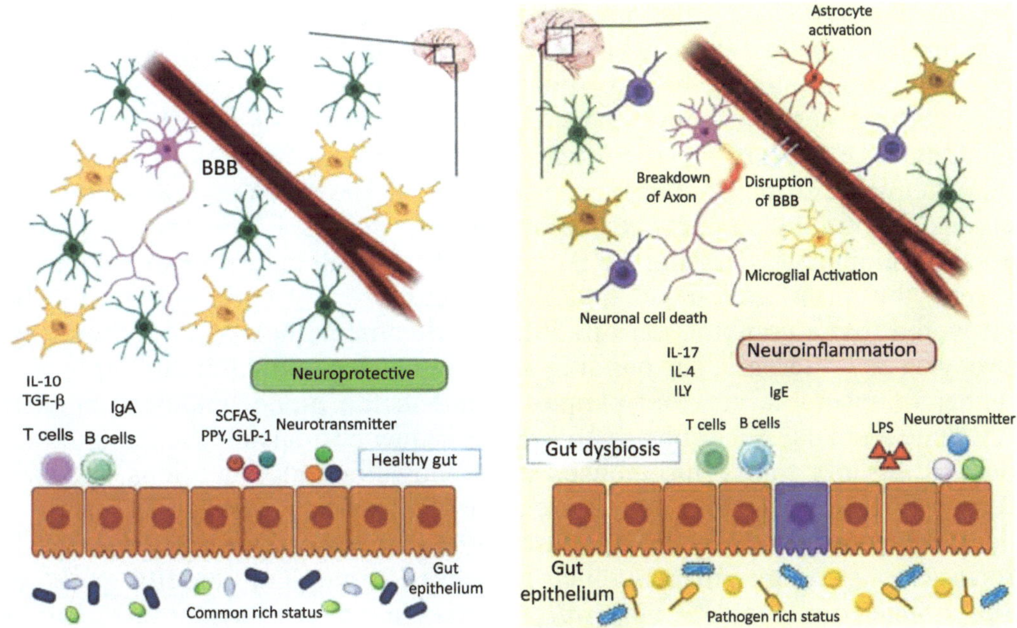

Fig. (2). By affecting both healthy and dysbiotic states *via* the gut-brain axis, the gut microbiota is essential for immunological and metabolic function. By interacting with intestinal immune cells, those on the left side promote the formation of gut-derived peptides, neurotransmitters, regulatory T and B cells, and short-chain fatty acids (SCFAs). Furthermore, they contribute to the preservation of intestinal permeability, lessen disruption of the blood-brain barrier (BBB), decrease the synthesis and translocation of lipopolysaccharides (LPS) to the periphery, stimulate brain immune and neuronal cells, and improve general brain function. In contrast, an inflammatory state is shifted by the gut microbiota during dysbiosis. They lower levels of SCFAs while raising those of inflammatory T and B cells, LPS, and proinflammatory cytokines. Increased BBB permeability, activation of astrocytes and microglia, and neuroinflammation result from this. Importantly, these processes also involve transforming growth factor- β (TGF-β), glucagon-like peptide-1 (GLP-1), and peptide YY (PYY) [51].

Alzheimer's Disease

Memory loss and decline in cognition are hallmarks of Alzheimer's disease (AD), which is brought on by nerve cell death. It is a type of dementia that usually hits older people [62]. Amyloid beta (Aβ) deposition in neurons and the dephosphorylation of tau protein-associated microtubules (t-protein) in cortical neurons' dendrites and axons are the hallmarks of the disease. These types of biomarkers have been determined to be exclusive to AD. Alzheimer's disease (AD) is also linked to mitochondrial dysfunction, resulting in abnormal mitophagy, impacts mitochondrial quality control, and causes oxidative stress and mitochondrial malfunction in AD patients' brains [63]. It has been demonstrated that microbial infections, including *spirochaetes*, fungal infections, and *Chlamydia pneumonia*, change the composition of the gut microbiota and raise blood levels of pro-inflammatory cytokines. In patients with cognitive impairment and brain amyloidosis, the presence of pro-inflammatory bacteria such as *Escherichia coli* and *Shigella*, along with anti-inflammatory bacteria, can disrupt the microbiota, exacerbating neurodegeneration and causing systemic inflammation. Research shows that when fumonisins (FBs), mycotoxins made by the fungus *Fusarium verticillioides*, are given to rats, they modify the neurochemical profile of enteric neurons, namely the myenteric and submucosal neurons, but do not impact the anatomy of the gut [64]. Fumonisins also alter neural development, affecting the B1 and B2 forms and their function in diets that prevent the proliferation of myenteric neurons. Furthermore, it has been discovered that a combination of antibiotic treatments decreases the number of astrocytes and microglia surrounding amyloid plaques, which in turn reduces the number of insoluble amyloid plaques found in the hippocampus of persisting transgenic animals. According to 16S rRNA sequence analysis, the gut microbiota composition in a transgenic mouse model shows notable variations in amyloid precursor protein (APP) levels relative to wildtype [65]. Research has demonstrated that Alzheimer's disease (AD) patients' brains contain hazardous proteases, such as gingipains, which are linked to tau and ubiquitin pathology. Mice infected orally with *P. gingivalis* experience increased synthesis of amyloid-β (Aβ1-42), a component of amyloid plaques, and brain colonization. For the treatment of *P. gingivalis* brain colonization and neurodegeneration, gingipain inhibition is essential. In addition to lowering the bacterial load during infection, it also lowers neuroinflammation, suppresses the manufacture of Aβ1-42, and safeguards hippocampal neurons [66]. About 108 old people participated in a clinical trial conducted in the United States; of these, 51 were free of dementia, 24 had AD, and 33 had other forms of dementia. Over the course of a 5-month follow-up period, the study assessed the expression of P-glycoprotein, a crucial regulator of intestinal homeostasis, using metagenomic analysis of stool samples and an in vitro assay for intestinal epithelial cells. In AD cases, the researchers found microbial taxa with a decreased prevalence of *Lachnoclostridium spp.* and a higher prevalence of *Bacteroides spp.*, *Alistipes spp.*, *Odoribacter spp.*, and *Barnesiella spp.* A possible detrimental effect on intestinal epithelial homeostasis *via* deregulation of the P-glycoprotein pathway is indicated by the lesser prevalence of the *Butyrivibrio* genus and other butyrate-producing bacteria in the

AD microbiome. Higher concentrations of the inflammasome proteins found in the gut microbiota also act as important precursors to the activation of inflammatory and cytotoxic mediators downstream. Treatment for genetic susceptibility to Alzheimer's disease (AD) and other neurological illnesses may involve altering gut microbiota (GM) since the NLRP3 protein in the gastrointestinal inflammasome may promote neuroinflammation [67]. In comparison to wild type, a study on AD mouse models revealed significant changes in microbial composition at different ages, decreased levels of fecal short-chain fatty acids (SCFA), and an increase in Proteobacteria and Verrucomicrobia. These changes suggested disruptions in at least 30 metabolic pathways. Research indicates that implementing dietary modifications such as switching to a ketogenic diet and taking probiotics may help to slow down the onset of AD [68]. These results highlight the role of GM in AD and provide insight into the ways that GM may affect the pathophysiology and management of the condition. The pathophysiological role of GM in AD and its modulatory effects on the GBA are summarized in Fig. (**3**).

Parkinson's Disease

In the substantia nigra, a part of the brain's central nervous system (CNS), dopaminergic nerve cells accumulate α-synuclein (α-syn). This accumulation is the cause of Parkinson's disease (PD). One trait that distinguishes Parkinson's disease (PD) is the build-up of α-syn, which can pass through the vagus nerve from the gut to the brain. Studies have shown that protecting mice against Parkinson's disease (PD) in populations from Sweden and Denmark involves chopping off the vagus nerve's trunk. Complete or highly selective vagotomy, on the other hand, either does not exhibit a substantial relationship with Parkinson's disease (PD), or just a slight association is observed [70]. As people age, Parkinson's disease (PD) changes course and development, causing neurodegeneration and impacting several cellular pathways. PD primarily affects men and accounts for 5-35 new cases per 100,000 people annually [71]. It usually attacks those under 50 rarely, with the chance of having the disease rising 5- to 10-fold with age. Intestinal dysbiosis has been associated with gastrointestinal (GIT) problems in Parkinson's disease (PD) patients with the development of a-syn deposits in the enteric nervous system (ENS) [72]. Furthermore, through cytokine networking, the gut microbiota (GM) has been linked to promoting physiological interactions in Parkinson's disease (PD). In Parkinson's disease, idiopathic constipation is linked to ENS neurodegeneration [73]. There is dysbiosis in the gut microbiota of Parkinson's disease patients, as evidenced by studies that found a significant decrease in *Prevotellaceae species* and an increase in *Enterobacteriaceae* in stool samples. According to in vivo research employing a Parkinson's disease (PD) model, neuroinflammatory processes are driven by short-chain fatty acids (SCFA). By transplanting fecal microbiota from PD patients, mice can be colonized with PD-associated microbiota, leading to motor impairments and neuroinflammation [74]. Supplementing with antibiotics has been shown to improve behavioral symptoms in PD patients. Intestinal microbial tyrosine decarboxylases have been found to decrease plasma levodopa levels in a rat PD model. These findings underscore the critical role of GM alterations in the pathogenesis and treatment of PD (Fig. **4**).

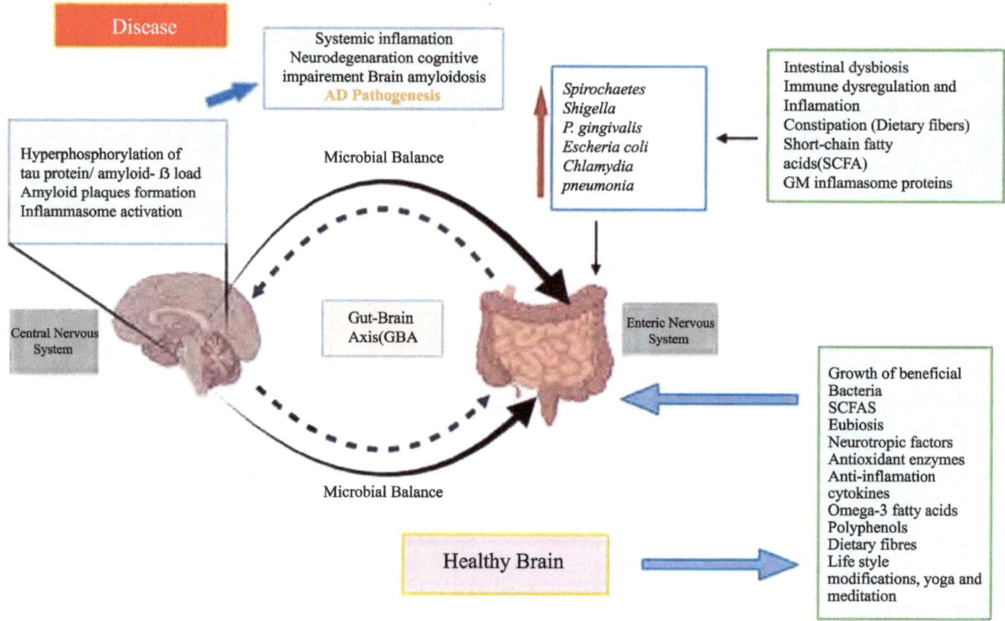

Fig. (3). Under both microbial balance and imbalance circumstances, the importance of gut microbiota (GM) in the pathogenesis of Alzheimer's disease (AD) is emphasized, notably *via* glucocerebrosidase (GBA). Maintaining a healthy brain requires a balanced microbial ecology in the intestine (left side). Numerous factors contribute to this balance: the growth of probiotics; the ideal concentrations of short-chain fatty acids (SCFAs); eubiotics; increased levels of neurotropic factors; the production of antioxidant enzymes; the consumption of polyphenols, dietary fibers, omega-3 fatty acids; and lifestyle changes like yoga and meditation. All of these factors support the health of the brain. On the other hand, infections may have a role in the onset of AD in a microbial imbalance situation (right side). Reduced SCFA levels, immunological dysregulation, inflammation, intestinal dysbiosis, and constipation (from a lack of dietary fiber) are possible outcomes of this imbalance. The development of AD is facilitated by GM-related inflammasome proteins, which are involved in tau protein hyperphosphorylation, the formation of amyloid plaques in the brain, and inflammasome activation. These events lead to systemic inflammation, neurodegeneration, cognitive decline, and brain amyloidosis [69].

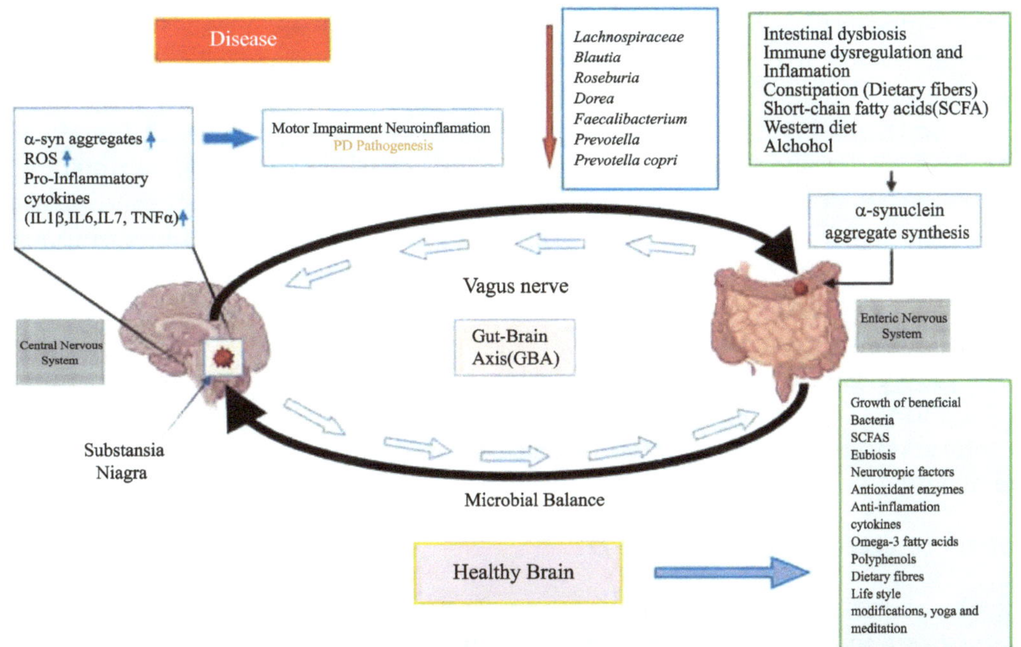

Fig. (4). The pathophysiology of Parkinson's disease (PD) is illustrated by the role of the gut microbiota (GM) within the gut-brain axis (GBA) under conditions of microbial balance and imbalance. The growth of beneficial bacteria, balanced short-chain fatty acids (SCFAs), protection against eubiosis, production of anti-inflammatory cytokines, synthesis of antioxidant enzymes, and an increase in omega-3 fatty acids, polyphenols, and dietary fibers are all factors that contribute to a balanced microbial environment and a healthy left side of the brain. The upkeep of the brain and general biological health is facilitated by these elements working together. Intestinal health can also be preserved by making lifestyle changes including exercising, practicing yoga, and practicing meditation. On the other hand, a right-sided microbial imbalance raises the pathogenicity of Parkinson's disease (PD) by processes such as immunological dysregulation, inflammation, constipation, decreased SCFA levels, consumption of a Western diet, and alcohol consumption. The vagus nerve carries pro-inflammatory cytokines (IL1β, IL6, IL17, and TNF-α) from the gut to the brain, and these factors can lead to the build-up of these substances in Parkinson's disease (PD) [75].

Multiple Sclerosis

Damaged axons, demyelination, and immune-mediated dysfunction are the hallmarks of multiple sclerosis (MS), which affect more than 2.3 million individuals globally, with a greater incidence rate in women. In the brain and spinal cord, demyelinated plaques develop in the grey or white matter. These plaques set off a neuro-inflammatory response that causes specialized cells, such as oligodendrocytes and neurodegeneration, to become demyelinated. CD4+ T cells are linked to the pathophysiology of multiple sclerosis (MS) in a mouse model of experimental autoimmune encephalomyelitis (EAE) [76]. EAE and validated animal models have shown in vivo that the pathophysiology of MS is associated with grey matter (GM). Moreover, CD4+ T cells that produce interleukin-10 are essential for immunological regulation processes. Th17 cells are activated by segmented filamentous bacteria that are gram-positive in the gastrointestinal tract, and this has a major effect on the severity of EAE [77]. As demonstrated by germ-free (GF) mice and pre-clinical antibiotic treatments in the mouse pre-frontal cortex, the microbiome affects the control of myelin production in multiple sclerosis. The blood-brain barrier's (BBB) integrity is maintained in part by GM, according to a study done on GF rats. In EAE, dietary modifications impact the makeup of GM [78]. Two months of twice-daily administration of a multispecies probiotic (*Lactobacillus species, Bifidobacterium species*, and *Streptococcus species*) can offset microbial alterations and have anti-inflammatory characteristics [79]. These results demonstrate the substantial influence of GM on MS physiopathology in both animal and human clinical investigations. The goal of current research is to successfully modify the GM as an intervention to reduce the likelihood of recurrence, minimize MS symptoms, and eventually treat the illness.

Autism Spectrum Disorder (ASD)

Social interaction, communication, and repetitive activities are among the neurodevelopmental symptoms of autism spectrum disorder (ASD) [80]. According to the Autism and Developmental Disabilities Monitoring (ADDM) network of the Centres for Disease Control and Prevention, one in every 44 children is affected with ASD [81]. Maternal autoantibodies against certain proteins in the developing brain, along with developmental abnormalities in infancy, infections, and malnutrition are among the many variables that contribute to the development of ASD. Autism is a neuropsychiatric condition, and recent research indicates that interactions between the gut microbiota (GM) and the brain may be involved. Furthermore, about 40 percent of those with ASD have digestive problems [82]. According to research, GM can affect behavioral changes and mood from childhood to maturity [83]. Soon after birth, the microbiome settles in the gut and begins to interact with the brain as the kid develops. Atypical behavior, mood and memory alterations, and cognitive impairment might result from any inflammation or disturbance during this process. The composition of the GM in animal models of ASD has been reported to be altered by established epidemiological risk factors for ASD, including maternal inflammation during pregnancy, maternal obesity, and maternal exposure to the anti-convulsant valproate [84]. Additionally, GM species that encourage an inflammatory state and are vancomycin-susceptible have been connected to ASD. Research has demonstrated that prebiotics, or non-digestible carbohydrates like fibers that are advantageous to the host and/or microbiota, and/or probiotics, which are helpful live microbial cultures, can influence an animal's social behavior [85]. These findings hold promise for the development of novel microbiota-based treatments for the treatment of ASD in humans.

Stroke and Brain Injury

Because they cause high rates of morbidity and mortality, stroke and brain injuries currently represent serious challenges to world health. Numerous illnesses, such as diabetes, arterial hypertension, dyslipidemia, atherosclerosis, and cerebrovascular disease, can cause these problems. The two primary types of acquired brain injury (ABI) are non-traumatic brain injury (non-TBI) and traumatic brain injury (TBI). ABI patients need thorough clinical management, improved pre-hospital care, and long-term rehabilitation assistance. Thus, it is essential to develop neuroprotective or neurorestorative tactics and treatments to avoid brain damage [86]. Moreover, the development of stroke and brain damage may be influenced by the gut microbiota (GM). Changes in GM composition, as well as impacts on gastrointestinal (GIT) motility and barrier permeability, have all been related to cerebral ischemia. Research indicates that the ischemia-induced brain damage and functional abnormalities in mice treated with antibiotics are worsened when the fecal microbiota of stroke patients is transplanted [87]. Additionally, research has linked the microbiota-derived metabolite trimethylamine n-oxide (TMAO), which is made from dietary choline to an increased risk of cardiovascular and cerebrovascular diseases, suggesting that it may play a role in the etiology of disease [88]. Due to the presence of gut bacteria, phosphatidylcholine metabolites (choline and TMAO) have been linked to atherosclerosis. Atherosclerotic lesion repair is greatly aided by a healthy microbiome. Opportunistic infections including *Desulfovibrio, Enterobacter, Megasphaera*, and *Oscillibacter* have been discovered to be present in patients with transient ischemic attack or stroke, but beneficial or commensal pathogens such as *Bacteroides, Fecalibacterium*, and *Prevotella* are less common [89]. There is evidence linking the severity of stroke to the abundance of *Peptococcaceae* and *Prevotellaceae*. Nonetheless, it is still unknown how exactly GM contributes to the development and course of brain damage and stroke. A greater understanding of the potential of microbial medicinal approaches requires more clinical research, even though animal models have yielded insightful information.

Epilepsy

A persistent neurological illness, epilepsy affects over 65 million people worldwide. About one-third of epilepsy patients experience refractory seizures that interfere with everyday life, even with anti-epileptic drug (AED) treatment [90]. Only 70% of epilepsy patients acquire complete seizure control. Due to the greater rates of morbidity and mortality associated with this illness, there is an urgent need for more effective and potentially curative therapies. These consequences have enormous socio-economic ramifications. A possible function for gut microbiota (GM) in the management of epilepsy has been suggested by recent research that has connected certain intestinal bacterial species to the condition [91]. A persistent neurological disease, epilepsy affects over 65 million people worldwide. About one-third of epilepsy patients experience refractory seizures that interfere with everyday life, even with anti-epileptic drug (AED) treatment. Only 70% of epilepsy patients acquire complete seizure control. Due to the greater rates of morbidity and mortality associated with this illness, there is an urgent need for more effective and potentially curative therapies. These consequences have enormous socio-economic ramifications. A possible function for gut microbiota (GM) in the management of epilepsy has been suggested by recent research that has connected certain intestinal bacterial species to the condition [92]. Manipulating genetic diversity may be a feasible therapy approach for uncontrolled epilepsy, as different therapeutic techniques have revealed variations in GM profiles when compared to healthy populations [93]. It has been discovered that firmicute bacteria affect neurotransmitter levels and that having more *Lactobacillus* and *Bifidobacterium* in the body is linked to fewer annual seizures. Patients with drug-resistant epilepsy show a notably greater α-diversity in GM when compared to drug-responsive patients, suggesting a possible involvement of uncommon gut bacterial species in epilepsy treatment. Remarkably, by altering zonisamide metabolism, the gut microbiota can function in a manner akin to that of anti-epileptic drugs. There may be a connection between dietary therapy and epilepsy treatment because the ketogenic diet (KD), which is known to lower seizure frequency in epilepsy patients, also modifies the content and structure of GM. Research conducted using the GF mouse model suggests that a KD mediates anti-seizure effects in the temporal lobe of epilepsy. Seizure thresholds were found to increase upon transplantation of KD microbiota species, including *Parabacteroides merdae, Akkermansia muciniphila*, and *Parabacteroides distasonis*. A greater understanding of how microbiota can impact the physiology and behavior of epilepsy disorders is necessary, as the data supporting the function of GM in epilepsy is weaker than that of other diseases [94].

Amyotrophic Lateral Sclerosis (ALS)

Motor neurons are impacted by amyotrophic lateral sclerosis (ALS), a severe neurodegenerative disease that usually appears later in life. Almost one person out of every 1000 is thought to be affected. Only 5-10% of ALS cases are familial; the majority of ALS cases are random. Degeneration of the cortical and spinal motor neurons is seen in both sporadic and familial ALS (FALS) cases, and this degeneration is frequently linked to mutations in superoxide dismutase [95]. Because it affects inter-individual differences and may affect ALS, the gut microbiota (GM) is critical to our general health. According to studies, ALS patients' guts contain less of the antimicrobial peptide defensin-5. There may be a connection between the development of ALS and the gut microbiome and intestinal epithelium because of this change in the microbiome, which is characterized by reduced levels of *Butyrivibriofibrisolvens*, *Escherichia coli*, and *Fermicus* in comparison to wild-type mice [96]. According to several studies, butyrate-producing bacteria are less prevalent in the GM of ALS patients than in mice in good condition, which may be related to modifications in the permeability of the gut [97]. Different gut microbial communities are found in ALS patients and healthy controls, indicating that GM manipulation—such as resolving deficiencies in Prevotella spp. or changing butyrate metabolism—may help treat ALS. When comparing ALS patients to healthy controls, clinical investigations utilizing 16S rDNA sequencing have revealed up-regulation of Bacteroidetes (at the phylum level) and many bacteria (at the genus level), but down-regulation of Firmicutes (at the phylum level) and Megamonas (at the genus level). Furthermore, reduced gene function in metabolic pathways is observed in ALS patients, suggesting that GM and its metabolic products may be useful therapeutic targets for subsequent research [98]. These results highlight the important role GM plays in ALS. To completely comprehend the part that microbiota plays in the etiology of ALS, more clinical study is nevertheless required.

Huntington's Disease (HD)

Three distinct clinical features—progressive motor, cognitive, and mental impairments—as well as involuntary weight loss—define Huntington's disease (HD), a neurodegenerative disorder that progresses over time [99]. The primary cause of the illness is the huntingtin (HTT) gene, which is expressed all over the brain, and its unstable trinucleotide (cytosine-adenine-guanine, or CAG) repeat. In both humans and animals, myelination deficiencies, white matter atrophy, and neuronal degeneration in the basal ganglia are early pathogenic characteristics of HD. Imperceptible weight loss is a typical clinical sign generated by gastrointestinal dysfunction in an HD mice model, and recent investigations have suggested that there may be gut dysbiosis in HD [100]. By the time the mice were 12 weeks old, significant alterations in the makeup of the microbiome had been seen, with *Bacteroidetes* being more prevalent and *Firmicutes* less common. In a bacterial artificial chromosome model of HD mice, callosal myelination and white matter plasticity were altered in the presence of germs, resulting in gut dysbiosis and motor impairments by the time the animals were 12 weeks old [101]. There were notable differences between the male groups in *Euryarchaeota, Firmicutes*, and *Verrucomicrobia* at the phylum level. There were also notable differences between the male groups in *Acidaminococcaceae, Akkermansiaceae, Bacteroidaceae, Bifidobacteraceae, Clostridiaceae, Christensenellaceae, Coriobacteriaceae, Eggerthellaceae, Enterobacteriaceae, Erysipelotrichaceae, Flavobacteriaceae, Lachnospiraceae, Methanobacteriaceae, Peptococcaceae, Peptostreptococcaceae,* and *Rikenellaceae.* In the HD gene expansion carrier group, correlations between gut microbiota, cognitive function, and clinical outcomes were also found.

LATEST TREATMENT APPROACHES

Given the link between NDDs and gut dysbiosis, dietary therapies aimed at addressing gut dysbiosis may be a viable means of addressing symptoms and slowing down the neuroinflammatory and degenerative processes associated with NDDs. To complement current therapeutic techniques, additional nutritional interventions can be used to change the composition of the gut microbiota and related metabolites, to create eubiosis and improve overall gut health. As shown in Fig (**5**), these therapies include various food regimens, probiotics, synbiotics, prebiotics, and faecal microbiota transplantation (FMT). Notably, these methods have demonstrated efficacy in promoting a healthy gut state and reversing gut dysbiosis [102].

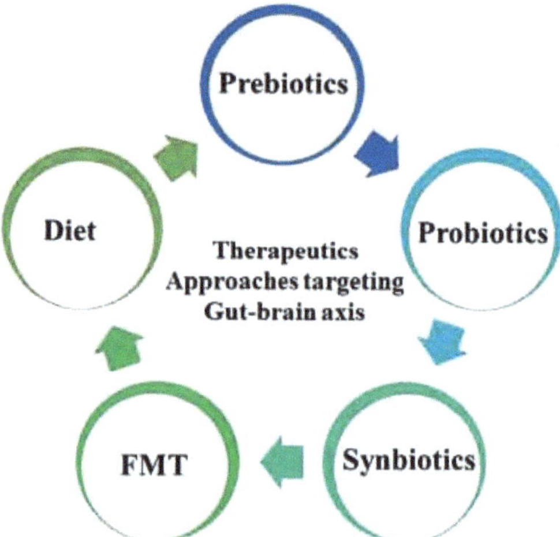

Fig. (5). A variety of approaches are used to enhance gut microbiota in the treatment of neurodegenerative illnesses. These include dietary changes that include probiotics—live bacteria that have been shown to provide health benefits—and prebiotics, which encourage the growth of beneficial microbes in the body. Synbiotics are a combination of probiotics and prebiotics that work together to increase the effects of both. Another strategy is Faecal Microbiota Transplantation (FMT), which introduces donor faecal microbiota that has undergone extensive screening to rebuild a healthy gut microbiome. To provide neuroprotective effects, these tactics mainly alter microbial populations and produce advantageous microbial metabolites, such as neurotransmitters and Short-Chain Fatty Acids (SCFAs). The goal of the suggested diet is to improve the composition and function of the gut microbiota by ingesting fruits, vegetables, legumes, and cereals [103].

Diet

The gut microbiota's makeup is significantly affected by dietary decisions, and this is an important aspect of preserving host homeostasis. The Mediterranean diet, or MD, is a prime example of a health-conscious eating plan that places a strong focus on fruits, vegetables, legumes, and cereals. Interestingly, research found that following the MD was associated with a 1.5–3.5-year slowdown in the progression of Alzheimer's disease (AD). The positive effects of MD seem associated with changes in gut microbiota and its anti-inflammatory characteristics.[194] Moreover, a plant-based diet that adheres to MD principles has been demonstrated to alter gut flora, increasing fecal short-chain fatty acids (SCFAs) and decreasing urine trimethylamine N-oxide (TMAO) [104]. Mice's intestinal barrier integrity, systemic inflammation, and gut dysbiosis all improved when microbiota-accessible carbohydrates, such as dietary fiber, were introduced through supplementation. Reductions in neuroglial activity and synaptic dysfunction were linked to these benefits. But when the supply of broad-spectrum antibiotics was reduced, these effects were reversed. Furthermore, eating a balanced diet reduces the chance of obesity and increases insulin resistance, both of which have been linked to an increased risk of neurodegenerative diseases (NDDs) like AD.

Rich in fruits and vegetables, polyphenols have a variety of functions. They control reactive oxygen species (ROS) to prevent oxidative stress, affect the autophagy pathway to reduce apoptosis, affect the gut microbiota to improve intestinal barrier integrity, and treat inflammation in the gut. Resveratrol is a polyphenol derived from grapes and wine that has been shown to improve cognition, reduce neuroinflammation, and potentially reduce pathological protein aggregation, such as Aβ plaques and neurofibrillary tangles (NFT), in animal models of Alzheimer's disease (AD). Resveratrol showed neuroprotective properties in a rat model of Parkinson's disease (PD) by reducing oxidative stress, lipid peroxidation, and protein carbonylation, as well as avoiding the death of dopaminergic neurons. On the other hand, alcohol consumption in addition to diets heavy in sugar and fat has a detrimental effect on neurodegenerative diseases (NDDs). Nonetheless, a few dietary elements are advantageous for health, including calorie restriction, curcumin, sulforaphane, resveratrol, blueberry polyphenols, polyunsaturated fatty acids, and antioxidants [105]. This suggests that there may be a relationship between dietary preferences and the chance of getting NDDs in a variety of populations. People following the Mediterranean diet (MD) had a 33% lower risk of AD and moderate cognitive impairment (MCI) than people following a different diet, according to a 2014 meta-analysis that included five prospective trials [106]. Further confirmation of the protective effect of MD adherence against dementia and cognitive decline was found in the

Hellenic Longitudinal Investigation of Ageing and Diet cohort, which included 1865 people [107].

Prebiotics

A prebiotic is a plant fiber supplement that will pass through the small intestine undigested and into the colon, where it will ferment as a substrate for the microbiome's beneficial bacteria. Prebiotics are not fibers that ferment, like cellulose. Prebiotics are characterized as fermentable fibers that are used by the microbiome and have a beneficial effect, such as inulin, fructans, galacto-oligosaccharides, and methylcellulose. To alter the composition of the microbiome and reverse dysbiosis, soluble fibers must be used as prebiotics, Prebiotics have been shown to have significant impacts in animal models, despite disagreements on the relative benefits of supplementation versus diet inclusion. For example, prebiotics can restore aberrant social behavior in a mouse model of ASD caused by a high-fat diet [108]. Inulin supplementation can suppress pro-inflammatory Proteobacteria in mice and promote the growth of advantageous bacteria like *Lactobacillus* (a bacteria that produces SCFA), *Akkermansia*, and *Bifidobacterium.* In contrast, psyllium fiber has less of an effect on the microbiome since it digests more slowly than other soluble fibers. Still, psyllium administration can alter the microbiota, lessen the severity of colitis, reverse inflammation, and improve rat model of diabetes symptoms. Because the gut microbiome is so diverse and research designs vary, it can be difficult and often impossible to determine the effects of prebiotics in humans. Prebiotic response varies significantly in human research for a variety of reasons, including starting microbiome, dose, duration of intervention, and diet. A systematic evaluation, for instance, of inulin-related clinical trials revealed that, although most of the studies reported increases in *Bifidobacterium*, *Lactobacillus*, and *Anaerostipes* and decreases in *Bacteroides*, this pattern did not align with the higher levels of SCFAs observed in animal studies. Prebiotics do not increase microbiome diversity; however, they can encourage the growth of particular bacterial populations [109].

Probiotics

Probiotics are recognized for their positive health effects and include bacteria such as *Lactobacillus*, *Bifidobacterium*, and yeasts, as well as more recently discovered *Akkermansia.* The potential of these bacteria, which are frequently found in the microbiome, has been investigated for several neurodegenerative illnesses, including PD, HD, ASD, MS, and MSA. Doses between 10^9 and 10^{10} colony-forming units (CFU) are usually given throughout 4 weeks in studies. Probiotic-related research has demonstrated notable enhancements in animal models of neurodegenerative and neurodevelopmental disorders, such as Parkinson's disease, Alzheimer's disease, ALS, and autism spectrum disorder [110]. Innovative probiotics like *Akkermansia* have shown promise in the treatment of diseases like depression and obesity. In animal models, the bacterium *Clostridium butyricum*, which generates short-chain fatty acids, has demonstrated potential for enhancing gut health and lowering inflammation. Research on animals has shown promise, but findings from trials on humans are less consistent. Probiotic therapy has been found in some studies to enhance metabolic indicators and cognitive performance in people with Parkinson's disease (PD) and Alzheimer's disease (AD) [111]. Other studies, meantime, have not discovered any appreciable advantages for AD patients' cognitive scores. Only one trial yielded good results in a review concentrating on ASD and ADHD; pregnant moms who took a *Lactobacillus* probiotic had a lower chance of their kid receiving an ASD or ADHD diagnosis by the time the child turned 13 years old [112]. Clinical investigations have not yet backed up the idea that probiotics can alleviate gastrointestinal symptoms in ASD, despite some pre-clinical and anecdotal data to the contrary.

Faecal Microbiome Transplant

Restoring a healthy mix of microbiota to a microbiome that exhibits dysbiosis would seem to be a sensible therapeutic approach, given the proven link of microbiomes with numerous diseases. Fecal microbiota transplantation (FMT) is the best treatment for recurrent or resistant *Clostridium difficile* infection (CDI), even if there isn't a set methodology in place at the moment [113]. FMT has been used since the early 1980s. The suggested course of treatment for CDI is FMT because of its high efficaciousness. The FDA in the US has approved FMT for the treatment of CDI, which causes colitis and diarrhoea, as well as for preventing its recurrence. Furthermore, FMT has been given more widespread approval for usage by the Australian Therapeutic Goods Administration (TMA) [114]. For different disorders, FMT is being studied in multiple open-label studies. In addition to metabolic disorders including metabolic syndrome and type 2 diabetes, it has the potential for treating gastrointestinal disorders like ulcerative colitis, Crohn's disease, irritable bowel syndrome, and inflammatory bowel disease (IBD). In a review of FMT, Wang *et al.* described how, between 2011 and 2021, it was used to treat 85 different disorders [115]. Animal models have been used extensively in early studies on neurodegenerative illnesses. A healthy animal's microbiota is either transplanted into a disease model of Alzheimer's disease (AD), Parkinson's disease (PD), multiple sclerosis (MS), amyotrophic lateral sclerosis (ALS), or autism spectrum disorder (ASD), or it is transplanted into a disease model of a human patient or an animal model that is diseased. The effectiveness of FMT in animal models has also been shown by this work, which further supports the robust microbiome-gut-brain axis relationship in neurogenerative and neurodevelopmental illnesses. It is less certain, nevertheless, if FMT is beneficial in human situations other than CDI [116]. Fecal microbiota transplantation (FMT) was performed on three MS patients to treat constipation. Every patient saw a dramatic improvement in their symptoms, and one even managed to walk again and maintain a 15-year remission. A single MS patient who underwent FMT for a Clostridium difficile infection (CDI) and kept consistent disability scores for ten years was the subject of another case study. In another single-subject case study, a bloating MS patient demonstrated better gait and walking after FMT. Following FMT, seven patients with autism spectrum disorder (ASD) showed some improvement in their symptoms, according to a 2016 case series [117]. Treatment with vancomycin for two weeks, followed by a colon cleanse and eight weeks of FMT, improved gastrointestinal symptoms, ASD behavioral symptoms, and microbiome diversity for the duration of the trial, according to an open-label study involving eighteen children with ASD. Following this medication, the metabolite profiles of patients with ASD also resembled those of the control group. Significantly, during a two-year follow-up, these symptom improvements remained and, in certain cases, even got better, with improvements also observed in the microbiota. Nevertheless, there are hazards associated with FMT, including transient side effects like fever, bloating, diarrhea, constipation, and nausea [118]. Longer-term negative effects could also occur, such as the transfer of pathogenic and infectious agents (bacteria, viruses, fungi), bacteria that are resistant to drugs, infectious material (like prions), and non-infectious materials (like antibiotics) from the donor to the recipient. There have been documented cases of obesity, irritable bowel syndrome (IBS), and rheumatoid arthritis disease transfer. A rate of major adverse events ranging from 2% to 6% was found in a systematic evaluation of FMT literature. The best method of preparation, the ideal dosage, the frequency of transplants, and the long-term health implications of FMT require more investigation. The caliber of the donor material has a direct impact on FMT's effectiveness. It is customary to screen for viruses, infections, and donors with recent or active illnesses, even if there isn't yet a standard for donor screening.

Traditional Chinese Medicine and Herbal Therapy

Numerous herbs and their combinations have been shown to have a good impact on the microbiome, according to recent research on the effects of herbal medications and traditional Chinese medicine (TCM). They could improve the intestinal barrier, lower inflammation, and diversify the microbiota [119]. The majority of research has concentrated on animal models of type 2 diabetes mellitus (T2DM), irritable bowel syndrome (IBS), and inflammatory bowel disease (IBD), but its conclusions may also apply to neurodegenerative and neurodevelopmental illnesses. Certain TCM therapies have shown promise in decreasing possible infections, boosting good bacteria that produce short-chain fatty acids (SCFAs), and relieving gastrointestinal complaints all while enhancing the intestinal barrier. Curcumin, aloe vera, slippery elm, guar gum, pectin, peppermint oil, and glutamine are combined in mouse models, and other treatments include a diallyl disulphide garlic extract, a gegen qinlian decoction, a Pi-Dan-Jian-Qing decoction, and a Qing-Fei-Pai-Du decoction [120]. In human studies, the microbiota and serum cholesterol levels of obese subjects were enhanced by konjaku flour. Furthermore, a Tanhuo infusion enhanced the microbiota and showed better results than Western therapy for individuals with acute ischemic stroke. With its diverse physiological effects, curcumin—a plant polyphenol with low systemic bioavailability—indicates a direct impact on the microbiome, maybe through translation into more bioactive forms [121]. There is evidence that curcumin helps strengthen the intestinal barrier, increase biodiversity, foster good bacteria, and lower pro-inflammatory cytokines. Moreover, curcumin has demonstrated efficacy in a mouse model of Parkinson's disease (PD) using 1-methyl-4-phenyl-1,2,3,6-tetrahydropyridine (MPTP), lowering α-synuclein aggregation and improving motor impairments [122]. Berberine has been shown to have impacts on a range of metabolic illnesses and to have a positive impact on the microbiome in a small number of human trials as well as animal models. Increases in mucin-degrading and SCFA-producing bacteria (*Akkermansia*) and decreases in LPS-producing bacteria (Proteobacteria and *Desulfovibrio*) are two examples of how this affects the microbiome. It was discovered that the combination of moxibustion and acupuncture improved the microbiome in a randomized controlled trial (RCT) for Crohn's disease, especially boosting the number of bacteria that produce short-chain fatty acids (SCFAs; *Faecalibacterium, Roseburia*) [123]. An enhanced intestinal barrier could be the cause of this improvement, as demonstrated in a model using rats. Numerous studies have shown that moxibustion and acupuncture treatment have a favorable impact on the microbiota in animal models of colitis and IBS. Furthermore, early research indicates that in animal models of Parkinson's disease, acupuncture may improve the gut flora. In an RCT (15 + 15), an 8-week course of electroacupuncture to the belly and scalp dramatically decreased pro-inflammatory microorganisms and ameliorated some Parkinson's disease symptoms. A mouse model of AD has demonstrated that acupuncture influences the microbiota [124].

Targeted Antibiotics

During infections, doctors use antibiotics to either eradicate or suppress dangerous microorganisms. Still, they can also have adverse effects on the microbiota, especially in the gut, where they can reduce beneficial SCFA-producing bacteria and increase potentially pathogenic bacteria. This disturbance may cause negative health outcomes, including infection with *C. difficile*, and may also be a factor in the development of diseases including autism spectrum disorder (ASD), Parkinson's disease (PD), and Alzheimer's disease (AD) [125]. The microbiome may not return to its pre-antibiotic state and may take months to fully recover, even if antibiotics are stopped. A small subset of antibiotics, referred to as "eubiotics," have distinct effects from this overall pattern. Beneficial *Bifidobacterium* and *Faecalibacterium* have been demonstrated to proliferate in the gut in response to the broad-spectrum antibiotic Nitrofurantoin, which is used to treat urinary tract infections [126]. Another antibiotic with unusual characteristics is rifaximin, which is better in the small intestine than the colon due to its slow absorption and ability to lower pro-inflammatory cytokines and strengthen the intestinal barrier, hence reducing inflammation. *Bifidobacterium, Lactobacillus*, and *Faecalibacterium* are more prevalent in the gut microbiota when rifaximin is used [127]. Originally prescribed to treat traveler's diarrhea, Rifaximin is currently preferred to treat small intestine bacterial overgrowth (SIBO). It has also demonstrated effectiveness in treating some symptoms of irritable bowel syndrome (IBS), ulcerative colitis, and moderately active Crohn's disease. More research is being done to see whether it can be used to treat neurodegenerative and neurodevelopmental illnesses, particularly in the early stages. Rifaximin can lessen inflammatory indicators, alter the microbiome, and alleviate Parkinson's disease symptoms, according to animal research [128]. However, a tiny human PD experiment only found that the bacterium *Flavonifractor,* which has been linked to Parkinson's disease—had increased. Rifaximin may raise the fraction of Firmicutes in AD and lower blood levels of phosphorylated tau and neurofilament-light, according to a limited trial, but it did not improve cognitive function. Targeting Gram-positive bacteria such as *Staphylococcus* and *Clostridium,* vancomycin is a narrow-spectrum antibiotic. Despite having some beneficial effects on the gut microbiome, it decreases the diversity of the microbiome and modifies its composition, reducing the generation of SCFA and bile acid conversion. Research has demonstrated that vancomycin can both delay the establishment of diabetes in a mouse model and increase the amount of *Akkermansia* [129]. According to certain accounts, treatment with vancomycin may be able to lessen the symptoms of ASD; however, these effects gradually wear off. Age-related senescence, PD, AD, ALS, and MS may be treated with β-lactam antibiotics like Ceftriaxone, according to some animal research. To sum up, while some antibiotics have shown promise in the treatment of neurodegenerative and neurodevelopmental illnesses, further study is required to confirm the effectiveness of targeted antibiotic regimens and to develop medicines that are specifically designed to target particular bacteria [130].

CONCLUSION

The chapter has elaborated on the various pathways that are involved in the development of neurological diseases due to changes in the gut microbiota. It is understood that gut microorganisms do not restrict themselves in the alimentary canal but are active participants in CNS disorders. So, correction and improvements in the microbiota are essential in the treatment of neurological diseases.

CONSENT FOR PUBLICATION

All authors have consented to publishing the book chapter "Neurological Disorders and the Gut-Brain Axis" in this book.

ACKNOWLEDGEMENTS

We the authors acknowledge Maulana Abul Kalam Azad University of Technology, W.B. Department of Pharmaceutical Technology, Haringhata, Nadia, 741249, West Bengal, India, and Adamas University, Barasat-Barrackpore Road, Barbaria, Jagannathpur, 24 Parganas (North), Kolkata-700 126, West Bengal, India for supporting us in writing the chapter.

REFERENCES

[1] Barko PC, McMichael MA, Swanson KS, Williams DA. The Gastrointestinal Microbiome: A Review. J Vet Intern Med 2018; 32(1): 9-25.
[http://dx.doi.org/10.1111/jvim.14875] [PMID: 29171095]

[2] Lyman CC, Holyoak GR, Meinkoth K, Wieneke X, Chillemi KA, DeSilva U. Canine endometrial and vaginal microbiomes reveal distinct and complex ecosystems. PLoS One 2019; 14(1): e0210157.
[http://dx.doi.org/10.1371/journal.pone.0210157] [PMID: 30615657]

[3] Hullar MAJ, Lampe JW, Torok-Storb BJ, Harkey MA. The canine gut microbiome is associated with higher risk of gastric dilatation-volvulus and high risk genetic variants of the immune system. PLoS One 2018; 13(6): e0197686.
[http://dx.doi.org/10.1371/journal.pone.0197686] [PMID: 29889838]

[4] Hugon P, Lagier JC, Colson P, Bittar F, Raoult D. Repertoire of human gut microbes. Microb Pathog 2017; 106: 103-12.
[http://dx.doi.org/10.1016/j.micpath.2016.06.020] [PMID: 27317857]

[5] Lloyd-Price J, Mahurkar A, Rahnavard G, *et al.* Strains, functions and dynamics in the expanded Human Microbiome Project. Nature 2017; 550(7674): 61-6.
[http://dx.doi.org/10.1038/nature23889] [PMID: 28953883]

[6] Cho I, Blaser MJ. The human microbiome: at the interface of health and disease. Nat Rev Genet 2012; 13(4): 260-70.
[http://dx.doi.org/10.1038/nrg3182] [PMID: 22411464]

[7] Lloyd-Price J, Abu-Ali G, Huttenhower C. The healthy human microbiome. Genome Med 2016; 8(1): 51.
[http://dx.doi.org/10.1186/s13073-016-0307-y] [PMID: 27122046]

[8] Arumugam M, Raes J, Pelletier E, Le Paslier D, Yamada T, Mende DR, Fernandes GR, Tap J, Bruls T, Batto JM, Bertalan M. Enterotypes of the human gut microbiome. nature. 2011; 473(7346): 174-80.

[9] Falk PG, Hooper LV, Midtvedt T, Gordon JI. Creating and maintaining the gastrointestinal ecosystem: what we know and need to know from gnotobiology. Microbiol Mol Biol Rev 1998; 62(4): 1157-70. [http://dx.doi.org/10.1128/MMBR.62.4.1157-1170.1998] [PMID: 9841668]

[10] Zhu X, Han Y, Du J, Liu R, Jin K, Yi W. Microbiota-gut-brain axis and the central nervous system. Oncotarget 2017; 8(32): 53829-38. [http://dx.doi.org/10.18632/oncotarget.17754] [PMID: 28881854]

[11] Bercik P, Collins SM, Verdu EF. Microbes and the gut-brain axis. Neurogastroenterol Motil 2012; 24(5): 405-13. [http://dx.doi.org/10.1111/j.1365-2982.2012.01906.x] [PMID: 22404222]

[12] Wu GD, Chen J, Hoffmann C, *et al.* Linking long-term dietary patterns with gut microbial enterotypes. Science 2011; 334(6052): 105-8. [http://dx.doi.org/10.1126/science.1208344] [PMID: 21885731]

[13] O'Mahony SM, Felice VD, Nally K, *et al.* Disturbance of the gut microbiota in early-life selectively affects visceral pain in adulthood without impacting cognitive or anxiety-related behaviors in male rats. Neuroscience 2014; 277: 885-901. [http://dx.doi.org/10.1016/j.neuroscience.2014.07.054] [PMID: 25088912]

[14] Deidda G, Biazzo M. Gut and brain: investigating physiological and pathological interactions between microbiota and brain to gain new therapeutic avenues for brain diseases. Front Neurosci 2021; 15: 753915. [http://dx.doi.org/10.3389/fnins.2021.753915] [PMID: 34712115]

[15] Ma Q, Xing C, Long W, Wang HY, Liu Q, Wang RF. Impact of microbiota on central nervous system and neurological diseases: the gut-brain axis. J Neuroinflammation 2019; 16(1): 53. [http://dx.doi.org/10.1186/s12974-019-1434-3] [PMID: 30823925]

[16] Bhattarai Y, Si J, Pu M, *et al.* Role of gut microbiota in regulating gastrointestinal dysfunction and motor symptoms in a mouse model of Parkinson's disease. Gut Microbes 2021; 13(1): 1866974. [http://dx.doi.org/10.1080/19490976.2020.1866974] [PMID: 33459114]

[17] Lee YK, Menezes JS, Umesaki Y, Mazmanian SK. Proinflammatory T-cell responses to gut microbiota promote experimental autoimmune encephalomyelitis. Proc Natl Acad Sci USA 2011; 108(Suppl 1) (Suppl. 1): 4615-22. [http://dx.doi.org/10.1073/pnas.1000082107] [PMID: 20660719]

[18] Braniste V, Al-Asmakh M, Kowal C, *et al.* The gut microbiota influences blood-brain barrier permeability in mice. Sci Transl Med 2014; 6(263): 263ra158. [http://dx.doi.org/10.1126/scitranslmed.3009759] [PMID: 25411471]

[19] Yin J, Liao SX, He Y, *et al.* Dysbiosis of gut microbiota with reduced trimethylamine-N-oxide level in patients with large-artery atherosclerotic stroke or transient ischemic attack. J Am Heart Assoc 2015; 4(11): e002699. [http://dx.doi.org/10.1161/JAHA.115.002699] [PMID: 26597155]

[20] Rhee SH, Pothoulakis C, Mayer EA. Principles and clinical implications of the brain–gut–enteric microbiota axis. Nat Rev Gastroenterol Hepatol 2009; 6(5): 306-14. [http://dx.doi.org/10.1038/nrgastro.2009.35] [PMID: 19404271]

[21] Cryan JF, O'Riordan KJ, Sandhu K, Peterson V, Dinan TG. The gut microbiome in neurological disorders. Lancet Neurol 2020; 19(2): 179-94. [http://dx.doi.org/10.1016/S1474-4422(19)30356-4] [PMID: 31753762]

[22] Hyland NP, Cryan JF. Microbe-host interactions: Influence of the gut microbiota on the enteric nervous system. Dev Biol 2016; 417(2): 182-7. [http://dx.doi.org/10.1016/j.ydbio.2016.06.027] [PMID: 27343895]

[23] Tremlett H, Bauer KC, Appel-Cresswell S, Finlay BB, Waubant E. The gut microbiome in human neurological disease: A review. Ann Neurol 2017; 81(3): 369-82. [http://dx.doi.org/10.1002/ana.24901] [PMID: 28220542]

[24] Tyler Patterson T, Grandhi R. Gut microbiota and neurologic diseases and injuries. Gut microbiota and pathogenesis of organ injury. 2020: 73-91. [http://dx.doi.org/10.1007/978-981-15-2385-4_6]

[25] McVey Neufeld KA, Mao YK, Bienenstock J, Foster JA, Kunze WA. The microbiome is essential for normal gut intrinsic primary afferent neuron excitability in the mouse. Neurogastroenterol Motil 2013; 25(2): 183-e88. [http://dx.doi.org/10.1111/nmo.12049] [PMID: 23181420]

[26] Neufeld KM, Kang N, Bienenstock J, Foster JA. Reduced anxiety-like behavior and central neurochemical change in germ-free mice. Neurogastroenterol Motil 2011; 23(3): 255-e119, e119. [http://dx.doi.org/10.1111/j.1365-2982.2010.01620.x] [PMID: 21054680]

[27] Park H, Poo M. Neurotrophin regulation of neural circuit development and function. Nat Rev Neurosci 2013; 14(1): 7-23. [http://dx.doi.org/10.1038/nrn3379] [PMID: 23254191]

[28] Kawase T, Nagasawa M, Ikeda H, Yasuo S, Koga Y, Furuse M. Gut microbiota of mice putatively modifies amino acid metabolism in the host brain. Br J Nutr 2017; 117(6): 775-83. [http://dx.doi.org/10.1017/S0007114517000678] [PMID: 28393748]

[29] Xu J, Kurup P, Zhang Y, *et al.* Extrasynaptic NMDA receptors couple preferentially to excitotoxicity *via* calpain-mediated cleavage of STEP. J Neurosci 2009; 29(29): 9330-43. [http://dx.doi.org/10.1523/JNEUROSCI.2212-09.2009] [PMID: 19625523]

[30] Hardingham GE, Bading H. Synaptic versus extrasynaptic NMDA receptor signalling: implications for neurodegenerative disorders. Nat Rev Neurosci 2010; 11(10): 682-96. [http://dx.doi.org/10.1038/nrn2911] [PMID: 20842175]

[31] De Vadder F, Grasset E, Mannerås Holm L, *et al.* Gut microbiota regulates maturation of the adult enteric nervous system *via* enteric serotonin networks. Proc Natl Acad Sci USA 2018; 115(25): 6458-63. [http://dx.doi.org/10.1073/pnas.1720017115] [PMID: 29866843]

[32] Israelyan N, Del Colle A, Li Z, *et al.* Effects of serotonin and slow-release 5-hydroxytryptophan on gastrointestinal motility in a mouse model of depression. Gastroenterology 2019; 157(2): 507-521.e4. [http://dx.doi.org/10.1053/j.gastro.2019.04.022] [PMID: 31071306]

[33] Yano JM, Yu K, Donaldson GP, *et al.* Indigenous bacteria from the gut microbiota regulate host serotonin biosynthesis. Cell 2015; 161(2): 264-76. [http://dx.doi.org/10.1016/j.cell.2015.02.047] [PMID: 25860609]

[34] Wilson KA, Han Y, Zhang M, *et al.* Inter-relations between 3-hydroxypropionate and propionate metabolism in rat liver: relevance to disorders of propionyl-CoA metabolism. Am J Physiol Endocrinol Metab 2017; 313(4): E413-28. [http://dx.doi.org/10.1152/ajpendo.00105.2017] [PMID: 28634175]

[35] Gavin PG, Mullaney JA, Loo D, *et al.* Intestinal metaproteomics reveals host-microbiota interactions in subjects at risk for type 1 diabetes. Diabetes Care 2018; 41(10): 2178-86. [http://dx.doi.org/10.2337/dc18-0777] [PMID: 30100563]

[36] Kasselman LJ, Vernice NA, DeLeon J, Reiss AB. The gut microbiome and elevated cardiovascular risk in obesity and autoimmunity. Atherosclerosis 2018; 271: 203-13. [http://dx.doi.org/10.1016/j.atherosclerosis.2018.02.036] [PMID: 29524863]

[37] Duan Y, Prasad R, Feng D, *et al.* Bone marrow-derived cells restore functional integrity of the gut epithelial and vascular barriers in a model of diabetes and ACE2 deficiency. Circ Res 2019; 125(11): 969-88.

[http://dx.doi.org/10.1161/CIRCRESAHA.119.315743] [PMID: 31610731]

[38] Braak H, Braak E. Neuropathological stageing of Alzheimer-related changes. Acta Neuropathol 1991; 82(4): 239-59.
[http://dx.doi.org/10.1007/BF00308809] [PMID: 1759558]

[39] Hampel H, Blennow K, Shaw LM, Hoessler YC, Zetterberg H, Trojanowski JQ. Total and phosphorylated tau protein as biological markers of Alzheimer's disease. Exp Gerontol 2010; 45(1): 30-40.
[http://dx.doi.org/10.1016/j.exger.2009.10.010] [PMID: 19853650]

[40] Nabi SU, Khan A, Siddiqui EM, *et al.* Mechanisms of mitochondrial malfunction in Alzheimer's disease: new therapeutic hope. Oxid Med Cell Longev 2022; 2022: 1-28.
[http://dx.doi.org/10.1155/2022/4759963] [PMID: 35607703]

[41] Fülöp T, Itzhaki RF, Balin BJ, Miklossy J, Barron AE. Role of microbes in the development of Alzheimer's disease: State of the art–An international symposium presented at the 2017 IAGG congress in San Francisco. Front Genet 2018; 9: 362.
[http://dx.doi.org/10.3389/fgene.2018.00362] [PMID: 30250480]

[42] Bairamian D, Sha S, Rolhion N, *et al.* Microbiota in neuroinflammation and synaptic dysfunction: a focus on Alzheimer's disease. Mol Neurodegener 2022; 17(1): 19.
[http://dx.doi.org/10.1186/s13024-022-00522-2] [PMID: 35248147]

[43] Kras K, Rudyk H, Muszyński S, *et al.* Morphology and chemical coding of rat duodenal enteric neurons following prenatal exposure to fumonisins. Animals (Basel) 2022; 12(9): 1055.
[http://dx.doi.org/10.3390/ani12091055] [PMID: 35565482]

[44] Sousa FC, Schamber CR, Amorin SSS, Natali MRM. Effect of fumonisin-containing diet on the myenteric plexus of the jejunum in rats. Auton Neurosci 2014; 185: 93-9.
[http://dx.doi.org/10.1016/j.autneu.2014.08.001] [PMID: 25183308]

[45] Meyer K, Lulla A, Debroy K, *et al.* Association of the gut microbiota with cognitive function in midlife. JAMA Netw Open 2022; 5(2): e2143941.
[http://dx.doi.org/10.1001/jamanetworkopen.2021.43941] [PMID: 35133436]

[46] Park JY, Choi J, Lee Y, *et al.* Metagenome analysis of bodily microbiota in a mouse model of Alzheimer disease using bacteria-derived membrane vesicles in blood. Exp Neurobiol 2017; 26(6): 369-79.
[http://dx.doi.org/10.5607/en.2017.26.6.369] [PMID: 29302204]

[47] Dominy SS, Lynch C, Ermini F, *et al. Porphyromonas gingivalis* in Alzheimer's disease brains: Evidence for disease causation and treatment with small-molecule inhibitors. Sci Adv 2019; 5(1): eaau3333.
[http://dx.doi.org/10.1126/sciadv.aau3333] [PMID: 30746447]

[48] Haran JP, Bhattarai SK, Foley SE, *et al.* Alzheimer's disease microbiome is associated with dysregulation of the anti-inflammatory P-glycoprotein pathway. MBio 2019; 10(3): e00632-19.
[http://dx.doi.org/10.1128/mBio.00632-19] [PMID: 31064831]

[49] Shen H, Guan Q, Zhang X, *et al.* New mechanism of neuroinflammation in Alzheimer's disease: The activation of NLRP3 inflammasome mediated by gut microbiota. Prog Neuropsychopharmacol Biol Psychiatry 2020; 100: 109884.
[http://dx.doi.org/10.1016/j.pnpbp.2020.109884] [PMID: 32032696]

[50] Zhang L, Wang Y, Xiayu X, *et al.* Altered gut microbiota in a mouse model of Alzheimer's disease. J Alzheimers Dis 2017; 60(4): 1241-57.
[http://dx.doi.org/10.3233/JAD-170020] [PMID: 29036812]

[51] Naomi R, Embong H, Othman F, Ghazi HF, Maruthey N, Bahari H. Probiotics for Alzheimer's disease: A systematic review. Nutrients 2021; 14(1): 20.
[http://dx.doi.org/10.3390/nu14010020] [PMID: 35010895]

[52] Holmqvist S, Chutna O, Bousset L, *et al.* Direct evidence of Parkinson pathology spread from the gastrointestinal tract to the brain in rats. Acta Neuropathol 2014; 128(6): 805-20. [http://dx.doi.org/10.1007/s00401-014-1343-6] [PMID: 25296989]

[53] Liu B, Fang F, Pedersen NL, *et al.* Vagotomy and Parkinson disease. Neurology 2017; 88(21): 1996-2002. [http://dx.doi.org/10.1212/WNL.0000000000003961] [PMID: 28446653]

[54] Svensson E, Horváth-Puhó E, Thomsen RW, *et al.* Vagotomy and subsequent risk of P arkinson's disease. Ann Neurol 2015; 78(4): 522-9. [http://dx.doi.org/10.1002/ana.24448] [PMID: 26031848]

[55] Miraglia F, Valvano V, Rota L, *et al.* Alpha-synuclein FRET biosensors reveal early alpha-synuclein aggregation in the endoplasmic reticulum. Life (Basel) 2020; 10(8): 147. [http://dx.doi.org/10.3390/life10080147] [PMID: 32796544]

[56] Benakis C, Brea D, Caballero S, *et al.* Commensal microbiota affects ischemic stroke outcome by regulating intestinal γδ T cells. Nat Med 2016; 22(5): 516-23. [http://dx.doi.org/10.1038/nm.4068] [PMID: 27019327]

[57] He W, Luo Y, Liu JP, *et al.* Trimethylamine N-oxide, a gut microbiota-dependent metabolite, is associated with frailty in older adults with cardiovascular disease. Clin Interv Aging 2020; 15: 1809-20. [http://dx.doi.org/10.2147/CIA.S270887] [PMID: 33061331]

[58] Farhangi MA, Vajdi M, Asghari-Jafarabadi M. Gut microbiota-associated metabolite trimethylamine N-Oxide and the risk of stroke: a systematic review and dose–response meta-analysis. Nutr J 2020; 19(1): 76. [http://dx.doi.org/10.1186/s12937-020-00592-2] [PMID: 32731904]

[59] Tu R, Xia J. Stroke and vascular cognitive impairment: the role of intestinal microbiota metabolite TMAO CNS & Neurological Disorders-Drug Targets. Formerly Current Drug Targets-CNS & Neurological Disorders 2023.

[60] Wang B, Qiu J, Lian J, Yang X, Zhou J. Gut metabolite trimethylamine-N-oxide in atherosclerosis: from mechanism to therapy. Front Cardiovasc Med 2021; 8: 723886. [http://dx.doi.org/10.3389/fcvm.2021.723886] [PMID: 34888358]

[61] Yin J, Liao SX, He Y, *et al.* Dysbiosis of gut microbiota with reduced trimethylamine-N-oxide level in patients with large-artery atherosclerotic stroke or transient ischemic attack. J Am Heart Assoc 2015; 4(11): e002699. [http://dx.doi.org/10.1161/JAHA.115.002699] [PMID: 26597155]

[62] Arulsamy A, Tan QY, Balasubramaniam V, O'Brien TJ, Shaikh MF. Gut microbiota and epilepsy: a systematic review on their relationship and possible therapeutics. ACS Chem Neurosci 2020; 11(21): 3488-98. [http://dx.doi.org/10.1021/acschemneuro.0c00431] [PMID: 33064448]

[63] Levira F, Thurman DJ, Sander JW, *et al.* Premature mortality of epilepsy in low- and middle-income countries: A systematic review from the Mortality Task Force of the International League Against Epilepsy. Epilepsia 2017; 58(1): 6-16. [http://dx.doi.org/10.1111/epi.13603] [PMID: 27988968]

[64] Chatzikonstantinou S, Gioula G, Kimiskidis VK, McKenna J, Mavroudis I, Kazis D. The gut microbiome in drug-resistant epilepsy. Epilepsia Open 2021; 6(1): 28-37. [http://dx.doi.org/10.1002/epi4.12461] [PMID: 33681645]

[65] Vezzani A. Epilepsy and inflammation in the brain: overview and pathophysiology. Epilepsy Curr 2014; 14(2_suppl) (Suppl.): 3-7. [http://dx.doi.org/10.5698/1535-7511-14.s2.3] [PMID: 24955068]

[66] Radulescu CI, Garcia-Miralles M, Sidik H, *et al.* Manipulation of microbiota reveals altered callosal

myelination and white matter plasticity in a model of Huntington disease. Neurobiol Dis 2019; 127: 65-75.
[http://dx.doi.org/10.1016/j.nbd.2019.02.011] [PMID: 30802499]

[67] Pradini GW, Fauziah N, Asarina S, Anggareni N, Widyastuti R, Syamsunarno MRAA. Prebiotic Effect of Cogon Grass Root Extract on Stimulating Lactic Acid Bacteria Growth in Mice Intestine. Journal of Medicine and Health 2024; 6(1): 34-44.
[http://dx.doi.org/10.28932/jmh.v6i1.7689]

[68] Costello E, Goodrich JA, Patterson WB, *et al.* Proteomic and Metabolomic Signatures of Diet Quality in Young Adults. Nutrients 2024; 16(3): 429.
[http://dx.doi.org/10.3390/nu16030429] [PMID: 38337712]

[69] Pant A, Chew D, Mamas M, Zaman S. Cardiovascular Disease and the Mediterranean Diet: Insights into Sex-Specific Responses. Nutrients 2024; 16(4): 570.
[http://dx.doi.org/10.3390/nu16040570] [PMID: 38398894]

[70] Ocampo-Anguiano PV, Victoria-Ruiz LL, Reynoso-Camacho R, *et al.* Ingestion of Bean Leaves Reduces Metabolic Complications and Restores Intestinal Integrity in C57BL/6 Mice with Obesity Induced by a High-Fat and High-Fructose Diet. Nutrients 2024; 16(3): 367.
[http://dx.doi.org/10.3390/nu16030367] [PMID: 38337654]

[71] Pérez LR, Lázaro JM, Puentes NC, Amador AÁ, Marrugo-Padilla A. Identification of proinflammatory pathways and promising bioactive polyphenols for the treatment of sickle cell anemia by in silico study and network pharmacology.
[http://dx.doi.org/10.21203/rs.3.rs-3961707/v1]

[72] Moftah HK, Mousa MHA, Elrazaz EZ, Kamel AS, Lasheen DS, Georgey HH. Novel quinazolinone Derivatives: Design, synthesis and in vivo evaluation as potential agents targeting Alzheimer disease. Bioorg Chem 2024; 143: 107065.
[http://dx.doi.org/10.1016/j.bioorg.2023.107065] [PMID: 38150939]

[73] Pandit N, Kulkarni S, Singhvi G. Effect of green tea on human brain health. InNutraceutical Fruits and Foods for Neurodegenerative Disorders. 2024; pp. 301-331. Academic Press.
[http://dx.doi.org/10.1016/B978-0-443-18951-7.00018-9]

[74] Jalanka J, Major G, Murray K, *et al.* The effect of psyllium husk on intestinal microbiota in constipated patients and healthy controls. Int J Mol Sci 2019; 20(2): 433.
[http://dx.doi.org/10.3390/ijms20020433] [PMID: 30669509]

[75] Bretin A, Zou J, San Yeoh B, *et al.* Psyllium fiber protects against colitis *via* activation of bile acid sensor farnesoid X receptor. Cell Mol Gastroenterol Hepatol 2023; 15(6): 1421-42.
[http://dx.doi.org/10.1016/j.jcmgh.2023.02.007] [PMID: 36828279]

[76] Le Bastard Q, Chapelet G, Javaudin F, Lepelletier D, Batard E, Montassier E. The effects of inulin on gut microbial composition: a systematic review of evidence from human studies. Eur J Clin Microbiol Infect Dis 2020; 39(3): 403-13.
[http://dx.doi.org/10.1007/s10096-019-03721-w] [PMID: 31707507]

[77] Roy Sarkar S, Banerjee S. Gut microbiota in neurodegenerative disorders. J Neuroimmunol 2019; 328: 98-104.
[http://dx.doi.org/10.1016/j.jneuroim.2019.01.004] [PMID: 30658292]

[78] Alipour Nosrani E, Tamtaji OR, Alibolandi Z, *et al.* Neuroprotective effects of probiotics bacteria on animal model of Parkinson's disease induced by 6-hydroxydopamine: A behavioral, biochemical, and histological study. J Immunoassay Immunochem 2021; 42(2): 106-20.
[http://dx.doi.org/10.1080/15321819.2020.1833917] [PMID: 33078659]

[79] Tang W, Zhu H, Feng Y, Guo R, Wan D. The impact of gut microbiota disorders on the blood–brain barrier. Infect Drug Resist 2020; 13: 3351-63.
[http://dx.doi.org/10.2147/IDR.S254403] [PMID: 33061482]

[80] Sugita S, Tahir P, Kinjo S. The effects of microbiome-targeted therapy on cognitive impairment and postoperative cognitive dysfunction—A systematic review. PLoS One 2023; 18(2): e0281049. [http://dx.doi.org/10.1371/journal.pone.0281049] [PMID: 36749772]

[81] Rianda D, Suradijono SHR, Setiawan EA, *et al.* Long-term benefits of probiotics and calcium supplementation during childhood, and other biomedical and socioenvironmental factors, on adolescent neurodevelopmental outcomes. J Funct Foods 2022; 91: 105014. [http://dx.doi.org/10.1016/j.jff.2022.105014]

[82] Pärtty A, Kalliomäki M, Wacklin P, Salminen S, Isolauri E. A possible link between early probiotic intervention and the risk of neuropsychiatric disorders later in childhood: a randomized trial. Pediatr Res 2015; 77(6): 823-8. [http://dx.doi.org/10.1038/pr.2015.51] [PMID: 25760553]

[83] Ng Q, Loke W, Venkatanarayanan N, Lim D, Soh A, Yeo W. A systematic review of the role of prebiotics and probiotics in autism spectrum disorders. Medicina (Kaunas) 2019; 55(5): 129. [http://dx.doi.org/10.3390/medicina55050129] [PMID: 31083360]

[84] Quraishi MN, Widlak M, Bhala N, *et al.* Systematic review with meta-analysis: the efficacy of faecal microbiota transplantation for the treatment of recurrent and refractory *Clostridium difficile* infection. Aliment Pharmacol Ther 2017; 46(5): 479-93. [http://dx.doi.org/10.1111/apt.14201] [PMID: 28707337]

[85] Mullish BH, Quraishi MN, Segal JP, *et al.* The use of faecal microbiota transplant as treatment for recurrent or refractory *Clostridium difficile* infection and other potential indications: joint British Society of Gastroenterology (BSG) and Healthcare Infection Society (HIS) guidelines. Gut 2018; 67(11): 1920-41. [http://dx.doi.org/10.1136/gutjnl-2018-316818] [PMID: 30154172]

[86] Ianiro G, Bibbò S, Scaldaferri F, Gasbarrini A, Cammarota G. Fecal microbiota transplantation in inflammatory bowel disease: beyond the excitement. Medicine (Baltimore) 2014; 93(19): e97. [http://dx.doi.org/10.1097/MD.0000000000000097] [PMID: 25340496]

[87] Sokol H, Landman C, Seksik P, *et al.* Fecal microbiota transplantation to maintain remission in Crohn's disease: a pilot randomized controlled study. Microbiome 2020; 8(1): 12. [http://dx.doi.org/10.1186/s40168-020-0792-5] [PMID: 32014035]

[88] Wang H, Lu Y, Yan Y, *et al.* Promising treatment for type 2 diabetes: fecal microbiota transplantation reverses insulin resistance and impaired islets. Front Cell Infect Microbiol 2020; 9: 455. [http://dx.doi.org/10.3389/fcimb.2019.00455] [PMID: 32010641]

[89] Wang Y, Zhang S, Borody TJ, Zhang F. Encyclopedia of fecal microbiota transplantation: a review of effectiveness in the treatment of 85 diseases. Chin Med J (Engl) 2022; 135(16): 1927-39. [http://dx.doi.org/10.1097/CM9.0000000000002339] [PMID: 36103991]

[90] Matheson JAT, Holsinger RMD. The role of fecal microbiota transplantation in the treatment of neurodegenerative diseases: A review. Int J Mol Sci 2023; 24(2): 1001. [http://dx.doi.org/10.3390/ijms24021001] [PMID: 36674517]

[91] Park SH, Lee JH, Shin J, *et al.* Cognitive function improvement after fecal microbiota transplantation in Alzheimer's dementia patient: a case report. Curr Med Res Opin 2021; 37(10): 1739-44. [http://dx.doi.org/10.1080/03007995.2021.1957807] [PMID: 34289768]

[92] Huang H, Xu H, Luo Q, *et al.* Fecal microbiota transplantation to treat Parkinson's disease with constipation. Medicine (Baltimore) 2019; 98(26): e16163. [http://dx.doi.org/10.1097/MD.0000000000016163] [PMID: 31261545]

[93] Xue LJ, Yang XZ, Tong Q, *et al.* Fecal microbiota transplantation therapy for Parkinson's disease. Medicine (Baltimore) 2020; 99(35): e22035. [http://dx.doi.org/10.1097/MD.0000000000022035] [PMID: 32871960]

[94] Kuai X, Yao X, Xu L, *et al.* Evaluation of fecal microbiota transplantation in Parkinson's disease

patients with constipation. Microb Cell Fact 2021; 20(1): 98.
[http://dx.doi.org/10.1186/s12934-021-01589-0] [PMID: 33985520]

[95] Borody T, Leis S, Campbell J, Torres M, Nowak A. Fecal microbiota transplantation (FMT) in multiple sclerosis (MS): 942. Official journal of the American College of Gastroenterology| ACG. 2011; 106: S352.

[96] Ward L, O'Grady HM, Wu K, Cannon K, Workentine M, Louie T. Combined oral fecal capsules plus fecal enema as treatment of late-onset autism spectrum disorder in children: report of a small case series. InOpen Forum Infectious Diseases. 2016; 3(1): p. 2219. Oxford University Press.
[http://dx.doi.org/10.1093/ofid/ofw172.1767]

[97] Kang DW, Adams JB, Gregory AC, *et al.* Microbiota Transfer Therapy alters gut ecosystem and improves gastrointestinal and autism symptoms: an open-label study. Microbiome 2017; 5(1): 10.
[http://dx.doi.org/10.1186/s40168-016-0225-7] [PMID: 28122648]

[98] Park SY, Seo GS. Fecal microbiota transplantation: is it safe? Clin Endosc 2021; 54(2): 157-60.
[http://dx.doi.org/10.5946/ce.2021.072] [PMID: 33827154]

[99] Wang S, Xu M, Wang W, *et al.* Systematic review: adverse events of fecal microbiota transplantation. PLoS One 2016; 11(8): e0161174.
[http://dx.doi.org/10.1371/journal.pone.0161174] [PMID: 27529553]

[100] Zhang B, Liu K, Yang H, Jin Z, Ding Q, Zhao L. Gut Microbiota: The Potential Key Target of TCM's Therapeutic Effect of Treating Different Diseases Using the Same Method—UC and T2DM as Examples. Front Cell Infect Microbiol 2022; 12: 855075.
[http://dx.doi.org/10.3389/fcimb.2022.855075] [PMID: 35433500]

[101] Fortea M, Albert-Bayo M, Abril-Gil M, *et al.* Present and future therapeutic approaches to barrier dysfunction. Front Nutr 2021; 8: 718093.
[http://dx.doi.org/10.3389/fnut.2021.718093] [PMID: 34778332]

[102] Huang JQ, Wei SY, Cheng N, *et al.* Chimonanthus nitens oliv. Leaf granule ameliorates DSS-induced acute colitis through Treg cell improvement, oxidative stress reduction, and gut microflora modulation. Front Cell Infect Microbiol 2022; 12: 907813.
[http://dx.doi.org/10.3389/fcimb.2022.907813] [PMID: 35832382]

[103] Wu G, Zhang W, Zheng N, *et al.* Integrated microbiome and metabolome analysis reveals the potential therapeutic mechanism of *Qing-Fei-Pai-Du* decoction in mice with coronavirus-induced pneumonia. Front Cell Infect Microbiol 2022; 12: 950983.
[http://dx.doi.org/10.3389/fcimb.2022.950983] [PMID: 36093201]

[104] Li Y, Kang Y, Du Y, *et al.* Effects of Konjaku flour on the gut microbiota of obese patients. Front Cell Infect Microbiol 2022; 12: 771748.
[http://dx.doi.org/10.3389/fcimb.2022.771748] [PMID: 35300378]

[105] Guo Q, Ni C, Li L, *et al.* Integrated traditional Chinese medicine improves functional outcome in acute Ischemic stroke: from clinic to mechanism exploration with gut microbiota. Front Cell Infect Microbiol 2022; 12: 827129.
[http://dx.doi.org/10.3389/fcimb.2022.827129] [PMID: 35223549]

[106] Jabczyk M, Nowak J, Hudzik B, Zubelewicz-Szkodzińska B. Curcumin and its potential impact on microbiota. Nutrients 2021; 13(6): 2004.
[http://dx.doi.org/10.3390/nu13062004] [PMID: 34200819]

[107] Cui C, Han Y, Li H, Yu H, Zhang B, Li G. Curcumin-driven reprogramming of the gut microbiota and metabolome ameliorates motor deficits and neuroinflammation in a mouse model of Parkinson's disease. Front Cell Infect Microbiol 2022; 12: 887407.
[http://dx.doi.org/10.3389/fcimb.2022.887407] [PMID: 36034698]

[108] Bao C, Wu L, Wang D, *et al.* Acupuncture improves the symptoms, intestinal microbiota, and inflammation of patients with mild to moderate Crohn's disease: A randomized controlled trial.

EClinicalMedicine 2022; 45: 101300.
[http://dx.doi.org/10.1016/j.eclinm.2022.101300] [PMID: 35198926]

[109] Bao CH, Wu LY, Shi Y, *et al.* Moxibustion down-regulates colonic epithelial cell apoptosis and repairs tight junctions in rats with Crohn's disease. World J Gastroenterol 2011; 17(45): 4960-70.
[http://dx.doi.org/10.3748/wjg.v17.i45.4960] [PMID: 22174545]

[110] Wei D, Xie L, Zhuang Z, Zhao N, Huang B, Tang Y, Yu S, Zhou Q, Wu Q. Gut microbiota: a new strategy to study the mechanism of electroacupuncture and moxibustion in treating ulcerative colitis. Evidence-Based Complementary and Alternative Medicine. 2019; 2019.
[http://dx.doi.org/10.1155/2019/9730176]

[111] Nazarova L, Liu H, Xie H, *et al.* Targeting gut-brain axis through scalp-abdominal electroacupuncture in Parkinson's disease. Brain Res 2022; 1790: 147956.
[http://dx.doi.org/10.1016/j.brainres.2022.147956] [PMID: 35660372]

[112] Yang B, He M, Chen X, *et al.* Acupuncture effect assessment in APP/PS1 transgenic mice: On regulating learning-memory abilities, gut microbiota, and microbial metabolites. Comput Math Methods Med 2022; 2022: 1-20.
[http://dx.doi.org/10.1155/2022/1527159] [PMID: 35432583]

[113] Kim M, Park SJ, Choi S, *et al.* Association between antibiotics and dementia risk: A retrospective cohort study. Front Pharmacol 2022; 13: 888333.
[http://dx.doi.org/10.3389/fphar.2022.888333] [PMID: 36225572]

[114] Mertsalmi TH, Pekkonen E, Scheperjans F. Antibiotic exposure and risk of Parkinson's disease in Finland: A nationwide case-control study. Mov Disord 2020; 35(3): 431-42.
[http://dx.doi.org/10.1002/mds.27924] [PMID: 31737957]

[115] Sun J, Zhan Y, Mariosa D, *et al.* Antibiotics use and risk of amyotrophic lateral sclerosis in Sweden. Eur J Neurol 2019; 26(11): 1355-61.
[http://dx.doi.org/10.1111/ene.13986] [PMID: 31087715]

[116] Jernberg C, Löfmark S, Edlund C, Jansson JK. Long-term impacts of antibiotic exposure on the human intestinal microbiota. Microbiology (Reading) 2010; 156(11): 3216-23.
[http://dx.doi.org/10.1099/mic.0.040618-0] [PMID: 20705661]

[117] Vervoort J, Xavier BB, Stewardson A, *et al.* Metagenomic analysis of the impact of nitrofurantoin treatment on the human faecal microbiota. J Antimicrob Chemother 2015; 70(7): 1989-92.
[http://dx.doi.org/10.1093/jac/dkv062] [PMID: 25766736]

[118] Ponziani FR, Zocco MA, D'Aversa F, Pompili M, Gasbarrini A. Eubiotic properties of rifaximin: Disruption of the traditional concepts in gut microbiota modulation. World J Gastroenterol 2017; 23(25): 4491-9.
[http://dx.doi.org/10.3748/wjg.v23.i25.4491] [PMID: 28740337]

[119] Sroka N, Rydzewska-Rosołowska A, Kakareko K, Rosołowski M, Głowińska I, Hryszko T. Show Me What You Have Inside—The Complex Interplay between SIBO and Multiple Medical Conditions—A Systematic Review. Nutrients 2022; 15(1): 90.
[http://dx.doi.org/10.3390/nu15010090] [PMID: 36615748]

[120] Prantera C, Lochs H, Grimaldi M, Danese S, Scribano ML, Gionchetti P. Rifaximin-extended intestinal release induces remission in patients with moderately active Crohn's disease. Gastroenterology 2012; 142(3): 473-481.e4.
[http://dx.doi.org/10.1053/j.gastro.2011.11.032] [PMID: 22155172]

[121] Hong CT, Chan L, Chen KY, *et al.* Rifaximin Modifies Gut Microbiota and Attenuates Inflammation in Parkinson's Disease: Preclinical and Clinical Studies. Cells 2022; 11(21): 3468.
[http://dx.doi.org/10.3390/cells11213468] [PMID: 36359864]

[122] Ianiro G, Tilg H, Gasbarrini A. Antibiotics as deep modulators of gut microbiota: between good and evil. Gut 2016; 65(11): 1906-15.

[http://dx.doi.org/10.1136/gutjnl-2016-312297] [PMID: 27531828]

[123] Obrenovich M, Jaworski H, Tadimalla T, *et al.* The role of the microbiota–gut–brain axis and antibiotics in ALS and neurodegenerative diseases. Microorganisms 2020; 8(5): 784. [http://dx.doi.org/10.3390/microorganisms8050784] [PMID: 32456229]

[124] Weng JC, Tikhonova MA, Chen JH, *et al.* Ceftriaxone prevents the neurodegeneration and decreased neurogenesis seen in a Parkinson's disease rat model: An immunohistochemical and MRI study. Behav Brain Res 2016; 305: 126-39. [http://dx.doi.org/10.1016/j.bbr.2016.02.034] [PMID: 26940602]

[125] Bicknell B, Liebert A, Borody T, Herkes G, McLachlan C, Kiat H. Neurodegenerative and Neurodevelopmental Diseases and the Gut-Brain Axis: The Potential of Therapeutic Targeting of the Microbiome. Int J Mol Sci 2023; 24(11): 9577. [http://dx.doi.org/10.3390/ijms24119577] [PMID: 37298527]

[126] Soliman YS, Elkhateb IT, Aly HZ. Neonatal Microbiome and the Gut–Brain Axis: Is It the Origin of Adult Diseases?. Journal of Pediatric Neurology. 2019; 17(3): 095-104.

[127] Suganya K, Koo BS. Gut–brain axis: role of gut microbiota on neurological disorders and how probiotics/prebiotics beneficially modulate microbial and immune pathways to improve brain functions. Int J Mol Sci 2020; 21(20): 7551. [http://dx.doi.org/10.3390/ijms21207551] [PMID: 33066156]

[128] Codagnone MG, Stanton C, O'Mahony SM, Dinan TG, Cryan JF. Microbiota and neurodevelopmental trajectories: role of maternal and early-life nutrition. Ann Nutr Metab 2019; 74 (Suppl. 2): 16-27. [http://dx.doi.org/10.1159/000499144] [PMID: 31234188]

[129] Tiwari P, Dwivedi R, Bansal M, Tripathi M, Dada R. Role of gut microbiota in neurological disorders and its therapeutic significance. J Clin Med 2023; 12(4): 1650. [http://dx.doi.org/10.3390/jcm12041650] [PMID: 36836185]

[130] Zheng Y, Bonfili L, Wei T, Eleuteri AM. Understanding the gut–brain axis and its therapeutic implications for neurodegenerative disorders. Nutrients 2023; 15(21): 4631. [http://dx.doi.org/10.3390/nu15214631] [PMID: 37960284]

CHAPTER 8

Gut Microbiota Modulation Strategies

Rudradeep Hazra[1], **Arijit Mallick**[1], **Soumyadeep Chattopadhyay**[1], **Sakuntala Gayen**[1] and **Souvik Roy**[1,*]

[1] *Department of Pharmaceutical Technology, NSHM Knowledge Campus, Kolkata-Group of Institutions, 124, B. L. Saha Road, Tara Park, Behala, Kolkata, West Bengal-700053, India*

Abstract: The gut microbiota plays a fundamental role in human health, influencing various physiological processes and contributing to overall welfare. This book chapter synthesizes current knowledge on the modulation of gut microbiota through key interventions, including prebiotics, probiotics, faecal microbiota transplantation (FMT), and dietary strategies. Prebiotics act as non-digestible fibers that selectively stimulate the growth and activity of primary three enterotypes like *Firmicutes*, *Bacteroidetes* and *Actinobacteria* that have emerged as promising contributors to gut health. Probiotics which are live microorganisms provide considerate health benefits and offer simultaneously, a direct means of manipulating microbial composition. FMT, a therapeutic approach involving the transfer of faecal material from a healthy donor to a recipient, has gained attention for its potential to restore gut microbiota equilibrium. Additionally, dietary interventions, such as high-fibrous diets, polyphenolic-rich foods, omega-3 fatty acids, and restricted sugar intake can exert profound effects on the gut microbial community. Understanding the intricate interplay between these interventions and the gut microbiota provides valuable insights into developing targeted strategies for promoting gastrointestinal health and managing various health conditions like obesity, IBD, and Type 2 diabetes. This chapter highlights recent advancements, challenges, and future directions in harnessing the potential of prebiotics, probiotics, FMT, and dietary interventions for modulating the gut microbiota and improving human health.

Keywords: Dietary intervention, Enterotypes, Fatty acids, Gastrointestinal health, Gut, Human health, Live-microorganisms, Microbiota, Obesity, Polyphenol-rich foods.

* **Corresponding author Souvik Roy:** Department of Pharmaceutical Technology, NSHM Knowledge Campus, Kolkata-Group of Institutions, 124, B. L. Saha Road, Tara Park, Behala, Kolkata, West Bengal-700053, India; E-mail: souvikroy35@gmail.com

Sandipan Dasgupta & Moitreyee Chattopadhyay (Eds.)

INTRODUCTION

Probiotics and Promoting a Healthy Gut Microbiome

A probiotic is defined as "a live microbial food ingredient that is beneficial to health" [1]. The probiotics extensively investigated to date are predominantly from the *Lactobacillus* and *Bifidobacterium* genera [2]. Probiotic therapy has shown great effectiveness in contrast to a wide range of alimentary diseases and ailments [2] as they colonise the human intestines and modify the composition of the gut flora in specific parts of the host thus, inhibiting the colonisation of pathogenic bacteria in the intestine. They assist the host in preserving a robust protective layer for the intestinal mucosa, thereby reinforcing immunity [3]. Probiotics also help enhance the bioavailability of micronutrients like calcium and iron from the ingested food [4]. This process is achieved by the release of short-chain fatty acids (SCFAs) from these probiotics during fermentation. Consequently, it leads to a reduction in intestinal pH, enhancing mineral solubility and expanding the surface area for enterocyte absorption [5]. Moreover, dairy products that we consume act as an outstanding food medium thus ensuring their stability, feasibility, and ideal expression of probiotic function [6].

Probiotics as a Relieving Agent Against Lactose Intolerance

Africans and Asians constitute the primary demographic population who experience such intolerance, while in Europe, the prevalence ranges from 2% to 70% [7]. Commonly observed symptoms include bloating, stomach pain, flatulence, loose stools, nausea, and borborygmi whereas, those with lactose intolerance can effectively tolerate and digest alternative sources of lactose, such as yogurt, kimchi, or sauerkraut, but struggle with the digestion of raw milk [8]. Yogurt and lactic acid bacteria in probiotics contain elevated levels of lactase, that are secreted into the enteric lumen. In this environment, lactase undergoes lysis facilitated by bile secretions [9]. Subsequently, lactase interacts with ingested lactose, alleviating symptoms associated with malabsorption. Additionally, fermented foods, including yogurt, contribute to a prolonged intestinal transit time, allowing for slower digestion of lactose and consequently mitigating symptoms.

Probiotics Help to Combat Diarrhoea

In instances of acute infantile diarrhoea, commonly associated with rotavirus infection, *Lactobacillus rhamnosus GG* consistently demonstrates the ability to decrease the period of diarrhoea by around 50% [10]. The potential mechanism through which this bacterium operates involves strengthening mucosal integrity and triggering the immune response, potentially through increased production of anti-rotavirus-specific immunoglobulin (Ig)A [10]. Another notable finding involves *Bifidobacterium bifidum*, administered alongside *Streptococcus thermophilus* present in standard milk formula, which has proved to be effective in reducing the occurrence of rotaviral diarrhoea [11].

Diarrhoea is a more prevalent issue in individuals undergoing antibiotic treatment [8]. Antibiotics can proximately disturb the native gut microbiota thereby diminishing colonization resistance and establishing a conducive environment for the development of disease-causing microorganisms like *Clostridium difficile* and *Klebsiella oxytoca* [12]. Probiotics are also advantageous in alleviating the complications linked to the 'triple therapy,' which entails the use of antibiotics to eradicate Helicobacter pylori from the stomach [13]. In particular, the administration of *Lactobacillus rhamnosus GG* has demonstrated effectiveness in reducing the frequency of diarrhoea, nausea, and alterations in taste among individuals undergoing *H. pylori* eradication with rabeprazole, clarithromycin, and tinidazole [13].

Probiotics for the Treatment of Inflammatory Bowel Disease (IBD)

Extensive research has been conducted on probiotics to explore their capacity to alleviate symptoms associated with chronic conditions such as Inflammatory Bowel Disease (IBD) and Colorectal Cancer. Inflammatory Bowel Disease (IBD) is a term that refers to a group of chronic inflammatory conditions of the gastrointestinal tract. The administration of probiotics either regulates or modulates the composition of the gut microbiome, providing relief from symptoms associated with IBD and preventing the recurrence of such inflammation [14]. The non-pathogenic strain E. coli Nissle 1917 and S. boulardii have demonstrated efficacy in individuals with Crohn's disease, showing a reduction in stool frequency and the severity of relapses when compared to a placebo [15]. VSL#3, a blend of four *Lactobacilli* (*L. acidophilus, Lactobacillus bulgaricus, Lactobacillus casei, and Lactobacillus plantarum*), three *Bifidobacteria* (*Bifidobacterium breve, Bifidobacterium infantis,* and *Bifidobacterium longum*), and *S. thermophilus* [16]. This combination has proven to be efficient in reducing the recurrence of chronic relapsing pouchitis [17]. VSL#3, given at a daily dosage of 6 g, exhibited a substantial decrease in the recurrence of relapses (15%) when contrasted with a placebo group (100%) throughout a 9-month duration [18]. Additionally, it was successful in preventing the onset of pouchitis in individuals who had undergone ileo-pouch anal anastomosis for ulcerative colitis (UC). Understanding the mechanisms underlying probiotic activity in treating inflammatory bowel disease (IBD) has primarily been derived from animal model studies. The suggested mechanism involves the engagement of probiotics with mucosal regulatory T cells and the control of cytokine transcription factors in the mucosa in reciprocation to invasive bacteria [19].

Probiotics for the Treatment of Colorectal Cancer (CRC)

About three-fourths of all CRCs occurring are irregular and continuously increase with age. The role of diet and its interactions with gut flora is significant, particularly as the diverse gut microbiome tends to diminish with age. Many faecal microorganisms are capable of producing carcinogens and promoting tumours from the diet that we consume but which species are proficient are yet to be identified. Common microorganisms like *Bifidobacteria* and *lactobacilli* produce non-toxic and non-carcinogenic metabolites. Additionally, probiotics can influence the favourable biomarkers associated with colorectal cancer (CRC). Specific bacterial species, such as Clostridia and Bacteroides, possess various enzymatic activities capable of transforming dietary components into harmful or carcinogenic substances like beta-glucuronidase, beta-glycosidase, azo-reductase, nitro-reductase, IO 'hydratase-dehydrogenase,' and nitrate/nitrite reductase. Various probiotics have demonstrated the ability to decrease the activity of harmful faecal enzymes. However, a clear connection between this reduction and a lowered risk of colorectal cancer (CRC) in humans has not been definitively established [20]. Pool-Zobel *et al.* investigated the protective capabilities of different probiotic strains, such as *L. acidophilus, Lactobacillus gasseri, Lactobacillus confuses, B. longum, B. breve,* and *S. thermophilus,* against DNA damage in rats [21]. Except for*S. thermophilus*, all strains exhibited dose-dependent protection. Furthermore, research involving rats has shown that particular probiotic strains, including *L. acidophilus, B. longum*, and *L. rhamnosus GG*, are associated with a decrease in the occurrence of colonic tumors when exposed to carcinogens or mutagens present in cooked food [20]. Epidemiological investigations in humans propose that probiotics, typically delivered through fermented dairy products like yogurt, may decrease the risk of large adenomas in the colon [20].

Impact of Probiotics on Immune Function

The gut microbiota plays a pivotal role in fortifying the intestinal defence barrier by initiating and maintaining particular immune responses while promoting tolerance to antigens. Specific bacterial species within the gastrointestinal tract release small peptides of low molecular weight that stimulate the immune system [22]. A recent investigation conducted by Chiang *et al.* emphasized the immune-boosting attributes of the *Bifidobacterium lactis HN019* strain. This strain enhances non-specific immune functions, such as the proliferation of leucocytes (lymphocytes and phagocytes), elevated phagocyte production, and the generation of proinflammatory cytokines (Fig. **1**) [23]. Several investigations have documented that the administration of *B. lactis HN019* to various groups, including the elderly, leads to increased peripheral blood leukocytes (Fig. **1**) and effective natural killer cells, contributing to the fight against tumors and viruses [24, 25].

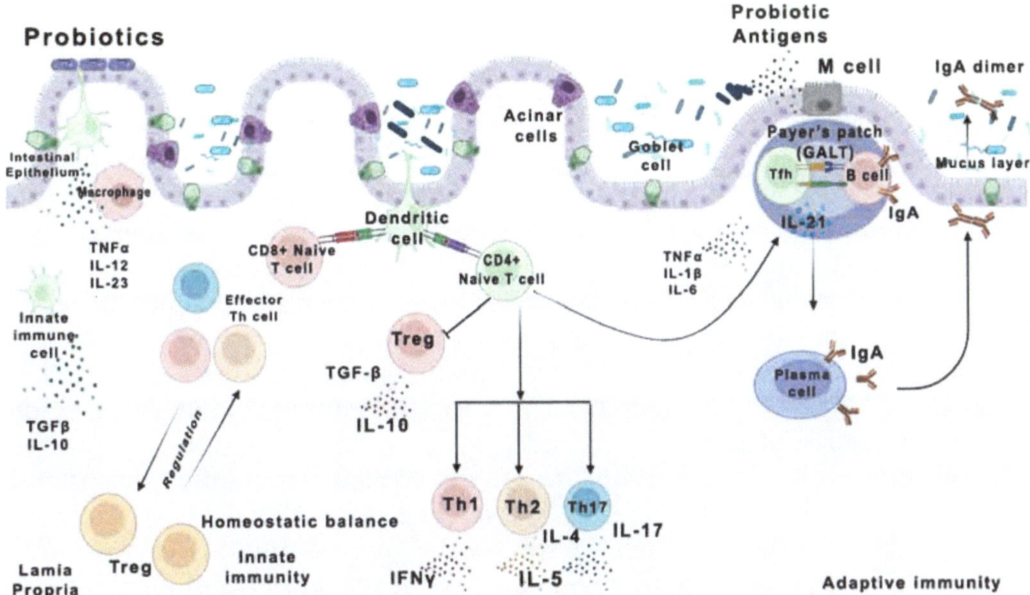

Fig. (1). Diagrammatic depiction of the probiotic-host intestinal immune cell interaction. Probiotics influence immune cells, which affects the host's innate and adaptive immunological responses.

By regulating the immune response, *L. rhamnosus GG* has shown effectiveness in preventing early onset atopic diseases in children at high risk [26]. Another study by Rosenfeldt *et al.* highlighted the therapeutic potential of a combination of *L. rhamnosus 19070-2* and *Lactobacillus reuteri DSM 122460* in managing atopic dermatitis in children [27]. The findings revealed that children treated with probiotics showed less severe eczema, with 56% exhibiting improvement compared to only 15% in the placebo group. Furthermore, research has shown that *Lactobacillus rhamnosus GG* can inhibit the immunoinflammatory responses in people with hypersensitivity to milk, while simultaneously acting as an immune stimulator in those who are healthy [28].

Mechanism of Action

The mechanism of action for probiotic strains is very complex and involves multiple factors. Current evidence indicates that the impact of probiotics differs across various strains. Consequently, probiotics play a pivotal role in situations where they have demonstrated the ability to decrease the occurrence and duration of gastroenteritis. This is primarily achieved through the fortification of colonization resistance and direct repressive effects against pathogens [29].

These mechanisms involve the production of inhibitory compounds such as bacteriocins, the reduction of luminal pH through the production of short-chain fatty acids (which can directly impede specific pathogens), competition for nutrients and attachment sites on the gut wall, modulation of the immune response, and regulation of gene expression in colonocytes (for instance, the regulation of genetic expression of mucin). To enhance our understanding of probiotic mechanisms, it is crucial to employ advanced molecular techniques with high resolution, such as transcriptomics assessed through DNA microarrays. This enables the exploration of the complex interplay between probiotics and mucosal cells. The precise mechanisms or the array of mechanisms utilized by probiotics in the human gut microbiota to improve overall health remain incompletely comprehended. Future investigations should adopt approaches driven by mechanisms, leveraging insights from in vitro and animal studies that elucidate the distinct modes of action of specific probiotic strains against well-defined pathological targets. To ascertain the effectiveness of probiotics in particular disease states such as Inflammatory Bowel Disease (IBD), colon cancer, and gastroenteritis, additional human feeding studies are essential. Given the strain-specific nature of probiotic activity and the multifaceted origins of these diseases, these studies should be designed to explore the specific mechanisms identified in *in-vitro* and animal studies, offering valuable perspectives into the potential applications of probiotics for targeted health advantages.

PREBIOTICS AND GUT MICROBIAL POPULATIONS (ROLE OF DIETARY FIBRES AND POLYPHENOLS AS PREBIOTICS, HIGHLIGHTING THEIR SIGNIFICANCE IN GUT HEALTH)

Several elements present in the food that we consume act as vital nutrients for gut bacteria. In reciprocation, commensal gut bacteria have the ability to metabolize these compounds into substances that contribute to inhibiting tumor growth. Prebiotics, are non-digestible or non-absorbable dietary fibers that are specifically utilized by gut microbes, have the potential to promote the colonization and growth of particular beneficial bacteria and their associated metabolites [30]. These metabolites, in turn, play a positive role in enhancing anti-tumour therapies [31]. However, the effectiveness of prebiotics is liable to the presence of commensal bacteria within the host's gut. Consequently, the combined use of probiotics and prebiotics, often referred to as a 'synbiotic,' holds great promise in this regard [32]. Both clinical trials and animal models have demonstrated that prebiotic supplementation can alter the quantity and makeup of specific gut bacteria [33].

Moreover, in various human studies, predominantly featuring conventional prebiotics such as inulin, FOS, and GOS, there was a notable rise in the overall abundance of gut bacteria within the *Actinobacteria* phylum following prebiotic intervention. Notably, *Bifidobacterium* constituted the majority of this observed enhancement [34]. Every study found a rise in *Bifidobacterium* at the genus level, and the majority of them also found a boost in *Lactobacillus* [35]. Following the consumption of prebiotics, the populations of some intestinal bacteria declined, presumably as a result of competitive suppression from other invading species that processed prebiotics in a more favourable manner [36].

One of the most utilized substrates as a prebiotic that help to replenish the gut microenvironment is polyphenols [37]. These polyphenols have the ability to affect host health therefore, the reciprocal relationship between gut microbiota and polyphenols is a well-known area of investigation. Polyphenols have the capacity to modify bacterial growth and metabolism, along with affecting the functionality of the cell membrane. This has a profound influence on the gut microbiota [37]. Through the inhibition of bacterial quorum sensing, most polyphenols can prevent the formation of biofilms and have important benefits [38]. For instance, flavanol and flavones classes of the genus *Staphylococcus* can prevent bacterial helicase activity while enhancing membrane cytoplasm permeability [37]. In another example, when segregated flavanones are combined with flavanone-rich citrus extract, it promotes a decline in biofilm development by obstructing the acyl-homoserine lactone-mediated quorum-sensing signal [39]. The production of acyl-homoserine lactone and its metabolites can also be inhibited by these flavanones. As a prebiotic substrate, polyphenols have two beneficial effects: on one side, they promote the growth and colonization of probiotic bacterial families like *Bifidobacteriaceae* and *Lactobacillaceae*; and on the other side, they decrease the number of pathogenic bacteria like *Escherichia coli, Clostridium perfringens*, and *Helicobacter pylori* [40, 41]. This reduction in pathogenic bacteria is related to a mechanism that alters the permeability and rigidity of the bacterial membrane through changes in the proportion of beneficial and pathogenic bacteria. Additionally, a shift in the composition of short-chain fatty acids (SCFAs) was noted, along with a decreased incidence of inflammation and obesity [42].

Fiber-rich Foods

It is widely recognised that dietary fiber is a vital component in food that promotes health. Compared to ancient patterns, modern dietary habits have resulted in a considerable decline in the consumption of fiber [43]. This has resulted in the rise of gastrointestinal disorders such as IBD, obesity, type II diabetes mellitus, and dysmetabolic syndrome in Western countries where fiber consumption is low and industrialization is at its peak [43]. Insulin resistance, intermittent fasting, postprandial glucose, elevated cholesterol levels in plasma, low-density lipoprotein (LDL) or bad cholesterol, and high-density lipoprotein (HDL) are the hallmark metabolic markers of these people. These populations also exhibit considerable changes in gut microbial profiles, pointing to a causal relationship between microorganisms, nutrition, and ailments. Thus, it has been hypothesized that dietary fiber ingestion can counteract these alterations [43]. They comprise a broad spectrum of carbohydrates and related molecules that are found in natural plant structures, as well as in molecules that have been isolated or synthesized [44]. In people with disorders linked to malfunctioning metabolism, dietary fibers can trigger microbial fermentation, which in turn produces short-chain fatty acids (SCFA), thus optimizing lipid and glucose limits. The original definition of dietary fiber was described as carbohydrate polymers found in plant cell walls that were incapable of being broken down and absorbed in the small intestine [45]. Shortly after, the term was broadened to encompass non-digestible polysaccharides that are not found inside plant cell walls, such as mucilages (ispaghula), exudates (gum arabic), and storage polysaccharides (galacto-mannans). Also, approximately 10% of the starch in the diet is also resistant to digestion (known as resistant starch) because it is either structurally unavailable to amylase in the stomach or is enclosed in the cellular structure of plants or seeds [46, 47]. Furthermore, food contains minute, non-digestible carbohydrates called oligosaccharides, which include those found in inulin. Additional indigestible carbohydrates, such as starch, can be artificially synthesized or altered from preexisting carbohydrates [48]. In addition, the gut flora influences and metabolizes non-carbohydrate compounds including lignin and non-extractable polyphenols, which are difficult to extract from fiber. The physiochemical characteristics of the fiber vary widely amongst multiple fiber types, including solubility, viscosity, and fermentation. This determines the precise effects of the fiber on its host metabolism [49].

Dietary fiber plays a crucial role in shaping the diversity, abundance, and structure of the microbiome (Table **1**). It provides a wide range of substrates that support the fermentation processes conducted by specific microorganisms equipped with the necessary enzymes to break down complex polysaccharides. In the large intestine, there are many microbiota species that are classified as fiber fermenters, which lead to the change in the intestine's nutritional preferences when dietary fiber intake rises, which permits these bacteria to proliferate [50]. People who consume low-fiber diets typically have fewer species of microbes [51] and provide residence to microorganisms that relish lipids and amino acids.

Animal proteins and fats are likely to replace the fibers in the diet. The consumption of diverse foods in varying geographic regions and socio-economic backgrounds has been shown in numerous studies to modify the microbial communities in the human gastrointestinal tract [52 - 54]. In 2015, Clemente *et al.* (2015) investigated the Yanomami tribe's microbiome in rural Venezuela. The study discovered that these individuals had greater *Prevotella* and lower *Bacteroides* abundances when correlated to people in the USA [52]. Furthermore, additional *Bacteroidetes* family members such as *Bacteroidales*, *Mollicutes*, and *Verrucomicrobia* were less common in this group. Finally, it was noted that these people have more *Phascolarctobacterium*, a genus known to produce SCFAs, in their bodies [55]. SCFAs are important in both the prevention and management of metabolic disorders [56]. They are essential for maintaining health and lowering the risk of disease development. The SCFAs stimulate and regulate a number of physiological processes in the gut, such as supplying colonocytes with energy, preserving their motility, regulating blood flow, and regulating the transport of nutrients and electrolytes throughout the lumen [57]. A variety of factors, including seasonality, lifestyle, stress, usage of antibiotics, disease state, and dietary preferences can dramatically alter an individual's food habits and the gut microbiome equilibrium, which can have a profound impact on the generation of SCFAs [58]. The Hadza tribe of Tanzania's microbiota was compared to that of Italians in a different study [59]. Numerous well-known bacteria that break down fiber were discovered to be present in both groups. These bacteria included members of the *Firmicutes* family, such as *Lachnospiraceae*, *Ruminococcaceae*, *Veillonellaceae*, *Clostridiales Incertae Sedis XIV*, and *Clostridiaceae*. *Prevotella* appeared to be more abundant in the microbiome of Hadza tribals, remains consistent throughout the results of other investigations. In contrast, *Bacteroides*were found to be less abundant in comparison to their Italian counterparts [59].

Polyphenolic-rich Foods

Polyphenols are plant-derived secondary metabolites and arguably the most abundant antioxidants necessary for daily well-being. Dietary polyphenols are presently categorized into four structural groups, namely phenolic acids, flavonoids, polyphenolic amides, and non-flavonoid compounds. Phenolic acids can be further divided into two main groups based on their C1–C6 and C3–C6 structures, namely derivatives of benzoic acid and cinnamic acid backbones [60]. Examples of flavonoids are anthocyanins, flavonoids, flavanones, isoflavones, chalcones, flavanols, flavonols, and flavanonols [61]. Avenanthramides and capsaicinoids are notable examples of nitrogen-containing functional substituents within polyphenolic amides. The non-flavonoids encompass stilbenes and lignans. Various non-flavonoid polyphenols, including resveratrol, ellagic acid, and its byproduct curcumin, *etc.*, present in food, play a significant role in human health, alongside phenolic acids, flavonoids, and phenolic amides. Fruits, vegetables, cereals, beans, tea, coffee, honey, and red wine are the primary dietary sources of polyphenols. Due to their biological significance for humans, these compounds are currently a subject of considerable scientific attention [61]. Studies conducted in vivo and in vitro have demonstrated their potential to promote health through various mechanisms, such as providing antioxidant effects, combating inflammation, displaying antibacterial properties, inhibiting adipogenesis, and offering neuroprotective benefits.

The structure and operational traits of the gut microbiota undergo substantial influence from dietary polyphenols. These compounds support the proliferation of beneficial bacteria like *Lactobacillus* and *Bifidobacterium*, both crucial for enhancing gastrointestinal health. They contribute to addressing gastrointestinal issues, mitigating symptoms of diarrhoea and constipation [62], and alleviating intolerance towards lactose [63]. According to a meta-analysis and methodical review conducted by Ma et al., polyphenol supplementation not only significantly enhanced the abundance of *Bifidobacterium* by 56% but also increased the abundance of *Lactobacillus* by 220%. Nevertheless, polyphenols possess the capability to inhibit the proliferation of harmful bacteria such as *Clostridium histolyticum* and *Clostridium perfringens*, both prevalent within the *Clostridium* genus. Inflammatory bowel illness is brought on by *Clostridium histolyticum* [64], while necrotizing enteritis and gastrointestinal disorders are linked to the production of many toxic substances and hydrolytic enzymes by *Clostridium perfringens* [65]. Polyphenols have the ability to regulate the production of short-chain fatty acids (SCFA)(Fig. **2**). Previous studies have demonstrated that the synthesis of propionate and acetate can be accelerated by the presence of *Akkermansia muciniphila*. Additionally, the nutritional interplay between butyrate-fabricating bacteria and *Akkermansia muciniphila* can stimulate the generation of butyrate [66]. McDougall's research revealed that the consumption of anthocyanin-rich raspberries significantly modified the bile acid concentration in the ideal fluid of individuals with ileostomies, leading to increased levels of glycine and taurine, byproducts of cholate and deoxycholate [67].

In-vitro studies have shown that polyphenolic-rich compounds can not only modulate but also inhibit the proliferation of specific disease-causing bacteria. Flavonoids in red wine demonstrated a modest suppression of *Clostridium* [68]. *Ruminococcus* growth may be inhibited by ellagic acid and anthocyanins, which are present in raspberry juices [69]. Grape polyphenols (Fig. **2**) have the ability to stop *Clostridium histolyticum* from proliferating [70]. On the flip side, polyphenols have the potential to promote the proliferation of beneficial gut bacteria, including *Bifidobacterium*. Tannin in pomegranates, gingerol in ginger, and grape polyphenols along with polyphenols in sorghum can stimulate the growth of *Bifidobacterium* [71 - 73].

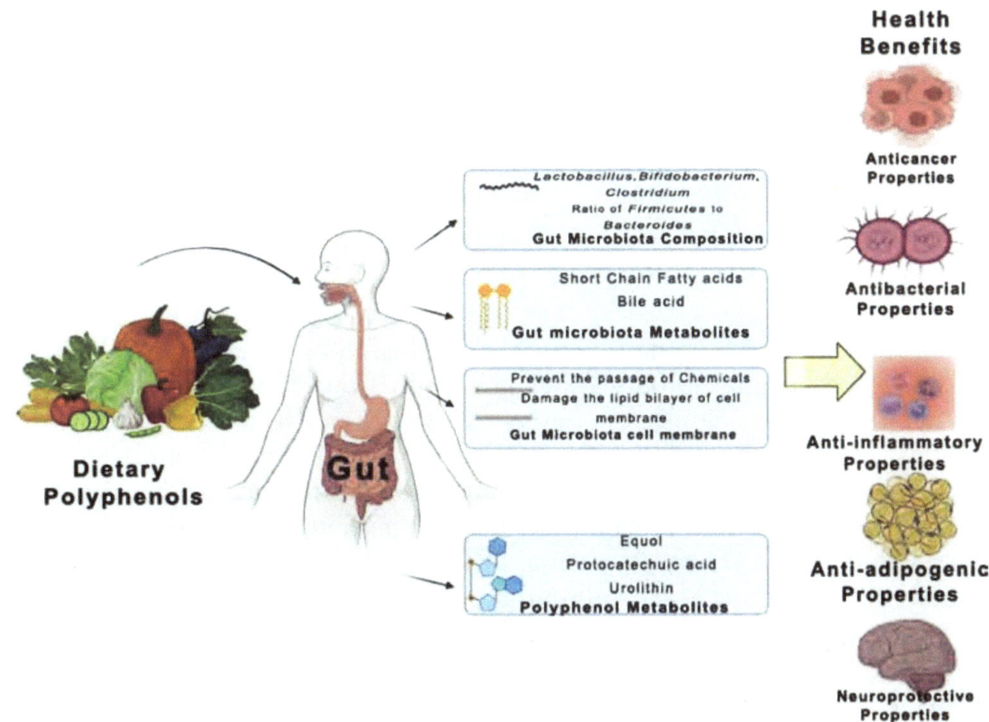

Fig. (2). Potential relationships between gut bacteria, dietary polyphenols, and host health.

Similarly, in vivo, research has demonstrated that supplementing with polyphenols can alter the microbiome of the gut in animal models by increasing the number of helpful bacteria and decreasing the number of notorious ones. Providing mice with a high-fat diet and supplementing it with mangoes can prevent the depletion of beneficial gut bacteria, including *Aldercrutzia*, *Akkermansia*, and *Bifidobacteria* [74]. When Orso was fed a diet, rich in tannins, extracted from a chestnut shell to a zebra fish with an inflamed intestine, he discovered that this encouraged the growth of good bacteria (*Pseudomonas* and *Enterobacteriaceae*) [75].

In-vivo studies on humans have shown that the addition of polyphenols, such as anthocyanins and flavonoids, can enhance the presence of protective agents in the intestines, such as *Lactobacillus* and *Bifidobacterium* [76, 77]. Anthocyanin which is abundant in blueberries has the ability to raise the quantity of lactic acid bacteria and Bifidobacteria in healthy individuals [78]. Moreno-Indias discovered the potency of polyphenols present in red wine and its ability to boost *Lactobacillus* and *Bifidobacteria* [79]. Yuan experimented with tea polyphenols in healthy participants and witnessed varying outcomes. In the fecal matter, there was an elevation in the abundance of *Firmicutes*, a reduction in the quantity of *Bacteroides*, and an increased ratio of *Firmicutes* to *Bacteroides* in the diet containing tea polyphenols [80]. Alcohol and polyphenols together have been shown by Queipo-Ortu to elevate the number of *Enterococcus*, *Prevotella*, *Bacteroides*, *Bifidobacterium*, *Bacteroides uniformis*, *Eggerthella lenta*, and *Blautia coccoides-Eubacterium*. However, no significant alterations were observed concerning *Lactobacillus* [81].

Healthy fat

Nuts are high in nutrients, have a number of health advantages, and effectively alter the intestinal microbiota. They have high fiber content, good lipids, and antioxidant qualities. Some nuts may have anti-inflammatory and prebiotic properties. Ingesting nuts can also help in the prevention of metabolic conditions such as type 2 diabetes (T2D), dyslipidemia, and cardiovascular diseases (CVD). It has been demonstrated that eating nuts can help prevent metabolic diseases such as type 2 diabetes (T2D), dyslipidemia, and cardiovascular disease (CVD) [82]. A new study conducted on 16,217 individuals suffering from T2D demonstrated that those who consumed approximately five servings of nuts per month as opposed to one serving per month had decreased incidence of total cardiovascular disease, coronary heart disease, death from CVD, and mortality from all causes (Fig. **2**) [83].

A positive shift regarding microbiota has been linked to the fermentation of fiber from nuts and the biotransformation of phytochemicals from other sources, giving rise to advantageous end products (such as butyric acid) [84]. Therefore, nuts may have prebiotic effects by enhancing microorganisms that may be advantageous for both lactic acid bacteria and *Bifidobacteria*. A significant portion of fats in nuts can enter the colon, demonstrating a significant effect on gut flora. A small amount of fat that is not fully masticated or that is inaccessible within cell structures cannot be absorbed upon digestion, and travels to the colon where it acts as a prebiotic [85, 86].

FECAL MICROBIOTA TRANSPLANTATION (FMT) AS A THERAPEUTIC OPTION

Faecal Microbial Transplantation (FMT) stands out as a promising therapeutic approach for the modulation of gut microbiota. This innovative technique involves the transfer of faecal material from a healthy donor to a recipient, aiming to restore or enhance the microbial balance in the recipient's gut. FMT has shown efficacy in addressing various gastrointestinal conditions, including recurrent *Clostridium difficile* infections. Researchers are actively exploring its potential to influence not only digestive health but also its impact on systemic conditions like inflammatory bowel diseases, metabolic disorders, and even neurological conditions. By introducing a diverse array of beneficial microorganisms, FMT serves as a targeted intervention to reshape the gut microbiota, emphasizing its role as a therapeutic strategy for promoting overall health and preventing or treating specific diseases.

Faecal Microbiota Transplantation in Ulcerative Colitis

The majority of research demonstrating the efficacy of faecal microbiota transplantation in conditions unrelated to recurrent *Clostridium difficile* infections, predominantly concentrates on inflammatory bowel diseases, particularly ulcerative colitis. This is due to the significant disruptions in the quantitative and qualitative conformation of the gut microbiota specific to this condition. Specifically, when comparing patients with ulcerative colitis to healthy individuals, the diversity of gut microbiota is reduced, and a discernible drop in the proportion of *Bacteroidetes* and *Firmicutes* is identified. As ulcerative colitis (UC) advanced, there was a marked rise in the abundance of *Proteobacteria* and *Actinobacteria*, coupled with a substantial decrease in the synthesis of butyrate by *Fecalibacterium prausnitzii* [87]. Intestinal dysbiosis leads to a diminished production of short-chain fatty acids (SCFAs), particularly butyrate. Butyrate is considered a crucial nutrient for colonocytes and exerts a substantial influence on immunological modulation. Five recognized randomized controlled studies (RCTs) have explored the effectiveness of fecal microbiota transplantation (FMT) in individuals with active ulcerative colitis (UC). Among these, three studies have reported promising results. In a single-blind randomized controlled trial, Moayyedi *et al.* examined seventy people with active UC who were given water enemas as the control group or allogeneic flexible mesh therapy (FMT) *via* enema (experimental group) [88]. Over a six-week period after the initiation of the randomized controlled trial (RCT), primary objectives which included, achieving a reduction in the overall Mayo score to less than three and endoscopic restoration (scoring 0 on an endoscopic Mayo scale), were observed in 24% of patients undergoing fecal microbiota transplantation (FMT) compared to 5% of patients who were administered a placebo. Notably, a substantial number of patients with exceptionally favorable outcomes (39% versus 10% from material obtained from other contributors) received FMT from a singular super donor, underscoring the significance of donor selection.

In order to evaluate the efficacy of FMT, Paramsothy *et al.* performed colonoscopies on patients who had minor to severe UC. The majority of these patients underwent FMT injections using donor material from three to seven different people [89]. Eleven out of forty patients (27%) who got active fecal material and three out of forty patients (8%) who received a placebo (saline) obtained steroid-free remission as well as an endoscopic response or remission. The absence of an effect was associated with a proportional rise in *Fusobacterium* representation, while the clinical effectiveness was correlated with an enhancement in the diversity of the gut microbiota. Additionally, Costello *et al.* used continuous enema delivery of frozen fecal material from multiple donors to examine the efficacy of FMT in individuals with minor to severe UC [90].

Fecal Microbiota Transplantation in Cancer Diseases

Various clinical studies have explored fecal microbiota transplantation (FMT) strategies in cancer patients, particularly those with melanoma, a type of skin cancer concerning melanocyte cells responsible for melanin production. Recently, innovative therapeutic methods have emerged to bolster a patient's immune system against tumors, utilizing immune checkpoint inhibitors in a treatment known as "cancer immunotherapy." Intriguingly, it has been discovered that this immune response is significantly regulated by the gut microbiome [91]. For instance, a noteworthy proportion of patients with metastatic melanoma exhibited enduring improvements when administered with monoclonal antibodies directed at the checkpoint regulator, programmed cell death protein 1 (PD-1) [92 - 94]. Studies have established that gut microbiota plays a role in influencing the response to anti-PD-1, thereby impacting the efficacy of this treatment. Human studies have revealed distinctions in the gut microbiota between individuals who respond positively to anti-PD-1 therapy and those who do not. In particular, individuals who positively respond to the treatment exhibit a superior alpha diversity and an increased presence of bacteria from the *Ruminococcaceae* family [95]. Moreover, they had raised levels of *Bifidobacterium longum, Collinsella aerofaciens*, and *Enterococcus faecium* [96], along with *Akkermansia muciniphila* [97]. Surprisingly, introducing stool samples from melanoma patients who responded well to anti-PD-1 therapy into germ-free mice amplifies the anticancer effects of PD-1 blocking. However, antiPD-1 is ineffective when FMT is carried out using stool samples from non-responders [97]. Therefore, the use of anti-PD-1 therapy fails to succeed in reaching its goal of preventing tumor growth when germ-free mice receiving stool samples from melanoma patients who responded favourably to the treatment are used to perform FMT (Fig. **3**) [97]. In contrast, when stool samples from non-responders are used in FMT, anti-PD-1 therapy is ineffective. In two clinical investigations, a subset of metastatic melanoma patients exhibited a positive response to anti-PD-1 immunotherapy when concurrently administered with faecal microbiota transplantation (FMT). This recent replication of pre-clinical results in mice [98, 99] suggests that a unique makeup of bacterial species in the gut microbiota, which may be transmitted through FMT is responsible for the feedback to anti-PD-1 treatment in melanoma patients.

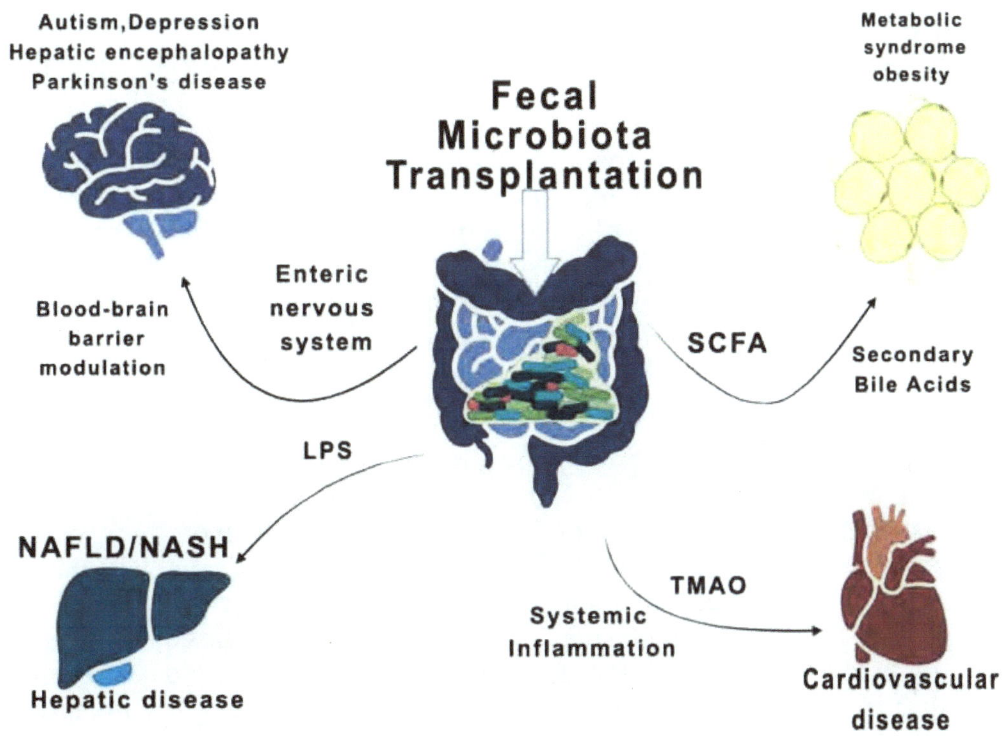

Fig. (3). Suggested mechanism of action faecal microbial transplantation.

Faecal Microbiota Transplantation in Cardiovascular Diseases

There exists a scarcity of information about the function of microbiota and FMT therapies in cardiovascular disorders, the majority of which is derived from animal models [100]. There is a proven cause-and-effect relationship between atherogenesis, the process that leads to the development of atherosclerotic plaques resulting in coronary artery heart disease, and the gut microbiome-produced metabolite called trimethylamine N-oxide (TMAO)(Fig. **3**) [101]. Due to their dietary choices, individuals who follow vegetarian or vegan diets generate lower levels of trimethylamine N-oxide (TMAO) compared to omnivorous individuals. In a study conducted by Smits *et al.* in the year 2018, faecal microbiota transplantation (FMT) was administered to individuals with metabolic syndrome using stools from lean vegan donors. However, no alterations in TMAO generation or factors linked to vasculitis were observed [102].

Zhang and colleagues (2021) have suggested that gut microbiota dysbiosis in geriatrics is a causative factor in the pathophysiology of atrial fibrillation, based on evidence from human and animal models. The researchers demonstrated that FMT between elderly atrial fibrillation rats and young rats increased the levels of LPS and vulnerability to the illness. The researchers have found that age-related dysbiosis causes a change in the microbiota-intestinal barrier-atrial orientation, which is linked to the disease.

They also found that elderly patients exhibited higher levels of circulating lipopolysaccharides (LPS) compared to their younger counterparts [103]. According to research, FMT gathered from control mice in the experimental autoimmune myocarditis (EAM) mouse model enhanced myocardial health by diminishing inflammation and augmenting microbial diversity, including an elevation in the *Firmicutes/Bacteroidetes* ratio [104].

Fecal Microbiota Transplantation in COVID-19 Diseases

Currently, no published randomized controlled trials have examined the efficacy or safety of FMT in patients with COVID-19. However in two clinical cases, physicians from Imperial College London and the Medical University of Warsaw provided the first indication that FMT could be helpful for COVID-19 patients [105]. In the first instance, a patient, who was 80 years old, was treated with remdesivir and "convalescent plasma," which included antibodies against SARS-CoV-2, for his blood poisoning and pneumonia. Surprisingly, two days following the transplant, his COVID-19 symptoms disappeared without his pneumonia getting any worse [105]. In another case, a 19-year-old patient, diagnosed with ulcerative colitis (UC), underwent immunosuppressive therapy. Hospital admission was prompted by recurrent *Clostridium difficile* infections. To prevent the recurrence of the infection, the patient received antibiotics and underwent a stool transplant. Approximately fifteen hours later, symptoms suggestive of a possible COVID-19 infection appeared, and a positive swab test confirmed the diagnosis. The next day, apart from experiencing two segregated episodes of fever, the patient's COVID-19 indications resolved. No specific medication was administered to address the COVID-19 in this second patient [105]. In the ongoing research, Zhang and colleagues are actively investigating the effects of a meticulously cleansed microbiota transplantation in individuals diagnosed with COVID-19. The objective is to not only assess its effectiveness in reducing mortality rates but also to optimise the overall well-being of patients wrestling with viral infection [106]. The design of this trial was both placebo-controlled and blinded. In addition to receiving normal care, patients who were recruited in the trial were given a placebo or a cleaned suspension of microbiota orally or by a nasogastric/nasojejunal tube [106].

Faecal Microbiota Transplantation in Brain Diseases

It is undeniable that the gut microbiome has an impact on both the proper and impaired functioning of the brain [107]. Probiotics and prebiotics have the potential to bring gut microbiota into equilibrium in cases of brain disorders [108], but FMT provides the larger benefit of transplanting the complete microflora. For instance, in a mouse model of Parkinson's disease, faecal microbiota transplantation (FMT) from healthy animals can reduce degenerative characteristics in the substantia nigra and ameliorate physical impairment (Fig. **3**) [109].

Furthermore, FMT obtained from individuals experiencing significant depression caused depressive-like behavioural and physiological characteristics in normal mice [110]. In human investigations, Faecal Microbiota Transplantation (FMT) has been explored in numerous clinical trials concerning neurological illnesses such as epilepsy, Parkinson's disease, multiple sclerosis, Alzheimer's disease, and autism spectrum disorders (ASD) (Fig. **3**) [111 - 113]. In one patient suffering from Parkinson's disease, FMT showed beneficial results by improving motor symptoms and constipation alleviation over the short term (two months) [114]. Also, it showed benefits in a broader patient group with respect to both motor and non-motor complaints, such as constipation [115]. A youngster with epilepsy along with Crohn's disease also showed improvement in neurological and gastrointestinal symptoms when FMT [116] was applied.

Additionally, GI symptoms [117] in both adults and children with ASD are correlated with gut microbiota dysbiosis [118 - 120] and ASD severity [121, 122]. FMT is a helpful strategy given the transitory effects of probiotics and their restricted availability in strains [108, 123]. Kang *et al.* (2017) enrolled eighteen children diagnosed with ASD, giving them a high FMT dosage at first, then progressively reduced doses every day for 7-8 weeks. In the final two months of therapy, there was an 80% reduction in GI symptoms. Interestingly, behavioral ASD symptoms were improved for up to two months. When the variety of bacteria was examined after FMT, more bacteria from the genera *Bifidobacterium*, *Prevotella*, and *Desulfovibrio* were discovered [124]. Two years after the therapy ended, the study team checked in with the same eighteen ASD children and discovered that most of the GI symptom improvements had persisted along with the elevation in ASD symptoms. The researchers also noted alterations triggered by faecal microbiota transplantation (FMT) in the gut microbiome, such as increased bacterial variety and higher proportions of *Bifidobacteria* and *Prevotella* [125].

Table 1. Dietary interventions for gut microbiota.

NCT Number	Intervention	Study Population	Outcomes Measures	Conclusion
NCT03330678	Probiotic (VSL#3)	14 healthy young women	Analysis of the gut microbiome of Indian women in good health and the impact of probiotic supplementation on gut flora composition.	Beneficial
NCT03760133	Duolac	100 participants (Bowel preparation before colonoscopy)	The influence of probiotics on the modification of gut microbiota following colon cleansing.	Beneficial
NCT04074421	Rifaximin+Probiotic	240 patients suffering from IBD	To evaluate the IBS symptom grade score and life score.	Beneficial
NCT02728414	Lactobacillus fermentum, TSF331, Lactobacillus reuteri, TSR332, Lactobacillus plantarum, TSP05	82 patients suffering from human metabolic syndrome	To evaluate blood biochemical indicators and changes in gut microbiota ratios and changes in gut aging index score.	Beneficial
NCT05273073	A probiotic sachet consisting of of 30 billion colony-forming units (CFU) of six viable probiotic strains.	166 patients suffering from Gestational Diabetes Mellitus	Mean difference of fasting blood glucose (FBG) and mean difference of (GLP -1).	Beneficial
NCT04120051	Fermented canola-seaweed	100 obese participants	Alterations in blood glucose levels 2 hours after an oral glucose tolerance test from the starting point to the conclusion.	Beneficial
NCT05239845	Mixture of bovine lactoferrin, bovine milk fat globule membrane (MFGM), and a prebiotic blend of (PDX/GOS).	68 healthy adults reported poor sleep quality.	Lab-recorded polysomnography- Sleep Quality	Beneficial
NCT04018066	Complex comprising soy protein isolates and grape polyphenols (GP-SPI).	34 healthy volunteers	Alteration in gut microbiota composition, comprehensive metabolic panel (CMP) Blood Test (ALP, AST, ALT)	Beneficial

(Table 1) cont.....

NCT Number	Intervention	Study Population	Outcomes Measures	Conclusion
NCT03800277	Cranberry, Agaves	122 overweight volunteers	Assess the number of lipopolysaccharides (LPS) and lipopolysaccharide-binding protein (LBP) in plasma to determine if metabolic endotoxemia has changed.	Beneficial
NCT04100200	Mixed berries and FOS	105 obese and overweight patients	Alterations in plasma biomarkers and levels of inflammation: Nrf2/NF-κB response.	Beneficial
NCT05463835	Rubus-Elite	32 stressed and anxious patients	Recovery of maximal isometric mid-thigh pull strength and recovery of self-reported muscle soreness	Beneficial
NCT03608800	Intermittent fasting	39 patients suffering from Metabolic Syndrome	Changes in BMI, body fat mass, serum LDL-cholesterol, serum HDL-cholesterol, serum triglyceride, serum Apo B/apo A1 levels.	Beneficial
NCT04223323	Almonds	84 participants who are overweight and obese	Changes in markers of systemic inflammation & metabolism, changes in adiposity, Changes in abundance of fecal *Roseburia* spp.	Beneficial
NCT03106844	FMT	50 participants suffering from Inflammatory Bowel Disorder and Clostridium Difficile Infection	Number of Participants with FMT Failure, Participants Colonized With *C.Difficile.*	Significant
NCT05821010	LFMT-capsules	48 patients suffering Non-Alcoholic Steatohepatitis	Alteration of liver histology in subjects with NASH and fibrosis stages 0-3, with an alteration defined as a change of steatohepatitis by $\geq$1 SAF-A point, or a change in $\geq$ 1 stage liver fibrosis.	Non-Significant

CONCLUSION

In conclusion, the gut microbiota is integral to human health, playing a vital role in numerous physiological processes and overall well-being. This chapter has provided a comprehensive overview of various interventions—prebiotics, probiotics, faecal microbiota transplantation (FMT), and dietary strategies—that can modulate gut microbiota composition and function. Prebiotics selectively promote the growth of beneficial bacteria such as *Firmicutes, Bacteroidetes,* and *Actinobacteria.* Probiotics offer a direct approach to enhancing microbial diversity and health benefits. FMT has emerged as a promising therapy for restoring microbial balance, while dietary interventions like high-fiber diets, polyphenolic-rich foods, omega-3 fatty acids, and reduced sugar intake have significant impacts on gut microbiota. A deeper understanding of the interactions between these interventions and the gut microbiota can inform the development of targeted strategies to promote gastrointestinal health and manage conditions such as obesity, inflammatory bowel disease (IBD), and Type 2 diabetes. This knowledge underscores the potential of gut microbiota modulation as a pivotal element in improving human health and treating various diseases.

ACKNOWLEDGEMENTS

The authors are highly grateful to NSHM Knowledge Campus, Kolkata for their continuous support and encouragement.

REFERENCES

[1] Scientific concepts of functional foods in Europe. Consensus document. Br J Nutr 1999; 81(4) (Suppl. 1): S1-S27.
[http://dx.doi.org/10.1017/S0007114599000471] [PMID: 10999022]

[2] Tuohy KM, Probert HM, Smejkal CW, Gibson GR. Using probiotics and prebiotics to improve gut health. Drug Discov Today 2003; 8(15): 692-700.
[http://dx.doi.org/10.1016/S1359-6446(03)02746-6] [PMID: 12927512]

[3] Wang X, Zhang P, Zhang X. Probiotics Regulate Gut Microbiota: An Effective Method to Improve Immunity. Molecules 2021; 26(19): 6076.
[http://dx.doi.org/10.3390/molecules26196076] [PMID: 34641619]

[4] Bielik V, Kolisek M. Bioaccessibility and Bioavailability of Minerals in Relation to a Healthy Gut Microbiome. Int J Mol Sci 2021; 22(13): 6803.
[http://dx.doi.org/10.3390/ijms22136803] [PMID: 34202712]

[5] Markowiak-Kopeć P, Śliżewska K. The Effect of Probiotics on the Production of Short-Chain Fatty Acids by Human Intestinal Microbiome. Nutrients 2020; 12(4): 1107.
[http://dx.doi.org/10.3390/nu12041107] [PMID: 32316181]

[6] Feeney EL, Mckinley MC. Milk and Dairy Foods IN: DIan Givens, Their Functionality in Human Health and Disease. Academic press 2020; pp. 205-25.
[http://dx.doi.org/10.1016/B978-0-12-815603-2.00008-5]

[7] Vesa TH, Marteau P, Korpela R. Lactose Intolerance. J Am Coll Nutr 2000; 19(sup2) (Suppl.): 165S-75S.
[http://dx.doi.org/10.1080/07315724.2000.10718086] [PMID: 10759141]

[8] Marteau P, Seksik P, Jian R. Probiotics and intestinal health effects: a clinical perspective. Br J Nutr 2002; 88(S1) (Suppl. 1): s51-7.
[http://dx.doi.org/10.1079/BJN2002629] [PMID: 12215185]

[9] Savaiano DA, Hutkins RW. Yogurt, cultured fermented milk, and health: a systematic review. Nutr

Rev 2021; 79(5): 599-614.
[http://dx.doi.org/10.1093/nutrit/nuaa013] [PMID: 32447398]

[10] Li YT, Xu H, Ye JZ, *et al.* Efficacy of *Lactobacillus rhamnosus* GG in treatment of acute pediatric diarrhea: A systematic review with meta-analysis. World J Gastroenterol 2019; 25(33): 4999-5016.
[http://dx.doi.org/10.3748/wjg.v25.i33.4999] [PMID: 31543689]

[11] Saavedra JM, Bauman NA, Perman JA, *et al.* Feeding of Bifidobacterium bifidum and Streptococcus thermophilus to infants in hospital for prevention of diarrhoea and shedding of rotavirus. Lancet 1994; 344(8929): 1046-9.
[http://dx.doi.org/10.1016/S0140-6736(94)91708-6] [PMID: 7934445]

[12] Pérez-Cobas A, Moya A, Gosalbes M, Latorre A. Colonization Resistance of the Gut Microbiota against Clostridium difficile. Antibiotics (Basel) 2015; 4(3): 337-57.
[http://dx.doi.org/10.3390/antibiotics4030337] [PMID: 27025628]

[13] Keikha M, Karbalaei M. Probiotics as the live microscopic fighters against Helicobacter pylori gastric infections. BMC Gastroenterol 2021; 21(1): 388.
[http://dx.doi.org/10.1186/s12876-021-01977-1] [PMID: 34670526]

[14] Haneishi Y, Furuya Y, Hasegawa M, Picarelli A, Rossi M, Miyamoto J. Inflammatory Bowel Diseases and Gut Microbiota. Int J Mol Sci 2023; 24(4): 3817.
[http://dx.doi.org/10.3390/ijms24043817] [PMID: 36835245]

[15] Sonnenborn U, Schulze J. The non-pathogenic Escherichia coli strain Nissle 1917 – features of a versatile probiotic. Microb Ecol Health Dis 2009; 21(3-4): 122-58.

[16] Chapman TM, Plosker GL, Figgitt DP. VSL#3 probiotic mixture: a review of its use in chronic inflammatory bowel diseases. Drugs 2006; 66(10): 1371-87.
[http://dx.doi.org/10.2165/00003495-200666100-00006] [PMID: 16903771]

[17] Mimura T, Rizzello F, Helwig U, *et al.* Once daily high dose probiotic therapy (VSL#3) for maintaining remission in recurrent or refractory pouchitis. Gut 2004; 53(1): 108-14.
[http://dx.doi.org/10.1136/gut.53.1.108] [PMID: 14684584]

[18] Gionchetti P, Rizzello F, Venturi A, *et al.* Oral bacteriotherapy as maintenance treatment in patients with chronic pouchitis: A double-blind, placebo-controlled trial. Gastroenterology 2000; 119(2): 305-9.
[http://dx.doi.org/10.1053/gast.2000.9370] [PMID: 10930365]

[19] Mazziotta C, Tognon M, Martini F, Torreggiani E, Rotondo JC. Probiotics Mechanism of Action on Immune Cells and Beneficial Effects on Human Health. Cells 2023; 12(1): 184.
[http://dx.doi.org/10.3390/cells12010184] [PMID: 36611977]

[20] Burns AJ, Rowland IR. Anti-carcinogenicity of probiotics and prebiotics. Curr Issues Intest Microbiol 2000; 1(1): 13-24.
[PMID: 11709850]

[21] Pool-Zobel BL, Neudecker C, Domizlaff I, *et al.* Lactobacillus- and bifidobacterium-mediated antigenotoxicity in the colon of rats. Nutr Cancer 1996; 26(3): 365-80.
[http://dx.doi.org/10.1080/01635589609514492] [PMID: 8910918]

[22] Singh V, Singh K, Amdekar S, *et al.* Innate and specific gut-associated immunity and microbial interference. FEMS Immunol Med Microbiol 2009; 55(1): 6-12.
[http://dx.doi.org/10.1111/j.1574-695X.2008.00497.x] [PMID: 19077031]

[23] Li Y, Jin L, Chen T. The Effects of Secretory IgA in the Mucosal Immune System. BioMed Res Int 2020; 2020(1): 2032057.
[http://dx.doi.org/10.1155/2020/2032057] [PMID: 31998782]

[24] Chiang BL, Sheih YH, Wang LH, Liao CK, Gill HS. Enhancing immunity by dietary consumption of a probiotic lactic acid bacterium (Bifidobacterium lactis HN019): optimization and definition of cellular immune responses. Eur J Clin Nutr 2000; 54(11): 849-55.

[http://dx.doi.org/10.1038/sj.ejcn.1601093] [PMID: 11114680]

[25] Arunachalam K, Gill HS, Chandra RK. Enhancement of natural immune function by dietary consumption of Bifidobacterium lactis (HN019). Eur J Clin Nutr 2000; 54(3): 263-7. [http://dx.doi.org/10.1038/sj.ejcn.1600938] [PMID: 10713750]

[26] Gill HS, Rutherfurd KJ, Cross ML, Gopal PK. Enhancement of immunity in the elderly by dietary supplementation with the probiotic Bifidobacterium lactis HN019. Am J Clin Nutr 2001; 74(6): 833-9. [http://dx.doi.org/10.1093/ajcn/74.6.833] [PMID: 11722966]

[27] Du T, Lei A, Zhang N, Zhu C. The Beneficial Role of Probiotic *Lactobacillus* in Respiratory Diseases. Front Immunol 2022; 13: 908010. [http://dx.doi.org/10.3389/fimmu.2022.908010] [PMID: 35711436]

[28] Rosenfeldt V, Benfeldt E, Nielsen SD, *et al.* Effect of probiotic Lactobacillus strains in children with atopic dermatitis. J Allergy Clin Immunol 2003; 111(2): 389-95. [http://dx.doi.org/10.1067/mai.2003.389] [PMID: 12589361]

[29] Pelto L, Isolauri E, Lilius EM, Nuutila J, Salminen S. Probiotic bacteria down-regulate the milk-induced inflammatory response in milk-hypersensitive subjects but have an immunostimulatory effect in healthy subjects. Clin Exp Allergy 1998; 28(12): 1474-9. [http://dx.doi.org/10.1046/j.1365-2222.1998.00449.x] [PMID: 10024217]

[30] Wang X, Zhang P, Zhang X. Probiotics Regulate Gut Microbiota: An Effective Method to Improve Immunity. Molecules 2021; 26(19): 6076. [http://dx.doi.org/10.3390/molecules26196076] [PMID: 34641619]

[31] Hutkins RW, Krumbeck JA, Bindels LB, *et al.* Prebiotics: why definitions matter. Curr Opin Biotechnol 2016; 37: 1-7. [http://dx.doi.org/10.1016/j.copbio.2015.09.001] [PMID: 26431716]

[32] Wu M, Bai J, Ma C, Wei J, Du X. The Role of Gut Microbiota in Tumor Immunotherapy. J Immunol Res 2021; 2021: 1-12. [http://dx.doi.org/10.1155/2021/5061570] [PMID: 34485534]

[33] Pandey KR, Naik SR, Vakil BV. Probiotics, prebiotics and synbiotics- a review. J Food Sci Technol 2015; 52(12): 7577-87. [http://dx.doi.org/10.1007/s13197-015-1921-1] [PMID: 26604335]

[34] Bedu-Ferrari C, Biscarrat P, Langella P, Cherbuy C. Prebiotics and the Human Gut Microbiota: From Breakdown Mechanisms to the Impact on Metabolic Health. Nutrients 2022; 14(10): 2096. [http://dx.doi.org/10.3390/nu14102096] [PMID: 35631237]

[35] Wang S, Xiao Y, Tian F, *et al.* 2020.

[36] Arboleya S, Watkins C, Stanton C, Ross RP. Gut Bifidobacteria Populations in Human Health and Aging. Front Microbiol 2016; 7: 1204. [http://dx.doi.org/10.3389/fmicb.2016.01204] [PMID: 27594848]

[37] Guarino M, Altomare A, Emerenziani S, *et al.* Mechanisms of Action of Prebiotics and Their Effects on Gastro-Intestinal Disorders in Adults. Nutrients 2020; 12(4): 1037. [http://dx.doi.org/10.3390/nu12041037] [PMID: 32283802]

[38] Plamada D, Vodnar DC. Polyphenols—Gut Microbiota Interrelationship: A Transition to a New Generation of Prebiotics. Nutrients 2021; 14(1): 137. [http://dx.doi.org/10.3390/nu14010137] [PMID: 35011012]

[39] Nain Z, Mansur FJ, Syed SB, *et al.* Inhibition of biofilm formation, quorum sensing and other virulence factors in *Pseudomonas aeruginosa* by polyphenols of *Gynura procumbens* leaves. J Biomol Struct Dyn 2022; 40(12): 5357-71. [http://dx.doi.org/10.1080/07391102.2020.1870563] [PMID: 33403919]

[40] Slobodníková L, Fialová S, Rendeková K, Kováč J, Mučaji P. Antibiofilm Activity of Plant

Polyphenols. Molecules 2016; 21(12): 1717.
[http://dx.doi.org/10.3390/molecules21121717] [PMID: 27983597]

[41] Dias R, Pereira CB, Pérez-Gregorio R, Mateus N, Freitas V. Recent advances on dietary polyphenol's potential roles in Celiac Disease. Trends Food Sci Technol 2021; 107: 213-25.
[http://dx.doi.org/10.1016/j.tifs.2020.10.033]

[42] Gowd V, Karim N, Shishir MRI, Xie L, Chen W. Dietary polyphenols to combat the metabolic diseases *via* altering gut microbiota. Trends Food Sci Technol 2019; 93: 81-93.
[http://dx.doi.org/10.1016/j.tifs.2019.09.005]

[43] Nash V, Ranadheera CS, Georgousopoulou EN, *et al.* The effects of grape and red wine polyphenols on gut microbiota – A systematic review. Food Res Int 2018; 113: 277-87.
[http://dx.doi.org/10.1016/j.foodres.2018.07.019] [PMID: 30195522]

[44] Cronin P, Joyce SA, O'Toole PW, O'Connor EM. Dietary Fibre Modulates the Gut Microbiota. Nutrients 2021; 13(5): 1655.
[http://dx.doi.org/10.3390/nu13051655] [PMID: 34068353]

[45] Thomson C, Garcia AL, Edwards CA. Interactions between dietary fibre and the gut microbiota. Proc Nutr Soc 2021; 80(4): 398-408.
[http://dx.doi.org/10.1017/S0029665121002834] [PMID: 34551829]

[46] Trowell HC, Burkitt DP. The development of the concept of dietary fibre. Mol Aspects Med 1987; 9(1): 7-15.
[http://dx.doi.org/10.1016/0098-2997(87)90013-6] [PMID: 3031417]

[47] Englyst HN, Kingman SM, Hudson GJ, Cummings JH. Measurement of resistant starch *in vitro* and *in vivo*. Br J Nutr 1996; 75(5): 749-55.
[http://dx.doi.org/10.1079/BJN19960178] [PMID: 8695601]

[48] Gallant DJ, Bouchet B, Buléon A, Pérez S. Physical characteristics of starch granules and susceptibility to enzymatic degradation. Eur J Clin Nutr 1992; 46(2) (Suppl. 2): S3-S16.
[PMID: 1330527]

[49] Laurentin A, Edwards CA. Differential fermentation of glucose-based carbohydrates in vitro by human faecal bacteria. Eur J Nutr 2004; 43(3): 183-9.
[http://dx.doi.org/10.1007/s00394-004-0457-3] [PMID: 15168041]

[50] Bijkerk CJ, Muris JWM, Knottnerus JA, Hoes AW, De Wit NJ. Systematic review: the role of different types of fibre in the treatment of irritable bowel syndrome. Aliment Pharmacol Ther 2004; 19(3): 245-51.
[http://dx.doi.org/10.1111/j.0269-2813.2004.01862.x] [PMID: 14984370]

[51] Walter J. Murine gut microbiota-diet trumps genes. Cell Host Microbe 2015; 17(1): 3-5.
[http://dx.doi.org/10.1016/j.chom.2014.12.004] [PMID: 25590753]

[52] Makki K, Deehan EC, Walter J, Bäckhed F. The Impact of Dietary Fiber on Gut Microbiota in Host Health and Disease. Cell Host Microbe 2018; 23(6): 705-15.
[http://dx.doi.org/10.1016/j.chom.2018.05.012] [PMID: 29902436]

[53] Clemente JC, Pehrsson EC, Blaser MJ, *et al.* The microbiome of uncontacted Amerindians. Sci Adv 2015; 1(3): e1500183.
[http://dx.doi.org/10.1126/sciadv.1500183] [PMID: 26229982]

[54] Martínez I, Stegen JC, Maldonado-Gómez MX, *et al.* The gut microbiota of rural papua new guineans: composition, diversity patterns, and ecological processes. Cell Rep 2015; 11(4): 527-38.
[http://dx.doi.org/10.1016/j.celrep.2015.03.049] [PMID: 25892234]

[55] De Filippo C, Di Paola M, Ramazzotti M, *et al.* Diet, Environments, and Gut Microbiota. A Preliminary Investigation in Children Living in Rural and Urban Burkina Faso and Italy. Front Microbiol 2017; 8: 1979.
[http://dx.doi.org/10.3389/fmicb.2017.01979] [PMID: 29081768]

[56] Wu F, Guo X, Zhang J, Zhang M, Ou Z, Peng Y. *Phascolarctobacterium faecium* abundant colonization in human gastrointestinal tract. Exp Ther Med 2017; 14(4): 3122-6. [http://dx.doi.org/10.3892/etm.2017.4878] [PMID: 28912861]

[57] Tirosh A, Calay ES, Tuncman G, *et al.* The short-chain fatty acid propionate increases glucagon and FABP4 production, impairing insulin action in mice and humans. Sci Transl Med 2019; 11(489): eaav0120. [http://dx.doi.org/10.1126/scitranslmed.aav0120] [PMID: 31019023]

[58] Tazoe H, Otomo Y, Kaji I, Tanaka R, Karaki SI, Kuwahara A. Roles of short-chain fatty acids receptors, GPR41 and GPR43 on colonic functions. J Physiol Pharmacol 2008; 59 (Suppl. 2): 251-62. [PMID: 18812643]

[59] King DE, Mainous AG III, Lambourne CA. Trends in dietary fiber intake in the United States, 1999-2008. J Acad Nutr Diet 2012; 112(5): 642-8. [http://dx.doi.org/10.1016/j.jand.2012.01.019] [PMID: 22709768]

[60] Schnorr SL, Candela M, Rampelli S, *et al.* Gut microbiome of the Hadza hunter-gatherers. Nat Commun 2014; 5(1): 3654. [http://dx.doi.org/10.1038/ncomms4654] [PMID: 24736369]

[61] Papuc C, Goran GV, Predescu CN, Nicorescu V, Stefan G. Plant Polyphenols as Antioxidant and Antibacterial Agents for Shelf-Life Extension of Meat and Meat Products: Classification, Structures, Sources, and Action Mechanisms. Compr Rev Food Sci Food Saf 2017; 16(6): 1243-68. [http://dx.doi.org/10.1111/1541-4337.12298] [PMID: 33371586]

[62] Wang X, Qi Y, Zheng H. Dietary Polyphenol, Gut Microbiota, and Health Benefits. Antioxidants 2022; 11(6): 1212. [http://dx.doi.org/10.3390/antiox11061212] [PMID: 35740109]

[63] Lye HS, Kuan CY, Ewe JA, Fung WY, Liong MT. The improvement of hypertension by probiotics: effects on cholesterol, diabetes, renin, and phytoestrogens. Int J Mol Sci 2009; 10(9): 3755-75. [http://dx.doi.org/10.3390/ijms10093755] [PMID: 19865517]

[64] Pelletier X, Laure-Boussuge S, Donazzolo Y. Hydrogen excretion upon ingestion of dairy products in lactose-intolerant male subjects: importance of the live flora. Eur J Clin Nutr 2001; 55(6): 509-12. [http://dx.doi.org/10.1038/sj.ejcn.1601169] [PMID: 11423928]

[65] Ma G, Chen Y. Polyphenol supplementation benefits human health *via* gut microbiota: A systematic review *via* meta-analysis. 2020. [http://dx.doi.org/10.1016/j.jff.2020.103829]

[66] Kleessen B, Kroesen AJ, Buhr HJ, Blaut M. Mucosal and invading bacteria in patients with inflammatory bowel disease compared with controls. Scand J Gastroenterol 2002; 37(9): 1034-41. [http://dx.doi.org/10.1080/003655202320378220] [PMID: 12374228]

[67] Zhai Q, Feng S, Arjan N, Chen W. A next generation probiotic, *Akkermansia muciniphila*. Crit Rev Food Sci Nutr 2019; 59(19): 3227-36. [http://dx.doi.org/10.1080/10408398.2018.1517725] [PMID: 30373382]

[68] McDougall GJ, Allwood JW, Pereira-Caro G, *et al.* Nontargeted LC-MS " Profiling of Compounds in Ileal Fluids That Decrease after Raspberry Intake Identifies Consistent Alterations in Bile Acid Composition. J Nat Prod 2016; 79(10): 2606-15. [http://dx.doi.org/10.1021/acs.jnatprod.6b00532] [PMID: 27643821]

[69] Sánchez-Patán F, Cueva C, Monagas M, *et al.* In vitro fermentation of a red wine extract by human gut microbiota: changes in microbial groups and formation of phenolic metabolites. J Agric Food Chem 2012; 60(9): 2136-47. [http://dx.doi.org/10.1021/jf2040115] [PMID: 22313337]

[70] Wu T, Chu X, Cheng Y, *et al.* Modulation of Gut Microbiota by *Lactobacillus casei* Fermented Raspberry Juice In Vitro and In Vivo. Foods 2021; 10(12): 3055.

[http://dx.doi.org/10.3390/foods10123055] [PMID: 34945605]

[71] Zhou L, Wang W, Huang J, *et al.* *In vitro* extraction and fermentation of polyphenols from grape seeds (Vitis vinifera) by human intestinal microbiota. Food Funct 2016; 7(4): 1959-67. [http://dx.doi.org/10.1039/C6FO00032K] [PMID: 26980065]

[72] Bialonska D, Ramnani P, Kasimsetty SG, Muntha KR, Gibson GR, Ferreira D. The influence of pomegranate by-product and punicalagins on selected groups of human intestinal microbiota. Int J Food Microbiol 2010; 140(2-3): 175-82. [http://dx.doi.org/10.1016/j.ijfoodmicro.2010.03.038] [PMID: 20452076]

[73] Wang J, Chen Y, Hu X, Feng F, Cai L, Chen F. Assessing the Effects of Ginger Extract on Polyphenol Profiles and the Subsequent Impact on the Fecal Microbiota by Simulating Digestion and Fermentation In Vitro. Nutrients 2020; 12(10): 3194. [http://dx.doi.org/10.3390/nu12103194] [PMID: 33086593]

[74] Sost MM, Ahles S, Verhoeven J, Verbruggen S, Stevens Y, Venema K. A Citrus Fruit Extract High in Polyphenols Beneficially Modulates the Gut Microbiota of Healthy Human Volunteers in a Validated In Vitro Model of the Colon. Nutrients 2021; 13(11): 3915. [http://dx.doi.org/10.3390/nu13113915] [PMID: 34836169]

[75] Ojo B, El-Rassi GD, Payton ME, *et al.* Mango Supplementation Modulates Gut Microbial Dysbiosis and Short-Chain Fatty Acid Production Independent of Body Weight Reduction in C57BL/6 Mice Fed a High-Fat Diet. J Nutr 2016; 146(8): 1483-91. [http://dx.doi.org/10.3945/jn.115.226688] [PMID: 27358411]

[76] Orso G, Solovyev MM, Facchiano S, *et al.* Chestnut Shell Tannins: Effects on Intestinal Inflammation and Dysbiosis in Zebrafish. Animals (Basel) 2021; 11(6): 1538. [http://dx.doi.org/10.3390/ani11061538] [PMID: 34070355]

[77] Molan AL, Liu Z, Plimmer G. Evaluation of the effect of blackcurrant products on gut microbiota and on markers of risk for colon cancer in humans. Phytother Res 2014; 28(3): 416-22. [http://dx.doi.org/10.1002/ptr.5009] [PMID: 23674271]

[78] Tzounis X, Rodriguez-Mateos A, Vulevic J, Gibson GR, Kwik-Uribe C, Spencer JPE. Prebiotic evaluation of cocoa-derived flavanols in healthy humans by using a randomized, controlled, double-blind, crossover intervention study. Am J Clin Nutr 2011; 93(1): 62-72. [http://dx.doi.org/10.3945/ajcn.110.000075] [PMID: 21068351]

[79] Vendrame S, Guglielmetti S, Riso P, Arioli S, Klimis-Zacas D, Porrini M. Six-week consumption of a wild blueberry powder drink increases bifidobacteria in the human gut. J Agric Food Chem 2011; 59(24): 12815-20. [http://dx.doi.org/10.1021/jf2028686] [PMID: 22060186]

[80] Moreno-Indias I, Sánchez-Alcoholado L, Pérez-Martínez P, *et al.* Red wine polyphenols modulate fecal microbiota and reduce markers of the metabolic syndrome in obese patients. Food Funct 2016; 7(4): 1775-87. [http://dx.doi.org/10.1039/C5FO00886G] [PMID: 26599039]

[81] Yuan X, Long Y, Ji Z, *et al.* Green Tea Liquid Consumption Alters the Human Intestinal and Oral Microbiome. Mol Nutr Food Res 2018; 62(12): 1800178. [http://dx.doi.org/10.1002/mnfr.201800178] [PMID: 29750437]

[82] Queipo-Ortuño MI, Boto-Ordóñez M, Murri M, *et al.* Influence of red wine polyphenols and ethanol on the gut microbiota ecology and biochemical biomarkers. Am J Clin Nutr 2012; 95(6): 1323-34. [http://dx.doi.org/10.3945/ajcn.111.027847] [PMID: 22552027]

[83] Muralidharan J, Galiè S, Hernández-Alonso P, Bulló M, Salas-Salvadó J. Plant-Based Fat, Dietary Patterns Rich in Vegetable Fat and Gut Microbiota Modulation. Front Nutr 2019; 6: 157. [http://dx.doi.org/10.3389/fnut.2019.00157] [PMID: 31681786]

[84] Liu G, Guasch-Ferré M, Hu Y, *et al.* Nut Consumption in Relation to Cardiovascular Disease

Incidence and Mortality Among Patients With Diabetes Mellitus. Circ Res 2019; 124(6): 920-9. [http://dx.doi.org/10.1161/CIRCRESAHA.118.314316] [PMID: 30776978]

[85] Holscher HD. Dietary fiber and prebiotics and the gastrointestinal microbiota. Gut Microbes 2017; 8(2): 172-84. [http://dx.doi.org/10.1080/19490976.2017.1290756] [PMID: 28165863]

[86] Cassady BA, Hollis JH, Fulford AD, Considine RV, Mattes RD. Mastication of almonds: effects of lipid bioaccessibility, appetite, and hormone response. Am J Clin Nutr 2009; 89(3): 794-800. [http://dx.doi.org/10.3945/ajcn.2008.26669] [PMID: 19144727]

[87] Ellis PR, Kendall CWC, Ren Y, *et al.* Role of cell walls in the bioaccessibility of lipids in almond seeds. Am J Clin Nutr 2004; 80(3): 604-13. [http://dx.doi.org/10.1093/ajcn/80.3.604] [PMID: 15321799]

[88] Frank DN, St Amand AL, Feldman RA, Boedeker EC, Harpaz N, Pace NR. Molecular-phylogenetic characterization of microbial community imbalances in human inflammatory bowel diseases. Proc Natl Acad Sci USA 2007; 104(34): 13780-5. [http://dx.doi.org/10.1073/pnas.0706625104] [PMID: 17699621]

[89] Moayyedi P, Surette MG, Kim PT, *et al.* Fecal Microbiota Transplantation Induces Remission in Patients With Active Ulcerative Colitis in a Randomized Controlled Trial. Gastroenterology 2015; 149(1): 102-109.e6. [http://dx.doi.org/10.1053/j.gastro.2015.04.001] [PMID: 25857665]

[90] Paramsothy S, Kamm MA, Kaakoush NO, *et al.* Multidonor intensive faecal microbiota transplantation for active ulcerative colitis: a randomised placebo-controlled trial. Lancet 2017; 389(10075): 1218-28. [http://dx.doi.org/10.1016/S0140-6736(17)30182-4] [PMID: 28214091]

[91] Costello SP, Waters O, Bryant RV, *et al.* Short Duration, Low Intensity, Pooled Fecal Microbiota Transplantation Induces Remission in Patients with Mild-Moderately Active Ulcerative Colitis: A Randomised Controlled Trial. Gastroenterology 2017; 152(5): S198-9. [http://dx.doi.org/10.1016/S0016-5085(17)30969-1]

[92] Finlay BB, Goldszmid R, Honda K, Trinchieri G, Wargo J, Zitvogel L. Can we harness the microbiota to enhance the efficacy of cancer immunotherapy? Nat Rev Immunol 2020; 20(9): 522-8. [http://dx.doi.org/10.1038/s41577-020-0374-6] [PMID: 32661409]

[93] Robert C, Ribas A, Schachter J, *et al.* Pembrolizumab versus ipilimumab in advanced melanoma (KEYNOTE-006): post-hoc 5-year results from an open-label, multicentre, randomised, controlled, phase 3 study. Lancet Oncol 2019; 20(9): 1239-51. [http://dx.doi.org/10.1016/S1470-2045(19)30388-2] [PMID: 31345627]

[94] Robert C, Long GV, Brady B, *et al.* Nivolumab in previously untreated melanoma without BRAF mutation. N Engl J Med 2015; 372(4): 320-30. [http://dx.doi.org/10.1056/NEJMoa1412082] [PMID: 25399552]

[95] Zarour HM. Reversing T-cell Dysfunction and Exhaustion in Cancer. Clin Cancer Res 2016; 22(8): 1856-64. [http://dx.doi.org/10.1158/1078-0432.CCR-15-1849] [PMID: 27084739]

[96] Gopalakrishnan V, Spencer CN, Nezi L, *et al.* Gut microbiome modulates response to anti–PD-1 immunotherapy in melanoma patients. Science 2018; 359(6371): 97-103. [http://dx.doi.org/10.1126/science.aan4236] [PMID: 29097493]

[97] Matson V, Fessler J, Bao R, *et al.* The commensal microbiome is associated with anti–PD-1 efficacy in metastatic melanoma patients. Science 2018; 359(6371): 104-8. [http://dx.doi.org/10.1126/science.aao3290] [PMID: 29302014]

[98] Routy B, Le Chatelier E, Derosa L, *et al.* Gut microbiome influences efficacy of PD-1–based immunotherapy against epithelial tumors. Science 2018; 359(6371): 91-7.

[http://dx.doi.org/10.1126/science.aan3706] [PMID: 29097494]

[99] Baruch EN, Youngster I, Ben-Betzalel G, *et al.* Fecal microbiota transplant promotes response in immunotherapy-refractory melanoma patients. Science 2021; 371(6529): 602-9. [http://dx.doi.org/10.1126/science.abb5920] [PMID: 33303685]

[100] Davar D, Dzutsev AK, McCulloch JA, *et al.* Fecal microbiota transplant overcomes resistance to anti–PD-1 therapy in melanoma patients. Science 2021; 371(6529): 595-602. [http://dx.doi.org/10.1126/science.abf3363] [PMID: 33542131]

[101] Tang WHW, Hazen SL. The Gut Microbiome and Its Role in Cardiovascular Diseases. Circulation 2017; 135(11): 1008-10. [http://dx.doi.org/10.1161/CIRCULATIONAHA.116.024251] [PMID: 28289004]

[102] Wang Z, Klipfell E, Bennett BJ, *et al.* Gut flora metabolism of phosphatidylcholine promotes cardiovascular disease. Nature 2011; 472(7341): 57-63. [http://dx.doi.org/10.1038/nature09922] [PMID: 21475195]

[103] Smits LP, Kootte RS, Levin E, *et al.* Effect of Vegan Fecal Microbiota Transplantation on Carnitine- and Choline-Derived Trimethylamine-N-Oxide Production and Vascular Inflammation in Patients With Metabolic Syndrome. J Am Heart Assoc 2018; 7(7): e008342. [http://dx.doi.org/10.1161/JAHA.117.008342] [PMID: 29581220]

[104] Zhang Y, Zhang S, Li B, *et al.* Gut microbiota dysbiosis promotes age-related atrial fibrillation by lipopolysaccharide and glucose-induced activation of NLRP3-inflammasome. Cardiovasc Res 2022; 118(3): 785-97. [http://dx.doi.org/10.1093/cvr/cvab114] [PMID: 33757127]

[105] Hu XF, Zhang WY, Wen Q, *et al.* Fecal microbiota transplantation alleviates myocardial damage in myocarditis by restoring the microbiota composition. Pharmacol Res 2019; 139: 412-21. [http://dx.doi.org/10.1016/j.phrs.2018.11.042] [PMID: 30508676]

[106] Biliński J, Winter K, Jasiński M, *et al.* Rapid resolution of COVID-19 after faecal microbiota transplantation. Gut 2022; 71(1): 230-2. [http://dx.doi.org/10.1136/gutjnl-2021-325010] [PMID: 34230217]

[107] Nejadghaderi SA, Nazemalhosseini-Mojarad E, Asadzadeh Aghdaei H. Fecal microbiota transplantation for COVID-19; a potential emerging treatment strategy. Med Hypotheses 2021; 147: 110476. [http://dx.doi.org/10.1016/j.mehy.2020.110476] [PMID: 33482620]

[108] Deidda G, Bozarth IF, Cancedda L. Modulation of GABAergic transmission in development and neurodevelopmental disorders: investigating physiology and pathology to gain therapeutic perspectives. Front Cell Neurosci 2014; 8: 119. [http://dx.doi.org/10.3389/fncel.2014.00119] [PMID: 24904277]

[109] Deidda G, Biazzo M. Gut and Brain: Investigating Physiological and Pathological Interactions Between Microbiota and Brain to Gain New Therapeutic Avenues for Brain Diseases. Front Neurosci 2021; 15: 753915. [http://dx.doi.org/10.3389/fnins.2021.753915] [PMID: 34712115]

[110] Sun MF, Zhu YL, Zhou ZL, *et al.* Neuroprotective effects of fecal microbiota transplantation on MPTP-induced Parkinson's disease mice: Gut microbiota, glial reaction and TLR4/TNF-α signaling pathway. Brain Behav Immun 2018; 70: 48-60. [http://dx.doi.org/10.1016/j.bbi.2018.02.005] [PMID: 29471030]

[111] Kelly JR, Borre Y, O' Brien C, *et al.* Transferring the blues: Depression-associated gut microbiota induces neurobehavioural changes in the rat. J Psychiatr Res 2016; 82: 109-18. [http://dx.doi.org/10.1016/j.jpsychires.2016.07.019] [PMID: 27491067]

[112] Evrensel A, Ceylan ME. Fecal Microbiota Transplantation and Its Usage in Neuropsychiatric Disorders. Clin Psychopharmacol Neurosci 2016; 14(3): 231-7.

[http://dx.doi.org/10.9758/cpn.2016.14.3.231] [PMID: 27489376]

[113] Vendrik KEW, Ooijevaar RE, de Jong PRC, *et al.* Fecal Microbiota Transplantation in Neurological Disorders. Front Cell Infect Microbiol 2020; 10: 98. [http://dx.doi.org/10.3389/fcimb.2020.00098] [PMID: 32266160]

[114] Xu HM, Huang HL, Zhou YL, *et al.* Fecal Microbiota Transplantation: A New Therapeutic Attempt from the Gut to the Brain. Gastroenterol Res Pract 2021; 2021: 1-20. [http://dx.doi.org/10.1155/2021/6699268] [PMID: 33510784]

[115] Huang H, Xu H, Luo Q, *et al.* Fecal microbiota transplantation to treat Parkinson's disease with constipation. Medicine (Baltimore) 2019; 98(26): e16163. [http://dx.doi.org/10.1097/MD.0000000000016163] [PMID: 31261545]

[116] Segal A, Zlotnik Y, Moyal-Atias K, Abuhasira R, Ifergane G. Fecal microbiota transplant as a potential treatment for Parkinson's disease – A case series. Clin Neurol Neurosurg 2021; 207: 106791. [http://dx.doi.org/10.1016/j.clineuro.2021.106791] [PMID: 34237681]

[117] He Z, Cui BT, Zhang T, *et al.* Fecal microbiota transplantation cured epilepsy in a case with Crohn's disease: The first report. World J Gastroenterol 2017; 23(19): 3565-8. [http://dx.doi.org/10.3748/wjg.v23.i19.3565] [PMID: 28596693]

[118] Molloy CA, Manning-Courtney P. Prevalence of chronic gastrointestinal symptoms in children with autism and autistic spectrum disorders. Autism 2003; 7(2): 165-71. [http://dx.doi.org/10.1177/1362361303007002004] [PMID: 12846385]

[119] Krajmalnik-Brown R, Lozupone C, Kang DW, Adams JB. Gut bacteria in children with autism spectrum disorders: challenges and promise of studying how a complex community influences a complex disease. Microb Ecol Health Dis 2015; 26: 26914. [PMID: 25769266]

[120] Tomova A, Husarova V, Lakatosova S, *et al.* Gastrointestinal microbiota in children with autism in Slovakia. Physiol Behav 2015; 138: 179-87. [http://dx.doi.org/10.1016/j.physbeh.2014.10.033] [PMID: 25446201]

[121] Cao X, Lin P, Jiang P, Li C. Characteristics of the gastrointestinal microbiome in children with autism spectrum disorder: a systematic review. Shanghai Jingshen Yixue 2013; 25(6): 342-53. [PMID: 24991177]

[122] Chaidez V, Hansen RL, Hertz-Picciotto I. Gastrointestinal problems in children with autism, developmental delays or typical development. J Autism Dev Disord 2014; 44(5): 1117-27. [http://dx.doi.org/10.1007/s10803-013-1973-x] [PMID: 24193577]

[123] Adams JB, Johansen LJ, Powell LD, Quig D, Rubin RA. Gastrointestinal flora and gastrointestinal status in children with autism – comparisons to typical children and correlation with autism severity. BMC Gastroenterol 2011; 11(1): 22. [http://dx.doi.org/10.1186/1471-230X-11-22] [PMID: 21410934]

[124] Żebrowska P, Łaczmańska I, Łaczmański Ł. Future Directions in Reducing Gastrointestinal Disorders in Children With ASD Using Fecal Microbiota Transplantation. Front Cell Infect Microbiol 2021; 11: 630052. [http://dx.doi.org/10.3389/fcimb.2021.630052] [PMID: 33718277]

[125] Kang DW, Adams JB, Gregory AC, *et al.* Microbiota Transfer Therapy alters gut ecosystem and improves gastrointestinal and autism symptoms: an open-label study. Microbiome 2017; 5(1): 10. [http://dx.doi.org/10.1186/s40168-016-0225-7] [PMID: 28122648]

[126] Kang DW, Adams JB, Coleman DM, *et al.* Long-term benefit of Microbiota Transfer Therapy on autism symptoms and gut microbiota. Sci Rep 2019; 9(1): 5821. [http://dx.doi.org/10.1038/s41598-019-42183-0] [PMID: 30967657]

CHAPTER 9

Gut Microbial Metabolites as Diagnostic Biomarkers

Mohamad Taleuzzaman[1,*], **Anupam**[2], **Manjari Verma**[2], **Kajal Chaudhary**[2] and **Rohit Choudhary**[3]

[1] *Department of Pharmaceutical Chemistry, Faculty of Pharmacy, Maulana Azad University, Village Bujhawar, Tehsil Luni, Jodhpur-342008, Rajasthan, India*

[2] *Rameesh Institute of Vocational & Technical Education, Greater Noida, U.P., 201310, India*

[3] *Kalka Institute for Research and Advanced Studies, Meerut, U.P., 250103, India*

Abstract: Metabolites that originate from the human host and microbiota significantly alter host physiology and metabolism, which is a key factor in disease susceptibility and development. The gastrointestinal tract's gut microbiota, a community of bacteria, produces vital signalling metabolites that are essential to the hosts' physiological well-being. However, disruptions in the production of these metabolites can result in a variety of diseases, including cancer, neurological diseases, gastrointestinal disorders, metabolic diseases, and cardiovascular diseases. The understanding of gut microbiota metabolites, encompasses their various forms and mechanisms of action on targets. Furthermore, we enumerate their physiological and pathologic roles in both health and illness, including influencing the gut microbiota's composition and providing nourishment. In order to fight microbial-driven disorders and promote health, this study can be useful in understanding the roles of gut microbiota metabolites as it provides suggestions for designing appropriate therapeutic options. Many of these metabolites may be used in conjunction with intestinal microbiota dysbiosis as diagnostic biomarkers to track disease states.

Keywords: Autoimmune disease, Cancer, Cardiovascular disease, Diabetes, Food interaction, Gut microbiota, Immune response, Metabolites, Metabolite profiling, Neurological disorders.

INTRODUCTION

The gastrointestinal system of humans houses a wide range of microorganisms, including viruses, bacteria, fungi, archaea, and protozoa. This group of organisms (gut microbiota) has a significant adaptable genome that benefits the host and res-

* **Corresponding author Mohamad Taleuzzaman:** Department of Pharmaceutical Chemistry, Faculty of Pharmacy, Maulana Azad University, Village Bujhawar, Tehsil Luni, Jodhpur-342008, Rajasthan, India; E-mail: zzaman007@gmail.com

Sandipan Dasgupta & Moitreyee Chattopadhyay (Eds.)

ponds to the intestinal environment and also located both inside and outside the body, such as the conjunctiva, saliva, oral, vaginal, and cutaneous mucosa [1]. The extensive range of roles that the microbiome has provided includes the metabolism of xenobiotics, vitamin synthesis, pathogen defence, fermentation of dietary fibres, and immune maturation. These functions demonstrate how the microbiome is intricately linked to human biology [2]. In the human digestive system, the microbial parasitic organ that lives in the gut is called the microbiota [3]. Ninety-five percent of the human microbiota is found in the gastrointestinal system, and each person has a different microbiota composition that may operate as a fingerprint [4].

A wide range of biological tissues, including the liver, kidney, urine, faeces, and cerebrospinal fluid, are frequently reported to contain microbial metabolites [2]. With 10 microbial cells and more than 22 million microbial genes, the gut microbiota can produce an extensive number of flexible enzymes to ferment many kinds of substances that are indigestible or difficult for human enzymes to break down, such as fibres. Thus, the gut microbiota is capable of producing a wide spectrum of metabolites with various bioactivities.

Based on their origin, the gut microbiota's metabolites can be broadly classified into three categories (a) Microbiota produced directly from diets, like SCFAs and indole derivatives; (b) Host and the gut microbiota that perform modification , like secondary bile acids, and (c) Produced de novo, like polysaccharide A [5].

Byproducts produced by the gut bacteria have a role in mediating their systemic effects. These microbial metabolites can either diffuse easily or are absorbed by the gut mucosa. The gut liver, gut brain, gut bone, gut kidney, gut lung, and gut heart axes are the channels *via* which the gut microbiota and various organs communicate with one another in a bidirectional fashion. Certain groups of metabolites derived from microbiota, including branched-chain amino acids, short-chain fatty acids, trimethylamine N-oxide, and tryptophan derivatives, have been linked to the etiology of neurological and cardiovascular diseases, metabolic disorders, and lifespan [3] as indicated in Fig. (**1**). There may be two ways in which these differential metabolites and disease are related: a) Metabolites from the gut microbiota change as the result of disease. Thus, these modified metabolites can serve as disease biomarkers. b) Because gut microbes produce chemicals that promote disease, they are considered risk factors for specific illnesses [6].

The biomedical literature provides data that the physiological and compositional shifts of gut flora may have a close relationship with variations in host immunity [4]. A biomarker can identify a disease's kind or identify and verify the existence of an illness [7]. Biomarkers might originate from imaging data or biological material. Artificial intelligence and machine learning are capable of identifying highly predictive illness biomarkers [8].

Gut microbiota has been linked to both the promotion of health and the development or maintenance of various gastrointestinal and non-gastrointestinal disorders, in part because of high-resolution observational studies that have made use of next-generation sequencing technologies and metabolite profiling.

As we approach the post-metagenomic era, we must shift from using basic observations to distinguish between causal relationships and correlations and concentrate our efforts and resources on the latter. The goal is to include a person's microbiota in some type of customized healthcare and, *via* a deeper comprehension of its function, more effectively and precisely treat a person's illnesses. One will be able to classify various disease states more precisely and ascertain whether or not the gut microbiota is a viable therapeutic target that we may modify to treat particular diseases if we have a deeper understanding of the disease process [9]. Many studies demonstrate that treatments including medication, nutrition, and surgery alter gut microbial populations, which in turn influences the development and course of the disease. Investigators have shown an intense curiosity in the involvement of gut microorganisms and diseases related to the digestive system recently to understand the processes by which these microbes affect intestinal homeostasis and human diseases [10].

From the metabolic viewpoint, studies have shown that dysbiosis of gut microbes can cause or exacerbate many diseases such as tumors, gastrointestinal diseases, metabolic diseases, cardiovascular diseases, and neurobiological diseases; likewise, the supplement of beneficial commensals may relieve symptoms. Trimethylamine N-oxide (TMAO), a metabolite produced from gut microbes, was found to be a novel biomarker for independently predicting the incidence of poor prognosis of cardiovascular disease. In addition, *Faecalibacterium prausnitzii*, one of the most abundant bacterial species found in the gut, is reduced in different intestinal diseases, which means that *F. prausnitzii* may therefore assist as a biomarker for intestinal disease diagnostics [11 - 13].

Ageing is characterized by an ongoing decrease in homeostasis, diminished function, and increased mortality risk. Fundamentally, the cellular and molecular characteristics of mammals are shown at age 25, but this coincides with alterations in the microbiome, which change in turn, thus, influencing the speed at which age-related decline occurs. Studies on the gut microbiome of the elderly can be broadly divided into two groups, those highlighting changes in the microbiome of the elderly that are connected to specific illnesses associated with advancing age, and those that describe variations in the gut microbiome composition related to age itself [14]. It is indicated in Fig. (**2**), how the age and microbiome are interrelated.

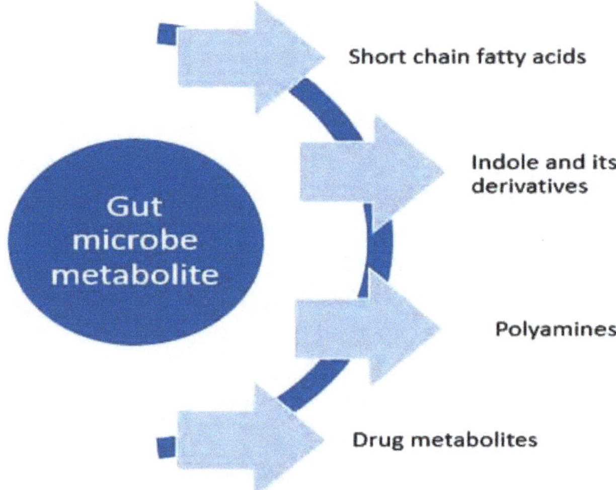

Fig. (1). Primary metabolites produced by Gut microbiomes.

Gestation	**Infancy**	**Parturition**
•Gestational health/ diabetes •Maternal food habits • Pregnancy weight gain •Antibiotics & probiotics •Bacteria in amniotic fluid and placenta •lifestyle and personal hygiene	•Mode of feeding •Fatty acid composition of breastmilk •composition and type of infant formula •Weaning •Type of solid food •Siblings & Pets •Environment & Medication	•Gestational age & Mode of delivery •Birth weight • Host physiology • Hospital environment and length of stay •Medications •Maternal vaginal, faecal and skin microflora
Puberty •Diet •Geographical and environmental influences •Personal hygine •Siblings, friends and pets •Probiotics & fermented foods •childhood illness •Medications & Malnutrition	**Adulthood** •Diet •Lifestyle •Disease & Medications •Probiotics/prebiotics •physical activities & Travelling •Sleep and mental health •Pregnancy	**Old age** •Diet •Lifestyle •Disease old-age •Types of disease •Medications •Probiotics/prebiotics •Hospital stays •Hygiene •Menopause

Fig. (2). Age-related factors affecting gut microbiota.

In a study that also examined the relationship between gut microbiota composition and ageing, the studies were divided into four general categories: (A) the gut microbiota composition of very long-lived people (such as nonagenarians and centenarians); (B) changes and transitions in gut microbiota that accompany ageing across the lifespan; (C) the gut microbiota's relationship with older adults' cognitive function; and (D) changes to the gut microbiota after interventions targeting the microbiome in older adults [15].

It was discovered that extreme ageing was connected to a higher abundance of gut microbiota genes related to xenobiotic degradation. One characteristic that distinguishes these general age-related changes is the disappearance of notable commensal taxa, such as the health-associated species *Bifidobacterium, Prevotella, Faecalibacterium, Eubacterium rectale, Lachnospira,* and *Coprococcus*.

Microbiome changes similar to those generally associated with frailty have also been found in research on the microbiome in other disorders linked to an unhealthy ageing pattern, such as decreased physical activity, cognitive decline, migraine, obesity, reduced bone mass density, metabolic syndrome and related comorbidities, chronic kidney disease, and pre-mortality [16].

Consuming dietary fibre is essential for preserving the variety of gut flora. Numerous chronic inflammatory diseases, including obesity, diabetes, and inflammatory bowel disease (IBD), have been linked to low microbial diversity. Dietary fibre can be categorized into four groups based on their chemical structures, (a) Nondigestible polysaccharides (b) Resistant starches (RS) (c) Nondigestible oligosaccharides, and (d) Chemically generated carbohydrates [17].

The essential component for preserving the variety of gut microbiota is dietary fibre. Numerous chronic inflammatory illnesses, including obesity, diabetes, and inflammatory bowel disease (IBD), are linked to low microbial diversity. One of the main causes of the decrease in fiber-degrading microorganisms in populations in industrialized countries is a diet high in fat, high in protein, and low in fibre. A meal heavy in fat, high in protein, and low in fat can limit the diversity of the gut microbiota in healthy adults in as little as one day. While there are many different plant-based foods that include dietary fibres, including grains, legumes, nuts, tubers, vegetables, and fruits. According to their chemical structures, dietary fibre can be divided into four categories: nondigestible polysaccharides, resistant starches (RS), nondigestible oligosaccharides, and chemically produced carbohydrates. Polymers such as cellulose, hemicellulose, polyfructoses, gums and mucilages, and pectins are examples of nondigestible polysaccharides. Certain dietary fibres cannot be fermented [17].

Metabolites Resulting from the Host's Gut Microbiota and Food Interaction

Short-chain Fatty Acids

Gut bacteria generate a wide range of metabolic end products as a result of their process of surviving on the host's food, including trimethylamine-N-oxide (TMAO), an extended number of tryptophan catabolites, and short-chain fatty acids (acetate, propionate, and butyrate). The bacteria in the colon consume fermentable dietary fibre which passes by the small intestine undigested or absorbed. As a result of fermentation, gases (H_2 and CO_2), butyrate, acetate, and propionate are produced. While 90-99% of the acetate, propionate, and butyrate produced are consumed by the stomach, the proportions for all are 60:20:20 [18].

Acetate plays a role in metabolic disorders, particularly type 2 diabetes mellitus (T2DM), and this discovery is significant. Because acetate acts with GPR41/43, some study links it to increased appetite and weight reduction; yet, because acetate is a building block for hepatic and adipocyte lipogenesis, other research suggests that acetate has obesogenic properties [19].

Probably the most studied and beneficial to human health is butyrate. The acetyl-CoA pathway is the principal of the four known pathways for butyrate synthesis [5]. Butyrate facilitates mucosal integrity and speeds up β-oxidation and oxygen consumption in the gut by activating the peroxisome proliferator-activated receptor-γ (PPARγ), which in turn creates a rich luminal anaerobic environment. By permitting the transformation of proinflammatory M1 macrophages into resolution-phase M2 macrophages, it enhances antimicrobial activity even further [20].

Propionate is produced by microorganisms fermenting indigestible fibres *via* the succinate pathway, with the acrylate and propanediol pathways playing a minor role. Once produced, propionate is either absorbed into the portal system and transported to the liver, where it is used as a substrate in hepatic gluconeogenesis, or it is used at the level of the colonocytes as a substrate for intestinal gluconeogenesis *via* the FFAR3 signalling pathway [21]. Propionate has been shown in human trials to have a general anti-obesity effect. Daily consumption of 10g of propionate was found to significantly reduce weight gain, intra-abdominal adipose tissue distribution, intrahepatocellular lipid content, and the development of insulin sensitivity observed in the control group. Additionally, the study was randomized and controlled [22]. Propionate has also been shown to have anti-inflammatory properties by decreasing the levels of interleukin-8 and TNF-α release from neutrophils [23, 24].

Butyrate is probably the most researched and advantageous to human health. There are four known mechanisms for the production of butyrate, with the acetyl-CoA pathway being the main one. The lysine, glutamate, and succinate pathways are the other three [25]. Not only is butyrate the preferred energy molecule in luminal colonocytes, but it also has extensive therapeutic benefits at the systemic level. These advantages include preserving mucosal integrity, regulating systemic and local immunity, and preventing cellular neoplastic alterations [26, 27]. By activating the peroxisome proliferator-activated receptor-γ (PPARγ), butyrate promotes mucosal integrity and accelerates β-oxidation and oxygen consumption in the gut, creating a rich luminal anaerobic environment [28]. Furthermore, it boosts the synthesis of immunoglobulins, boosts the release of antimicrobial peptides, and causes goblet cells to produce more mucin [29, 30]. By permitting the transformation of proinflammatory M1 macrophages into resolution-phase M2 macrophages, it enhances antimicrobial activity even further [31]. Apart from the significant immunity role, butyrate has been shown to support a strong anti-neoplastic effect.

Tryptophan Metabolites

The key metabolites produced by proteolysis have not gotten as much attention as the SCFA and TMAO metabolites produced by the microbiota, which have been researched for more than a century. Proteolysis-related products have historically been linked to harmful effects, but more recent research indicates that tryptophan metabolites may be beneficial for intestinal homeostasis. These tryptophan metabolites have a variety of roles, such as immune system modulation, antibacterial activity, and mucosal homeostasis maintenance through systemic hormone secretion regulation and antioxidant characteristics. Research on indole shows that it has antibacterial properties. It has antibacterial properties against Salmonella, Lactobacillus, E. Coli, B. cereus, and Staphylococcus aureus. Moreover, indole ethanol stops the growth of parasitic protozoa and bacteriophage replication in specific bacterial strains [5].

Polyamines

All living things require these non-protein amino acids, which also play a role in a variety of physiological processes, including the regulation of the activity of enzymes, the control of genes and stress responses, and cell division and proliferation. Since they affect the host's overall health, putrescine, spermidine, and spermine rank among the most important metabolites produced by the gut microbiota. Increased levels of PA from probiotic therapy can decrease chronic low-grade inflammation, which can extend the host's lifespan and increase its resilience to oxidative damage [32]. Increased consumption of PA, particularly spermidine, has been linked to a decrease in cardiovascular events and mortality, according to recent epidemiological research [33 - 35]. Low spermidine and spermine levels have been shown in recent research to enhance dazomet accumulation and thus lower DNA methylation levels.

Bile Acids

The gut microbiota transforms saturated hydroxylated C-24 sterols, which are first generated by hepatocytes, into bile acids that are water-soluble, amphipathic metabolites of cholesterol. An alternative pathway in the liver uses cholesterol to make primary bile acids, with the former being more important. The enzyme that limits the synthesis of primary bile acids in the traditional pathway is 7 α-hydroxylase [36]. The two primary hepatic bile acids that humans manufacture are cholic acid and chenodeoxycholic acid. These acids can conjugate with taurine or glycine to form bile salts. The liver produces the primary bile salts, which are then stored in the gallbladder and expelled into the duodenum. To keep the bile acid pool intact, the host can reabsorb primary bile acids from the intestinal tract and return them to the liver through a process known as enterohepatic circulation [37].

Bacterial Vitamins

These include necessary vitamins that the gut flora can produce. The gut microbiota is primarily responsible for producing vitamin K2 and several vitamins belonging to the B family. Although it is less common, recent research has also demonstrated that the gut bacteria produce ascorbate or vitamin C. Although the exact metabolic mechanisms that microbes use in the intestinal microbiota to create ascorbic acid are unknown, people with IBD have been shown to have reduced levels of ascorbate in their inflamed mucosa [38]. In addition, ascorbate was reported to suppress T-effector cells and inhibit T-cell activation [39]. A recent study by Pham *et. al.* demonstrated that colon-delivered vitamin C results in significantly increased microbial alpha diversity and faecal SCFAs [40]. Further investigation is needed to determine both the metabolic pathways and the effect of ascorbate levels on preventing microbiota-related human diseases.

Functions of Gut Microbiota Metabolites

Fundamental processes of bacterial metabolism and the metabolic and physiological processes of mammals rely on vitamin K and B groups. By functioning as complementary endogenous vitamin sources, the amino acid metabolites produced by the gut microbiota, such as isoleucine, valine, leucine, and tryptophan, are precursors to metabolites that have a major impact on mammalian physiology and are necessary for protein synthesis [41].

Impacting the Systemic Immune Response

Apart from regulating the intestinal immunity in the vicinity, the gut microbiota has the ability to impact the innate and adaptive immune responses in several extraintestinal organs by interacting with a wide range of immune cells, including B cells, T cells, and macrophages. Through modulating metabolic sensors and raising acetyl-CoA, SCFAs help spleen B cells produce antibodies. In the lungs, the defence against allergies and asthma is provided by gut microbiota metabolites, primarily SCFAs. Treatment with antibiotics increases allergic lung inflammation, while SCFAs decrease it by influencing T helper type 2 cells and lowering immunoglobulin E levels in the blood [42].

Influencing the nervous system: The ability of the central nervous system (CNS) to influence gut motility, production of digestive juice, immunological response, blood flow, and nociception has long been known. Furthermore, through the intestinal immune system, signals from the brain to the gut can further influence the makeup and functionality of the gut microbiota [43].

Affecting drug efficacy and toxicity: Gut microbiota plays important roles in the modification of the toxicity and efficacy of drugs and herbal compounds such as metformin, berberine, and aconitine [44]. Drug efficacy and toxicity can be adjusted by gut microbiota metabolites, which can also influence the expression of drug transporters and hepatic drug-metabolizing enzymes. These metabolites can compete with drug-metabolizing enzymes. Firmicutes, Bacteroidetes, Actinobacteria, and Fusobacteria phyla produce p-Cresol by microbial conversion of tyrosine and phenylalanine [45, 46].

One common non-steroidal anti-inflammatory medication used to alleviate pain and fever is acetaminophen. In a clinical setting, an acetaminophen overdose can result in severe and occasionally deadly hepatotoxicity [47].

GUT MICROBIAL METABOLITES AS BIOMARKERS

Gut microbial metabolites have gained significant attention in recent years due to their diverse roles in human health and disease. These metabolites, produced by the complex microbial community residing in the gastrointestinal tract, can influence various physiological processes and serve as potential biomarkers for monitoring health status and disease progression. The human gut microbiota, comprising trillions of microorganisms, plays a fundamental role in host physiology and metabolism. One of the key contributions of this microbial community is the production of various metabolites through the breakdown of dietary components and endogenous substrates. The ideal characteristics of biomarkers are given in Fig. (**3**).

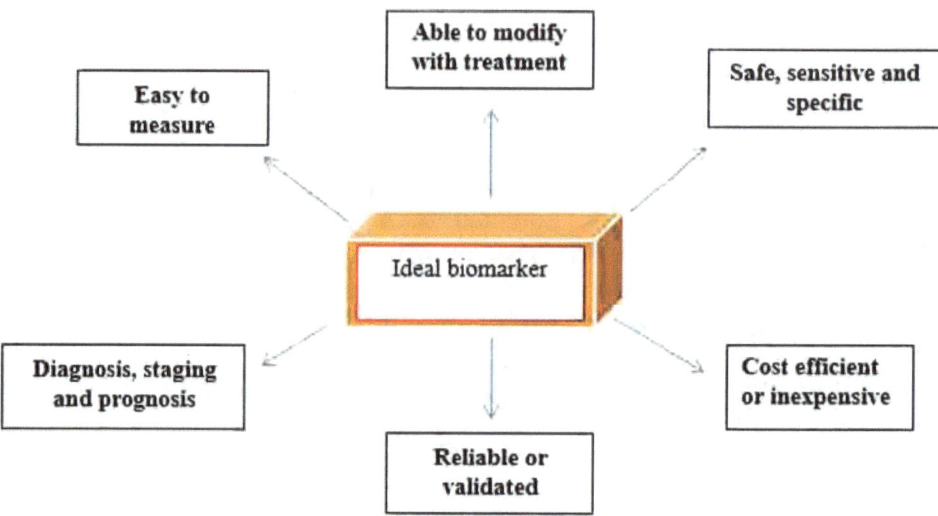

Fig. (3). Ideal characteristics of biomarkers.

Metabolism-Related Disturbance Of The Gut Microbiome-Host Interactions

Gut microbiota is essential to the preservation of the host's physiological processes. Numerous metabolic illnesses might arise as a result of a disturbance in the delicate host-microbiota interaction balance. These metabolites may originate directly from microorganisms or may be transformed from substrates derived from food or hosts [48].

Inflammatory Bowel Disease (IBD)

The phrase "inflammatory bowel disease" (IBD) refers to a collection of intricate, recurrent, long-term inflammatory disorders that harm the gastrointestinal system. IBD is extremely common in Western nations, but because of the quick rise in both its incidence and prevalence in Asia, IBD is progressively becoming more widespread around the world and expanding into both developed and developing nations [49]. Traditional diagnostic methods for IBD, such as endoscopy and histological analysis, are invasive and costly. Gut microbial biomarkers offer a promising alternative for early diagnosis and monitoring of disorder activity [50].

In IBD investigations, microbiota-derived metabolites such as tryptophan, short-chain fatty acids (SCFA), and other small compounds have garnered a lot of interest. Dysbiosis of the gut microbial population and its byproducts is linked to IBD. The significance of gut microbiota in IBD pathogenesis has been made clear by recent advancements in the field of gut microbiota research. Due to its effects on intestinal permeability and the immune system, the microbiota and its metabolites are essential in the progress of IBD [2].

Obesity and Metabolic Syndrome

The causes of overweight and obesity are positive energy balances resulting from biological, behavioural, and environmental processes that require further research and understanding [51]. By regulating several metabolic pathways in the host, the gut microbiome appears to have a dynamic metabolic potential, which at least partially explains the emergence of metabolic diseases and obesity. The amount of research on gut microbiota and obesity has increased dramatically in recent years. This knowledge has made it easier to identify the microbial characteristics linked to obesity in many populations and to understand how those characteristics interact with host genetics, age, and nutrition. Obesity and metabolic problems have continuously been linked to poor diversity in gene count and microbial makeup [52].

Diabetes

Emerging evidence suggests that the gut microbiota contributes to the pathogenesis of diabetes through its effects on energy metabolism, inflammation, and insulin sensitivity. Gut microbial biomarkers, such as changes in the ratio of butyrate-producing bacteria to opportunistic pathogens, have been associated with diabetes risk [53].

Cancer

A paradigm change in cancer therapy is underway as a result of the long-lasting clinical responses that tumour immunotherapies have demonstrated. One of the main components of tumour immunity is CD8+ T cells. Poor clinical outcomes with several cancer therapies are caused by reduced CD8+ T cell infiltration or malfunction in the tumour microenvironment (TME). Consequently, encouraging CD8+ T cell infiltration and activity in the TME may assist in increasing the effectiveness of cancer treatments [54].

Dendritic cells and CD4+ T-cells can be regulated by the gut microbiota to improve cancer immunosurveillance and support treatment effectiveness. Dysbiosis, characterized by alterations in microbial composition and function, may promote carcinogenesis through inflammation, genotoxicity, and immune modulation. Gut microbial biomarkers have the potential to aid in cancer diagnosis, prognosis, and treatment response prediction. Additionally, microbial metabolites, such as secondary bile acids and polyamines, may serve as biomarkers for cancer risk stratification and therapeutic targeting [55].

Biomarkers Used for Different Diseases

There are three types of biomarkers:

- Type 0 biomarker- It is an indicator of a disease's natural course that shows a longitudinal correlation with established clinical standards.
- Type I biomarker- An indicator that records the outcomes of a treatment intervention in line with its therapeutic effects, mode of action, and toxicological effects of a drug.
- Type II biomarker is a surrogate biomarker that is used to predict how a treatment intervention will be received and is thought to be an alternative to clinical outcome assessments of disease.

Classification of Biomarkers

Biomarkers can be classified in various ways based on their characteristics, origin, function, and application. Here is a classification of biomarkers based on different criteria-

Based on Origin

- Genetic Biomarkers: The most often utilized biomarkers for illness diagnosis are genetic (DNA mutation, DNA single nucleotide polymorphism, and karyotypic) differences. The majority of indicators linked to over 319 diseases or ailments are DNA-based [56].
- Protein Biomarkers: They could function as indicators of the emergence of anxiety, swelling, and immunology along with associated diseases like Type 2 diabetes, cancer, heart issues, and additional disorders.
- Metabolic Biomarkers: Small molecules involved in metabolic pathways.
- Cellular Biomarkers: Cellular biomarkers are quantifiable and biological indicators that can be employed in laboratory and clinical procedures. Cellular biomarkers are frequently assessed in soft tissue, bodily fluids, or blood to determine how they will react to a certain course of treatment. These kinds of biomarkers enable the separation, classification, measurement, and description of cells based on their morphological and physiological characteristics.
- Inflammatory Biomarkers: Molecules associated with inflammation. *e.g.* C-reactive protein (CRP), cytokines [interleukin (IL)-1, IL-6, IL-8, monocyte chemoattractant protein-1 (MCP-1)], soluble CD40 ligand, serum amyloid A (SAA), and selectins (E-selectin, P-selectin).
- Neurological Biomarkers: Biomarkers related to brain function or structure.

Based on Function

- Diagnostic Biomarkers: *e.g.* Cardiac troponin, 3-hydroxy-fatty acids, glycosaminomers, glutamate, cate statin, cystatin-C, liver-type fatty acid-binding protein (L-FABP).
- Prognostic biomarkers: Prognostic biomarkers include blood pressure, cholesterol, N-acetyl-beta-glucosaminidase, serine, and ketamine reaction. They are used to identify cardiovascular illnesses, heart failure, renal impairment, bone and skeletal metastases, and anti-depressant responses to ketamine.
- Therapeutic biomarkers: These biomarkers are helpful in assessing how therapy affects sickness or stress as well as the clinical response. D-serine's efficacy as a therapeutic biomarker in individuals with depression and schizophrenia was demonstrated by clinical research. As a serum tumor biomarker, CA15-3 is helpful in tracking the effectiveness of breast cancer treatment. HbA1c was employed to track the effectiveness of anti-diabetic medication.

Based on Clinical Application

- Cardiovascular Biomarkers: Biomarkers associated with cardiovascular diseases [57 - 61, 65, 69].
- Neurological Biomarkers: Biomarkers used in the diagnosis and monitoring of neurological disorders.
- Infectious Disease Biomarkers: Biomarkers associated with infectious agents and immune responses.
- Autoimmune Biomarkers: Biomarkers associated with autoimmune diseases.

Based on Sample Type

- Blood Biomarkers: Biomarkers detected in blood samples.
- Urine Biomarkers: Biomarkers detected in urine samples [70, 71].
- Cerebrospinal Fluid Biomarkers: Biomarkers detected in cerebrospinal fluid.
- Tissue Biomarkers: Biomarkers detected in tissue samples.

Numerous other important uses for biomarkers include early disease diagnosis, risk prediction, prognosis evaluation, and health status monitoring (including staging). They can be applied to prognostic indicators, personalized therapeutic interventions, drug reaction prediction and treatment, cell type identification, pharmacodynamics and dose-response investigations, illness screening, diagnosis, characterization, and monitoring (Table **1**).

Different roles of biomarkers:

- Antecedent: Identifying the risk of developing an illness.
- Prognostic: Predicting future disease course /response to therapy.

- Diagnostic: Recognising overt diseases and categorising disease severity.
- Screening: Screening for subclinical disease.

Table 1. Biomarkers for the detection of various diseases.

S. No.	Diseases	Biomarkers	References
1	Cancer	RS/DJ-1, HSP60, HSP90, CA 15-3, RS/DJ-1, Lipophilin B, beta-globin, Hemopexin, RS/DJ-1.	[59, 61]
2	Cardiovascular Diseases	Brain natriuretic peptide (BNP), N-terminal proBNP (NT-proBNP), Troponin	[57, 62]
3	Diabetes	Hemoglobin A1c (HbA1c), C-peptide	[63, 68]
4	Neurological Disorders	Amyloid Beta and Tau Proteins, Alpha-Synuclein'Neurofilament Light Chain (NfL)	[61]
5	Alzheimer's disease	Amyloid Beta and Tau Proteins	[58, 64]
6	Parkinson's Disease	(RT-QuIC), protein misfolding cyclic amplification (PMCA)	[60]
7	Infectious diseases	Viral load for HIV,HBsAg for Hepatitis B, and PCR tests for various infectious agents	[66]
8	Autoimmune diseases	Anti-CCP antibodies, anti-dsDNA, TNF-alpha and IL-6.	[67, 69]

Biomarkers are quantifiable markers of biological states, techniques, or therapeutic reactions. They play a crucial role in diagnosing diseases, monitoring disease progression, predicting treatment responses, and developing new therapies. Here are some examples of biomarkers used for different diseases:

Cancer

When a cancer begins to grow, tumor markers may be generated. Proteins, hormone/hormone metabolites, enzymes, and antigens are examples of tumor markers that can be found in cells, tissues, and bodily fluids [59].

- CA-125 for ovarian and fallopian tube cancer and CEA (Carcinoembryonic Antigen) for colorectal, gastric, pancreatic, and lungs cancer.
- Genetic mutations such as BRCA1 and BRCA2, CA 15-3 for breast and ovarian cancers.
- Circulating tumor cells (CTCs) and cell-free DNA (cfDNA) for monitoring disease progression and treatment response.
- ALP in bone metastasis of many malignancies and chromogranin A in neuroendocrine tumors.
- Calcitonin in medullary thyroid cancer, bronchogenic carcinoma.

Cardiovascular Diseases

Cardiac biomarkers' functions are:

- Troponin levels for diagnosing myocardial infarction.
- Lipid profile including cholesterol levels for assessing cardiovascular risk.
- Brain natriuretic peptide (BNP) and N-terminal pro-b-type natriuretic peptide (NT-proBNP) for heart failure [57].

Diabetes

Diabetes mellitus is a chronic illness that is complicated and results in elevated blood glucose levels. Biomarkers may indicate the existence and degree of vascular problems associated with diabetes or hyperglycemia, or diabetes itself.

- Blood glucose levels for diagnosing and monitoring diabetes.
- Glycated hemoglobin (HbA1c) for long-term blood sugar control.
- C-peptide levels for assessing insulin production [63].

Alzheimer's Disease and Neurodegenerative Disorders

Common neuropathological pathway that is typified by brain deposits of extracellular fibrillar beta-amyloid (Aβ), intracellular neurofibrillary tangles (NFT), and degeneration of both neurons and axons.

- Amyloid beta and tau proteins in cerebrospinal fluid for diagnosing Alzheimer's disease.
- Neurofilament light chain (NfL) for monitoring neurodegeneration and disease progression [64]

Infectious Diseases

In the past 20 years, bloodborne viruses known as the hepatitis B and hepatitis C viruses (HBV) have become the primary cause of liver cancer-related death and morbidity. HIV is a member of the family Retroviridae, which is also responsible for AIDS.

- Viral load for diseases like HIV and hepatitis.
- Antibody levels for diagnosing infections and assessing immune response, such as in COVID-19 serology testing.

Autoimmune Diseases

Autoimmune illnesses are defined by the generation of autoantibodies, immune cell activation, elevated pro-inflammatory cytokine expression, and type I interferon activation [66].

- Autoantibodies like rheumatoid factor (RF) and anti-cyclic citrullinated peptide (anti-CCP) for rheumatoid arthritis.
- Antinuclear antibodies (ANA) for systemic lupus erythematosus (SLE).

Kidney Diseases

Kidney disease usually develops gradually over many years, with a protracted latent phase during which the illness is clinically quiet. As a result, biomarkers that measure kidney function are primarily used in the diagnosis, evaluation, and therapy of kidney disease.

- Serum creatinine and estimated glomerular filtration rate (eGFR) for assessing kidney function.
- Urine albumin-to-creatinine ratio for detecting early signs of kidney damage [70]

Liver Diseases

The liver is involved in the synthesis of proteins, the production of digestive enzymes, and the first detoxification of different metabolites. The liver is also important for metabolism, red blood cell (RBC) control, and the synthesis and storage of glucose.

- Liver enzymes like ALT (Alanine Aminotransferase) and AST (Aspartate Aminotransferase) for assessing liver function and detecting liver damage.
- Bilirubin levels for assessing liver health and function [71].

CONCLUSION

The gut microbiota, a microbial population found in the gastrointestinal system, generates critical signalling chemicals that are necessary for the hosts' physiological health. A disruption in the delicate equilibrium of the host-microbiota connection could lead to a variety of metabolic disorders. Secondary bile acids and polyamines are examples of microbial metabolites that may be used as biomarkers for cancer risk assessment and treatment targeting. Biomarkers have many other significant applications, such as monitoring health status, prognosis evaluation, risk prediction, and early illness detection.

ACKNOWLEDGEMENTS

The authors acknowledge the Department of Pharmaceutical Chemistry, Faculty of Pharmacy, Maulana Azad University, Village Bujhawar, Tehsil Luni, Jodhpur 342008, Rajasthan, India, Rameesh Institute of Vocational & Technical Education, Greater Noida, U.P, 201310. India, 201310 and Kalka Institute for Research and Advanced Studies, Meerut, U.P. 250103 India for supporting them in writing the chapter.

REFERENCES

[1] Krautkramer KA, Fan J, Bäckhed F. Gut microbial metabolites as multi-kingdom intermediates. Nat Rev Microbiol 2021; 19(2): 77-94. [http://dx.doi.org/10.1038/s41579-020-0438-4] [PMID: 32968241]

[2] Lavelle A, Sokol H. Gut microbiota-derived metabolites as key actors in inflammatory bowel disease. Nat Rev Gastroenterol Hepatol 2020; 17(4): 223-37. [http://dx.doi.org/10.1038/s41575-019-0258-z] [PMID: 32076145]

[3] Gagnon E, Mitchell PL, Manikpurage HD, *et al.* Impact of the gut microbiota and associated metabolites on cardiometabolic traits, chronic diseases and human longevity: a Mendelian randomization study. J Transl Med 2023; 21(1): 60. [http://dx.doi.org/10.1186/s12967-022-03799-5] [PMID: 36717893]

[4] Hajjo R, Sabbah DA, Al Bawab AQ. Unlocking the potential of the human microbiome for identifying disease diagnostic biomarkers. Diagnostics (Basel) 2022; 12(7): 1742. [http://dx.doi.org/10.3390/diagnostics12071742] [PMID: 35885645]

[5] Liu J, Tan Y, Cheng H, Zhang D, Feng W, Peng C. Functions of gut microbiota metabolites, current status and future perspectives. Aging Dis 2022; 13(4): 1106-26. [http://dx.doi.org/10.14336/AD.2022.0104] [PMID: 35855347]

[6] Ma Y, Liu X, Wang J. Small molecules in the big picture of gut microbiome-host cross-talk. EBioMedicine 2022; 81: 104085. [http://dx.doi.org/10.1016/j.ebiom.2022.104085] [PMID: 35636316]

[7] Vostal JG, Buehler PW, Gelderman MP, *et al.* Proceedings of the Food and Drug Administration's public workshop on new red blood cell product regulatory science. 255-66.

[8] Hajjo R, Sabbah DA, Bardaweel SK, Tropsha A. Identification of tumor-specific MRI biomarkers using machine learning (ML). Diagnostics (Basel) 2021; 11(5): 742. [http://dx.doi.org/10.3390/diagnostics11050742] [PMID: 33919342]

[9] Marchesi JR, Adams DH, Fava F, *et al.* The gut microbiota and host health: a new clinical frontier. Gut 2016; 65(2): 330-9. [http://dx.doi.org/10.1136/gutjnl-2015-309990] [PMID: 26338727]

[10] Qi C, Wang P, Fu T, *et al.* A comprehensive review for gut microbes: technologies, interventions, metabolites and diseases. Brief Funct Genomics 2021; 20(1): 42-60. [http://dx.doi.org/10.1093/bfgp/elaa029] [PMID: 33554248]

[11] Lopez-Siles M, Duncan SH, Garcia-Gil LJ, Martinez-Medina M. *Faecalibacterium prausnitzii* : from microbiology to diagnostics and prognostics. ISME J 2017; 11(4): 841-52. [http://dx.doi.org/10.1038/ismej.2016.176] [PMID: 28045459]

[12] Li XS, Obeid S, Klingenberg R, *et al.* Gut microbiota-dependent trimethylamine N-oxide in acute coronary syndromes: a prognostic marker for incident cardiovascular events beyond traditional risk factors. Eur Heart J 2017; 38(11): ehw582. [http://dx.doi.org/10.1093/eurheartj/ehw582] [PMID: 28077467]

[13] Qu K, Guo F, Liu X, Lin Y, Zou Q. Application of machine learning in microbiology. Front Microbiol 2019; 10: 827.
[http://dx.doi.org/10.3389/fmicb.2019.00827] [PMID: 31057526]

[14] Ghosh TS, Shanahan F, O'Toole PW. The gut microbiome as a modulator of healthy ageing. Nat Rev Gastroenterol Hepatol 2022; 19(9): 565-84.
[http://dx.doi.org/10.1038/s41575-022-00605-x] [PMID: 35468952]

[15] Badal VD, Vaccariello ED, Murray ER, *et al.* The gut microbiome, aging, and longevity: a systematic review. Nutrients 2020; 12(12): 3759.
[http://dx.doi.org/10.3390/nu12123759] [PMID: 33297486]

[16] Nagpal R, Mainali R, Ahmadi S, *et al.* Gut microbiome and aging: Physiological and mechanistic insights. Nutr Healthy Aging 2018; 4(4): 267-85.
[http://dx.doi.org/10.3233/NHA-170030] [PMID: 29951588]

[17] Zhang P. Influence of foods and nutrition on the gut microbiome and implications for intestinal health. Int J Mol Sci 2022; 23(17): 9588.
[http://dx.doi.org/10.3390/ijms23179588] [PMID: 36076980]

[18] Cronin P, Joyce SA, O'Toole PW, O'Connor EM. Dietary fibre modulates the gut microbiota. Nutrients 2021; 13(5): 1655.
[http://dx.doi.org/10.3390/nu13051655] [PMID: 34068353]

[19] Galicia-Garcia U, Benito-Vicente A, Jebari S, *et al.* Pathophysiology of type 2 diabetes mellitus. Int J Mol Sci 2020; 21(17): 6275.
[http://dx.doi.org/10.3390/ijms21176275] [PMID: 32872570]

[20] Rahman S, O'Connor AL, Becker SL, Patel RK, Martindale RG, Tsikitis VL. Gut microbial metabolites and its impact on human health. Ann Gastroenterol 2023; 36(4): 360-8.
[http://dx.doi.org/10.20524/aog.2023.0809] [PMID: 37396009]

[21] Chambers ES, Byrne CS, Morrison DJ, *et al.* Dietary supplementation with inulin-propionate ester or inulin improves insulin sensitivity in adults with overweight and obesity with distinct effects on the gut microbiota, plasma metabolome and systemic inflammatory responses: a randomised cross-over trial. Gut 2019; 68(8): 1430-8.
[http://dx.doi.org/10.1136/gutjnl-2019-318424] [PMID: 30971437]

[22] De Vadder F, Kovatcheva-Datchary P, Goncalves D, *et al.* Microbiota-generated metabolites promote metabolic benefits *via* gut-brain neural circuits. Cell 2014; 156(1-2): 84-96.
[http://dx.doi.org/10.1016/j.cell.2013.12.016] [PMID: 24412651]

[23] Chambers ES, Viardot A, Psichas A, *et al.* Effects of targeted delivery of propionate to the human colon on appetite regulation, body weight maintenance and adiposity in overweight adults. Gut 2015; 64(11): 1744-54.
[http://dx.doi.org/10.1136/gutjnl-2014-307913] [PMID: 25500202]

[24] Vital M, Howe AC, Tiedje JM. Revealing the bacterial butyrate synthesis pathways by analyzing (meta)genomic data. MBio 2014; 5(2): e00889-14.
[http://dx.doi.org/10.1128/mBio.00889-14] [PMID: 24757212]

[25] Yip W, Hughes MR, Li Y, *et al.* Butyrate shapes immune cell fate and function in allergic asthma. Front Immunol 2021; 12: 628453.
[http://dx.doi.org/10.3389/fimmu.2021.628453] [PMID: 33659009]

[26] Li Q, Cao L, Tian Y, *et al.* Butyrate suppresses the proliferation of colorectal cancer cells *via* targeting pyruvate kinase M2 and metabolic reprogramming. Mol Cell Proteomics 2018; 17(8): 1531-45.
[http://dx.doi.org/10.1074/mcp.RA118.000752] [PMID: 29739823]

[27] Byndloss MX, Olsan EE, Rivera-Chávez F, *et al.* Microbiota-activated PPAR-γ signaling inhibits dysbiotic Enterobacteriaceae expansion. Science 2017; 357(6351): 570-5.
[http://dx.doi.org/10.1126/science.aam9949] [PMID: 28798125]

[28] Toni T, Alverdy J, Gershuni V. Re-examining chemically defined liquid diets through the lens of the microbiome. Nat Rev Gastroenterol Hepatol 2021; 18(12): 903-11.
[http://dx.doi.org/10.1038/s41575-021-00519-0] [PMID: 34594028]

[29] Chen J, Vitetta L. The role of butyrate in attenuating pathobiont-induced hyperinflammation. Immune Netw 2020; 20(2): e15.
[http://dx.doi.org/10.4110/in.2020.20.e15] [PMID: 32395367]

[30] Chen J, Vitetta L. The role of butyrate in attenuating pathobiont-induced hyperinflammation. Immune Netw 2020; 20(2): e15.
[http://dx.doi.org/10.4110/in.2020.20.e15] [PMID: 32395367]

[31] Tang WHW, Wang Z, Levison BS, *et al.* Intestinal microbial metabolism of phosphatidylcholine and cardiovascular risk. N Engl J Med 2013; 368(17): 1575-84.
[http://dx.doi.org/10.1056/NEJMoa1109400] [PMID: 23614584]

[32] Ding Y, Ting JP, Liu J, Al-Azzam S, Pandya P, Afshar S. Impact of non-proteinogenic amino acids in the discovery and development of peptide therapeutics. Amino Acids 2020; 52(9): 1207-26.
[http://dx.doi.org/10.1007/s00726-020-02890-9] [PMID: 32945974]

[33] Rothhammer V, Quintana FJ. The aryl hydrocarbon receptor: an environmental sensor integrating immune responses in health and disease. Nat Rev Immunol 2019; 19(3): 184-97.
[http://dx.doi.org/10.1038/s41577-019-0125-8] [PMID: 30718831]

[34] Qin HL, Liu J, Fang WY, Ravindar L, Rakesh KP. Indole-based derivatives as potential antibacterial activity against methicillin-resistance Staphylococcus aureus (MRSA). Eur J Med Chem 2020; 194: 112245.
[http://dx.doi.org/10.1016/j.ejmech.2020.112245] [PMID: 32220687]

[35] Chambers ES, Byrne CS, Morrison DJ, *et al.* Dietary supplementation with inulin-propionate ester or inulin improves insulin sensitivity in adults with overweight and obesity with distinct effects on the gut microbiota, plasma metabolome and systemic inflammatory responses: a randomised cross-over trial. Gut 2019; 68(8): 1430-8.
[http://dx.doi.org/10.1136/gutjnl-2019-318424] [PMID: 30971437]

[36] Winston JA, Theriot CM. Diversification of host bile acids by members of the gut microbiota. Gut Microbes 2020; 11(2): 158-71.
[http://dx.doi.org/10.1080/19490976.2019.1674124] [PMID: 31595814]

[37] Hossain KS, Amarasena S, Mayengbam S. B vitamins and their roles in gut health. Microorganisms 2022; 10(6): 1168.
[http://dx.doi.org/10.3390/microorganisms10061168] [PMID: 35744686]

[38] Poland JC, Flynn CR. Bile acids, their receptors, and the gut microbiota. Physiology (Bethesda) 2021; 36(4): 235-45.
[http://dx.doi.org/10.1152/physiol.00028.2020] [PMID: 34159805]

[39] Chang YL, Rossetti M, Vlamakis H, *et al.* A screen of Crohn's disease-associated microbial metabolites identifies ascorbate as a novel metabolic inhibitor of activated human T cells. Mucosal Immunol 2019; 12(2): 457-67.
[http://dx.doi.org/10.1038/s41385-018-0022-7] [PMID: 29695840]

[40] Pham VT, Fehlbaum S, Seifert N, *et al.* Effects of colon-targeted vitamins on the composition and metabolic activity of the human gut microbiome– a pilot study. Gut Microbes 2021; 13(1): 1875774.
[http://dx.doi.org/10.1080/19490976.2021.1875774] [PMID: 33615992]

[41] Pham VT, Dold S, Rehman A, Bird JK, Steinert RE. Vitamins, the gut microbiome and gastrointestinal health in humans. Nutr Res 2021; 95: 35-53.
[http://dx.doi.org/10.1016/j.nutres.2021.09.001] [PMID: 34798467]

[42] Schluter J, Peled JU, Taylor BP, *et al.* The gut microbiota is associated with immune cell dynamics in humans. Nature 2020; 588(7837): 303-7.

[http://dx.doi.org/10.1038/s41586-020-2971-8] [PMID: 33239790]

[43] Gwak MG, Chang SY. Gut-brain connection: microbiome, gut barrier, and environmental sensors. Immune Netw 2021; 21(3): e20.
[http://dx.doi.org/10.4110/in.2021.21.e20] [PMID: 34277110]

[44] Feng W, Liu J, Ao H, Yue S, Peng C. Targeting gut microbiota for precision medicine: Focusing on the efficacy and toxicity of drugs. Theranostics 2020; 10(24): 11278-301.
[http://dx.doi.org/10.7150/thno.47289] [PMID: 33042283]

[45] Selmer T, Andrei PI. p-*Hydroxyphenylacetate decarboxylase from* Clostridium difficile. Eur J Biochem 2001; 268(5): 1363-72.
[http://dx.doi.org/10.1046/j.1432-1327.2001.02001.x] [PMID: 11231288]

[46] Bone E, Tamm A, Hill M. The production of urinary phenols by gut bacteria and their possible ce:role in the causation of large bowel cancer. Am J Clin Nutr 1976; 29(12): 1448-54.
[http://dx.doi.org/10.1093/ajcn/29.12.1448] [PMID: 826152]

[47] Hodgman MJ, Garrard AR. A review of acetaminophen poisoning. Crit Care Clin 2012; 28(4): 499-516.
[http://dx.doi.org/10.1016/j.ccc.2012.07.006] [PMID: 22998987]

[48] Valdes AM, Walter J, Segal E, Spector TD. Role of the gut microbiota in nutrition and health. BMJ 2018; 361: k2179.
[http://dx.doi.org/10.1136/bmj.k2179] [PMID: 29899036]

[49] Saeid Seyedian S, Nokhostin F, Dargahi Malamir M. A review of the diagnosis, prevention, and treatment methods of inflammatory bowel disease. J Med Life 2019; 12(2): 113-22.
[http://dx.doi.org/10.25122/jml-2018-0075] [PMID: 31406511]

[50] Zhang YZ, Li YY. Inflammatory bowel disease: Pathogenesis. World J Gastroenterol 2014; 20(1): 91-9.
[http://dx.doi.org/10.3748/wjg.v20.i1.91] [PMID: 24415861]

[51] Romieu I, Dossus L, Barquera S, Blottiere HM, Franks PW, Gunter M, Hwalla N, Hursting SD, Leitzmann M, Margetts B, Nishida C. IARC working group on Energy Balance and Obesity (2017). Energy balance and obesity: what are the main drivers: 247-58.

[52] Wu J, Wang K, Wang X, Pang Y, Jiang C. The role of the gut microbiome and its metabolites in metabolic diseases. Protein Cell 2021; 12(5): 360-73.
[http://dx.doi.org/10.1007/s13238-020-00814-7] [PMID: 33346905]

[53] Sanmamed MF, Chen L. A paradigm shift in cancer immunotherapy: from enhancement to normalization. Cell 2018; 175(2): 313-26.
[http://dx.doi.org/10.1016/j.cell.2018.09.035] [PMID: 30290139]

[54] Shim JA, Ryu JH, Jo Y, Hong C. The role of gut microbiota in T cell immunity and immune mediated disorders. Int J Biol Sci 2023; 19(4): 1178-91.
[http://dx.doi.org/10.7150/ijbs.79430] [PMID: 36923929]

[55] Bodaghi A, Fattahi N, Ramazani A. Biomarkers: Promising and valuable tools towards diagnosis, prognosis and treatment of Covid-19 and other diseases. Heliyon 2023; 9(2): e13323.
[http://dx.doi.org/10.1016/j.heliyon.2023.e13323] [PMID: 36744065]

[56] Kaplan JM, Wong HR. Biomarker discovery and development in pediatric critical care medicine. Pediatr Crit Care Med 2011; 12(2): 165-73.
[http://dx.doi.org/10.1097/PCC.0b013e3181e28876] [PMID: 20473243]

[57] Cao Z, Jia Y, Zhu B. BNP and NT-proBNP as diagnostic biomarkers for cardiac dysfunction in both clinical and forensic medicine. Int J Mol Sci 2019; 20(8): 1820.
[http://dx.doi.org/10.3390/ijms20081820] [PMID: 31013779]

[58] Prvulovic D, Hampel H. Amyloid β (Aβ) and phospho-tau (p-tau) as diagnostic biomarkers in

Alzheimer's disease. cclm 2011; 49(3): 367-74.
[http://dx.doi.org/10.1515/CCLM.2011.087] [PMID: 21342022]

[59] Hanash SM, Baik CS, Kallioniemi O. Emerging molecular biomarkers—blood-based strategies to detect and monitor cancer. Nat Rev Clin Oncol 2011; 8(3): 142-50.
[http://dx.doi.org/10.1038/nrclinonc.2010.220] [PMID: 21364687]

[60] Henchcliffe C. Blood and cerebrospinal fluid markers in Parkinson's disease: current biomarker findings. Curr Biomark Find 2014; 1-1.
[http://dx.doi.org/10.2147/CBF.S50424]

[61] Misek DE, Kim EH. Protein biomarkers for the early detection of breast cancer. International journal of proteomics. 2011; 2011.
[http://dx.doi.org/10.1155/2011/343582]

[62] Taghdiri A. Cardiovascular biomarkers: exploring troponin and BNP applications in conditions related to carbon monoxide exposure. Egypt Heart J 2024; 76(1): 9.
[http://dx.doi.org/10.1186/s43044-024-00446-w] [PMID: 38282021]

[63] Ortiz-Martínez M, González-González M, Martagón AJ, Hlavinka V, Willson RC, Rito-Palomares M. Recent developments in biomarkers for diagnosis and screening of type 2 diabetes mellitus. Curr Diab Rep 2022; 22(3): 95-115.
[http://dx.doi.org/10.1007/s11892-022-01453-4] [PMID: 35267140]

[64] Jouanne M, Rault S, Voisin-Chiret AS. Tau protein aggregation in Alzheimer's disease: An attractive target for the development of novel therapeutic agents. Eur J Med Chem 2017; 139: 153-67.
[http://dx.doi.org/10.1016/j.ejmech.2017.07.070] [PMID: 28800454]

[65] Surguchov A. Biomarkers in Parkinson's disease. Neurodegenerative diseases biomarkers: Towards translating research to clinical practice. 2022: 155-80.
[http://dx.doi.org/10.1007/978-1-0716-1712-0_7]

[66] Yousefpouran S, Mostafaei S, Manesh PV, *et al.* The assessment of selected MiRNAs profile in HIV, HBV, HCV, HIV/HCV, HIV/HBV Co-infection and elite controllers for determination of biomarker. Microb Pathog 2020; 147: 104355.
[http://dx.doi.org/10.1016/j.micpath.2020.104355] [PMID: 32569788]

[67] Yousefpouran S, Mostafaei S, Manesh PV, *et al.* The assessment of selected MiRNAs profile in HIV, HBV, HCV, HIV/HCV, HIV/HBV Co-infection and elite controllers for determination of biomarker. Microb Pathog 2020; 147: 104355.
[http://dx.doi.org/10.1016/j.micpath.2020.104355] [PMID: 32569788]

[68] Lyons TJ, Basu A. Biomarkers in diabetes: hemoglobin A1c, vascular and tissue markers. Transl Res 2012; 159(4): 303-12.
[http://dx.doi.org/10.1016/j.trsl.2012.01.009] [PMID: 22424433]

[69] Fenton KA, Pedersen HL. Advanced methods and novel biomarkers in autoimmune diseases - a review of the recent years progress in systemic lupus erythematosus. Front Med (Lausanne) 2023; 10: 1183535.
[http://dx.doi.org/10.3389/fmed.2023.1183535] [PMID: 37425332]

[70] Lopez-Giacoman S, Madero M. Biomarkers in chronic kidney disease, from kidney function to kidney damage. World J Nephrol 2015; 4(1): 57-73.
[http://dx.doi.org/10.5527/wjn.v4.i1.57] [PMID: 25664247]

[71] Gowda S, Desai PB, Hull VV, Math AA, Vernekar SN, Kulkarni SS. A review on laboratory liver function tests. Pan Afr Med J 2009; 3: 17.
[PMID: 21532726]

CHAPTER 10

Therapeutic Approaches Targeting Gut Microbial Metabolites

Priyakshi Chutia[1], **Sabir Hussain**[1] and **Sailendra Kumar Mahanta**[1,*]

[1] *Department of Pharmacology, School of Pharmacy, The Assam Kaziranga University, Jorhat-785006, Assam, India*

Abstract: In recent years, there has been a lot of interest in studying gut microbial metabolites and their potential medicinal applications. This chapter gives a detailed review of therapeutic techniques that target gut microbial metabolites, including their role in health and illness, research methodologies, clinical applications, obstacles, and future directions. We begin with an overview of gut microbial metabolites, emphasizing their many roles and relevance in sustaining host physiology. We then investigate the complex link between gut microbiota and metabolism, explaining the processes by which microbial metabolites affect human health. The taxonomy of gut microbial metabolites, such as short-chain fatty acids, amino acid derivatives, bile acids, biogenic amines, and others, is thoroughly investigated, focusing on their functions and therapeutic possibilities.

To give insights into the instruments used in this discipline, methods for researching gut microbial metabolites are presented, including analytical techniques, metabolomics approaches, and microbiota profiling. The therapeutic potential of gut microbial metabolites is investigated, including targeting metabolites for disease management, modifying gut microbiota composition, and individualized treatments suited to particular patients. Clinical applications and case studies emphasize the importance of gut microbial metabolites in gastrointestinal problems, metabolic diseases, and neurological and immune system issues.

Challenges and future objectives in the area are discussed, highlighting the need to understand the complexities of gut microbial metabolite interactions, develop targeted therapeutics, and realize the translational potential of research discoveries. To summarize, pharmaceutical techniques targeting gut microbial metabolites provide intriguing options for enhancing human health and combating illness.

Keywords: Clinical applications, Gut microbial metabolites, Gut microbiota, Metabolomics, Personalized medicine, Short-chain fatty acids, Therapeutic approaches.

[*] **Corresponding author Sailendra Kumar Mahanta:** Department of Pharmacology, School of Pharmacy, The Assam Kaziranga University, Jorhat-785006, Assam, India; E-mails: sailendra04@gmail.com, sailendrakumar@kzu.ac.in

Sandipan Dasgupta & Moitreyee Chattopadhyay (Eds.)

INTRODUCTION TO GUT MICROBIAL METABOLITES

Gut microbial metabolites are critical in maintaining the delicate balance of the gut microbiome and impacting different physiological processes within the host. These metabolites, generated by the varied microbial community that lives in the gastrointestinal system, include a wide range of substances such as short-chain fatty acids (SCFAs), bile acids, trimethylamine N-oxide (TMAO), and neurotransmitters. SCFAs, notably acetate, propionate, and butyrate, are essential energy sources for colonic epithelial cells and have anti-inflammatory properties, which contribute to gut health. Bile acids, which are predominantly generated in the liver and then changed by gut bacteria, are essential for lipid metabolism and cholesterol balance. Furthermore, growing research demonstrates the importance of gut microbial metabolites in systemic health, including their role in metabolic disorders, immunological modulation, and even brain function. Understanding the complicated interplay between gut microbial populations and their metabolites has enormous therapeutic potential for treating a variety of health issues by targeted therapies that modulate these metabolites [1].

OVERVIEW OF GUT MICROBIOTA AND METABOLISM

The human gut microbiota, a complex ecology of billions of bacteria that live in the gastrointestinal tract, is critical for controlling host metabolism. Recent research has shown the complicated interplay between gut bacteria and many metabolic systems, providing light on their significant effect on human health and illness. Gut microorganisms create a wide range of metabolites from dietary components, including short-chain fatty acids (SCFAs), bile acids, and amino acid derivatives, all of which have different impacts on host physiology. These microbial metabolites act as signaling molecules, regulating immunological responses, energy metabolism, and neurobehavioral processes. Furthermore, the makeup and activity of the gut microbiota are regulated by a variety of factors, including nutrition, antibiotics, and host genetics, demonstrating the symbiotic relationship's dynamic character [2].

ROLE OF GUT MICROBIAL METABOLITES IN HEALTH AND DISEASES

The scientific community has given the function of gut microbial metabolites in health and illness a great deal of attention lately. Through complex metabolic interactions, the billions of bacteria that make up the human gut microbiota are essential to the preservation of host homeostasis. There is growing evidence that the microbial metabolites that are generated when food ingredients ferment play a major role in host physiology. Protonate, butyrate, and acetate are a few examples of short-chain fatty acids (SCFAs) that are produced by gut bacteria. The effects of these SCFAs on immunological response, intestinal barrier integrity, and host metabolism are varied. For example, butyrate has anti-inflammatory qualities and is an essential energy source for colonic epithelial cells, which helps to prevent inflammatory bowel disorders (IBD). Furthermore, some physiological processes, including lipid metabolism, immunological regulation, and neuronal function, have been linked to additional microbial metabolites, such as bile acids, derivatives of amino acids, and polyphenol metabolites.

Microbial metabolites resulting in various diseases are shown in Fig. (**1**).

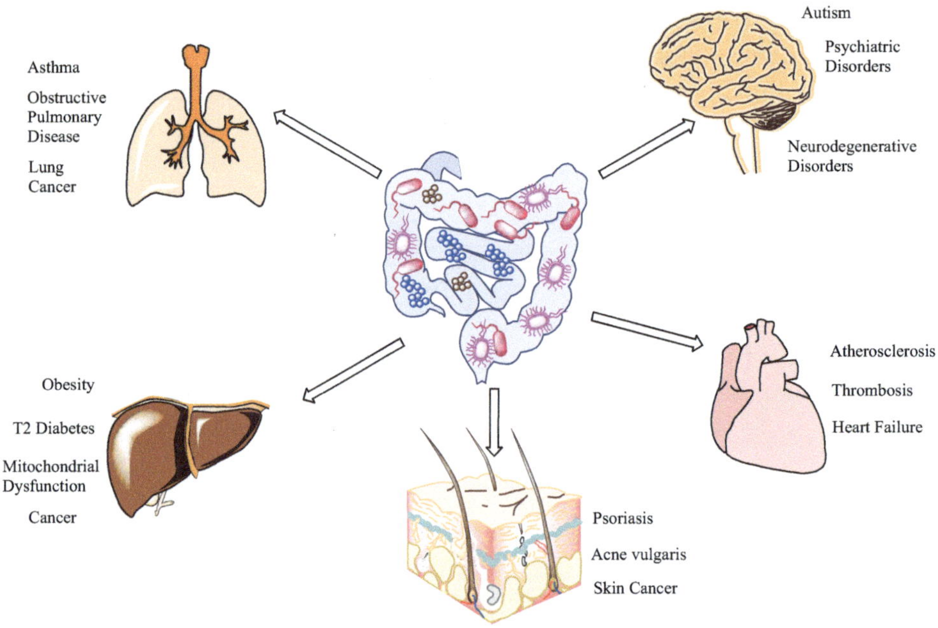

Fig. (1). Microbial metabolites and their association with various diseases.

Novel treatment approaches that target gut microbial metabolites have been made possible by recent research that has clarified the complex relationship between these metabolites and human health. The use of probiotics, prebiotics, or dietary modifications to alter the makeup of the gut microbiota has become a viable strategy for modifying microbial metabolite profiles and improving disease conditions. For example, it has been demonstrated that giving certain probiotic strains to people with IBD increases SCFA synthesis and improves gut barrier function. Additionally, dietary treatments high in fermentable fibers encourage gut bacteria to produce SCFAs, which protect against metabolic diseases including type 2 diabetes and obesity. Moreover, novel approaches to the therapeutic modification of gut microbiota metabolites are presented by developments in targeted drug delivery systems. The delivery of metabolite precursors or the modulation of microbial enzyme activity using nanoformulations presents enormous therapeutic promise for gastrointestinal diseases and metabolic syndrome. When taken as a whole, explaining the function of gut microbial metabolites in health and illness advances our knowledge of host-microbiota interactions and provides new treatment approaches to address a wide range of human conditions [3 - 5].

TYPES OF GUT MICROBIAL METABOLITES

Short-Chain Fatty Acids (SCFAs)

Gut microbial metabolites have a significant impact on human health, and short-chain fatty acids (SCFAs) are particularly important. SCFAs are organic fatty acids with less than six carbon atoms, notably acetate, propionate, and butyrate, that gut microbes create by fermenting food fibers and other undigested carbohydrates. These metabolites have received a lot of interest because of their many physiological effects on the host. For starters, SCFAs provide energy to colonocytes, which helps to maintain the gut epithelium's integrity and function. Butyrate, in particular, is important for colonic health because it promotes epithelial cell proliferation and differentiation while simultaneously having anti-inflammatory properties. Furthermore, SCFAs influence the immune system by increasing the production of regulatory T cells and decreasing the production of pro-inflammatory cytokines. Furthermore, these metabolites control hunger and metabolism by affecting the release of gut hormones such as glucagon-like peptide 1 (GLP-1) and peptide YY (PYY), which affects satiety and energy balance. Furthermore, SCFAs have been linked to metabolic balance, with studies indicating that they may have a role in the prevention of obesity, insulin resistance, and other metabolic diseases. The complex interaction between gut microbiota and host physiology, mediated by SCFAs, emphasizes the necessity of understanding these microbial metabolites in the context of human health and illness [6 - 8].

Amino Acid Derivatives

Amino acid-derived bacterial metabolites are substances that bacteria in the gut make by breaking down amino acids, which are the building blocks of proteins. These metabolites have a variety of roles in the gut, including microbial communication, metabolism, physiology, and growth. When bacteria degrade amino acids, they produce a variety of metabolites with different activities. Some of these metabolites function as signaling molecules, allowing bacteria to interact with one another and coordinate their actions. Others act as energy sources for bacteria or impact their development and spread. Importantly, amino acid-derived metabolites can influence the host's physiology. For example, certain metabolites can interact with gut lining receptors, influencing nutrition absorption or immunological activity. Furthermore, some metabolites may have systemic effects when they enter the circulation, possibly affecting distant organs and systems in the body. Understanding the functions of these metabolites is critical for deciphering the intricate connections between gut bacteria and their hosts. It also has the potential to lead to the development of novel medicines to boost gut health and cure various disorders [9, 10].

Bile Acids

Bile acids, which were previously recognized for their involvement in lipid absorption, have emerged as important modulators of gut microbiota composition and function. Research has progressively emphasized their varied impact on microbial populations in the gastrointestinal system. These metabolites, which are generated from cholesterol in the liver, go through substantial biotransformation by gut bacteria, so changing the microbiome. Studies [11] reveal the complicated interplay between bile acids and gut flora, emphasizing their mutualistic relationship. The presence of bile acids regulates not only microbial abundance but also the variety and metabolic activity of gut microorganisms, as demonstrated by [12]. Furthermore, bile acids function as signaling molecules, directing a variety of physiological processes critical to host health. Bile acids have a significant impact on digestive health *via* the processes described in [11]and [12], such as the control of gastrointestinal motility, immunological responses, and energy metabolism. Furthermore, gut microbial bile acid regulation has important implications for understanding and treating digestive disorders. Dysregulation of bile acid metabolism, which is frequently associated with changes in gut microbiota composition, has been related to inflammatory bowel disease (IBD), obesity, and colorectal cancer. A study [12] gives insight into the complex processes that underpin these relationships, indicating prospective therapeutic targets for bile acid-microbiota interactions in disease management. Furthermore, the findings from a study [11] highlight the bidirectional nature of bile acid-microbiota interaction, providing fresh techniques for restoring microbial equilibrium and enhancing gastrointestinal health. Bile acids are essential components of the gut microbial metabolome, with significant implications on microbial ecology, host physiology, and disease pathogenesis. Studies highlight the complex interaction between bile acids and gut microbiota, opening up new possibilities for therapeutic approaches targeted at exploiting the therapeutic potential of bile acid regulation in digestive health and illness [13].

Bio-genic Amines

Biogenic amines are a type of organic molecules generated by microbial metabolism. These molecules are formed from amino acids and can be found in a variety of foods and beverages. Biogenic amines can have both positive and negative impacts on human health. Biogenic amines are frequently created in food by the action of specific bacteria, yeast, and molds during the fermentation and spoiling processes. Common biogenic amines include histamine, tyramine, putrescine, and cadaverine. While low levels of biogenic amines are normally safe, large levels can produce headaches, nausea, and hypertension, particularly in people with limited tolerance or poor health. Histamine, for example, is linked to allergic reactions and is commonly found in fermented foods such as aged cheese, wine, and sauerkraut [14, 15]. Tyramine, which can cause migraines in sensitive people, is found in foods such as aged cheese, cured meats, and certain fermented items. However, biogenic amines have a crucial role in physiological processes such as neurotransmission, blood pressure regulation, and immunological responses. Understanding the formation and impact of biogenic amines is critical for food safety and avoiding potential health concerns from their ingestion [16, 17].

Other Metabolites

Microcins and TOMMs

Microcins are tiny antimicrobial peptides generated by some Gram-negative bacteria. They have a narrow-spectrum action against closely related bacterial species and are distinguished by distinct posttranslational alterations. One example is microcin B17, which converts cysteine and serine residues into thiazoles and oxazoles. Adenosine monophosphate is added to microcin C7, but microcin E492 has a siderophore linked to the C terminus. Microcin J25 displays internal amide cross-linking, resulting in a lasso-like structure. These changes improve the stability and antibacterial activity of microcins. Microcins play an important role in microbial competitiveness in complex ecosystems such as the human microbiome. Similar to lantibiotics in Gram-positive bacteria, microcins help to shape the makeup and dynamics of the microbial community. They are used as weapons to contend with closely similar bacterial strains for resources and niche colonization [18]. The study of microcins has sparked attention because of their potential as new antibacterial agents. Researchers hope to create novel treatment techniques for antibiotic-resistant bacteria by taking advantage of their narrow-spectrum activity and distinct mechanisms of action. Understanding the biosynthesis and mechanisms of action of microcins has led to the investigation of Tailored-Overproducing Microcins (TOMMs), a type of tailored microcin with improved antibacterial characteristics. TOMMs show potential as future alternatives to standard antibiotics, providing new routes for tackling infectious illnesses while reducing the possibility of resistance [19].

Ribosomally Synthesized, Posttranslationally Modified Peptides (RiPPs)

A ribosomally synthesized and post-translationally modified peptide (RiPP) is an intriguing class of natural products with various structures and bioactivities. RiPPs are distinguished by a distinct biosynthetic process that includes ribosomal synthesis followed by significant post-translational modifications. This procedure produces peptides with complex structures and functions that are difficult to achieve using typical synthetic methods. The analysis of RiPPs, focuses on structural diversity, biosynthetic processes, and bioactivities. RiPPs have received a lot of interest due to their potential as lead molecules in drug discovery and development. Researchers discovered and described a new RiPP with a β-amino acid and macrocyclic motif. This discovery highlights the ongoing research into RiPPs as a source of structurally varied and physiologically active chemicals. Overall, RiPPs are a diverse and exciting field of natural product chemistry study, having implications for both fundamental science and drug development [20a, 20b].

METHOD FOR STUDYING GUT MICROBIAL METABOLITES

Analytical Techniques

GC-MS

Sample Preparation

Serum

The serum volume utilized ranges from 40 to 200 µL. After diluting the serum with water, protein precipitation is frequently performed using either an organic solvent (*e.g.*, methanol (MeOH)) or an acidified solution (*e.g.*, H_2SO_4). Protein precipitation is a sample pretreatment method that removes proteins while preserving the metabolites of interest. This technique reduces interference from undesirable species while also extending the life of the column and mass detector. Protein precipitation, on the other hand, might reduce the repeatability or accuracy of analytical procedures if the metabolites of interest have a strong affinity for proteins. Following protein precipitation, simple extraction with MeOH or diethyl ether (DE) *via* liquid-liquid extraction or centrifugation is commonly advised. However, Pautova *et al.* used microextraction by packed sorbent (MEPS) to extract indolic acids, which are Trp gut microbial metabolites, from blood and cerebral fluid without protein precipitation. MEPS is a solid-phase extraction (SPE) technique for extracting and purifying tiny volumes of material. Unlike SPE columns, MEPS may be reused and completely automated before being analyzed using GC-MS or liquid chromatography (LC)-MS. This approach mitigates the serum matrix influence on indolic acid analysis. However, it adds extra stages to the conditions, such as washing and drying of the MEPS column, which requires further research and validation [21].

Faeces

Due to the variety of fecal samples, the sample pretreatment process is critical, and the volume of the sample must be regulated to minimize column overload and detector saturation. Zhao *et al.* used NaOH solution to homogenize 10 mg of freeze-dried human fecal samples before centrifugation. After collecting the supernatant, the sample was re-extracted with cold MeOH, and the two extracts were mixed in a series of tests to determine the optimal amount of rat feces and extraction solvent combinations. A multivariate study of fecal metabolite profiles revealed that a larger proportion of MeOH in the MeOH/chloroform extraction combination was better for gut microbial AAA metabolites, but a lower amount of MeOH was better for tricarboxylic cycle metabolites. Unfortunately, a mixture of MeOH, chloroform, and water (225:75:300, v/v/v) was used in their investigation since it is acceptable for a wide variety of metabolites; unfortunately, this may decrease the sensitivity of this approach [21].

Bacterial Cultures

Following untargeted or metabolite profiling research, significant AAA metabolites discovered in human samples can be validated using bacterial cultures to determine their roles in metabolic pathways. To accurately detect intracellular metabolites from bacteria or other organisms, samples must be quenched to minimize metabolite turnover and leakage. The most common quenching strategies for bacterial metabolomics include cold MeOH solution, cold glycerol-saline solution, and liquid nitrogen. The bulk of previous quenching techniques were designed for untargeted metabolomic analysis, rather than AAA metabolite analysis. However, a fast-quenching method that uses liquid nitrogen in combination with filter-based sampling has been shown to be useful for quantifying intracellular amino acids in bacteria. Zhao *et al.* quenched the bacterial cells by washing them in phosphate-buffered saline (PBS) before reconstituting them. Cell lysates were homogenized with water before being extracted with cold MeOH by centrifugation. Although this high-throughput GC-MS-based method detected AAA metabolites in blood, urine, and feces, no metabolites were discovered in the study's bacterial cells. Polar and nonvolatile metabolites, including AA, free fatty acids, and AAA microbiological metabolites, typically need chemical derivatization. LLOQ levels of metabolites were assessed in at least three studies. The SQ methodology outperformed the IT and TOF strategies. Overall, the GC-MS approaches had a dynamic range of one to two orders of magnitude, although, for some compounds, the TOF method exceeded three orders of magnitude (Table). Two-dimensional GC-MS (GC × GC-MS) improves peak capacity, metabolite detection rates, and identification accuracy. However, compared to standard GC-MS, it has not been widely used to assess AAA metabolites [22].

Metabolomics Approaches

Metabolomic approaches primarily entail the identification and measurement of metabolites, which provide information on metabolic pathways and their regulation. The two main analytical platforms utilized in metabolomics are nuclear magnetic resonance (NMR) spectroscopy and mass spectrometry (MS). NMR spectroscopy provides non-destructive, high-throughput analysis, allowing for the identification and measurement of metabolites in complicated mixtures. MS methods, such as Liquid Chromatography-Mass Spectrometry (LC-MS) and Gas Chromatography-Mass Spectrometry (GC-MS), have great sensitivity and selectivity, allowing for the identification of a large variety of metabolites. Metabolomic techniques may be used to study host-gut microbiota interactions by evaluating metabolic patterns in biological materials such as feces, urine, and blood. Researchers can discover metabolites related to certain physiological processes or microbiological activity by comparing metabolite profiles from healthy and sick states, as well as between experimental situations. Furthermore, metabolomic investigations allow for the explanation of metabolic pathways influenced by changes in gut microbiota composition or function. Overall, metabolomic methods contribute significantly to our understanding of host-gut microbiota interactions, providing vital insights into the intricate interplay between the host and its associated microbial populations. These approaches show significant potential for the discovery of biomarkers, therapeutic targets, and therapies that modulate the gut microbiota to improve health and disease prevention [22].

Microbiota Profiling

Microbial community profiling with 16S rRNA is seeing a revival as high-throughput methods such as barcoded pyrosequencing enable us to acquire comprehensive insights into hundreds of microbial communities at once. These investigations are made feasible by the extraordinary discovery that a short portion of the 16S rRNA gene may be used as a proxy for the full-length sequence in various community analyses, including those based on a phylogeny. Although the phylogenetic trees produced from 250-base reads from the current 454 Life Sciences (Roche) GS FLX instrument are relatively inaccurate, they are still vastly better than the so-called "star phylogeny," the phylogeny that assumes all species are equally related, that all nonphylogenetic methods for comparing communities implicitly use (Hamady & Knight, 2009). The microbiota profile of low-biomass materials, such as skin, presents a challenge for metagenomics. These samples are prone to DNA contamination from the host or external sources, which can override the DNA of interest. Thus, rather than undertaking metagenomics, the standard technique is to amplify and sequence particular genetic markers that are widespread in the investigated kingdom. Ribosomal marker genes are often used to characterize bacteria: 16S rRNA and 23S rRNA genes, and ITS1 and ITS2 sections for fungi [23]. The gut microbiota influences signaling pathways involved in intestinal mucosal homeostasis *via* metabolite production/fermentation. When a balanced relationship between the gastrointestinal (GI) tract and the resident microbiota is disturbed, intestinal and extraintestinal gut Microbiota Metabolome illnesses include allergies, inflammatory bowel disease (IBD), obesity, cancer and diabetes, metabolic disorders, cardiovascular dyslipidemia, and neuropathology. The emergence of the omics-based systems biology era has created a new paradigm for understanding the gut ecosystem by providing light on its form, regulation, and interaction with bacteria, food functioning, and the role of nutrients in health [24].

THERAPEUTIC IMPLICATIONS OF GUT MICROBIAL METABOLITES

The emerging field of study into the therapeutic implications of gut microbial metabolites has the potential to revolutionize our knowledge and treatment of a wide range of health issues. Recent research has shed light on the complex interplay between gut microbiota and host physiology, emphasizing the critical role of microbial metabolites in influencing immune function, neurotransmission, and metabolism. For example, short-chain fatty acids (SCFAs) such as acetate, propionate, and butyrate, which are formed by microbial fermentation of dietary fibers, have emerged as important mediators of gut-brain communication and inflammatory control. Furthermore, secondary bile acids, which are produced by microbial metabolism of primary bile acids, have a variety of impacts on host metabolism and may play an important role in the prevention of metabolic diseases such as obesity and type 2 diabetes [25]. Over the last five years, researchers have found convincing evidence for the therapeutic potential of targeting gut microbial metabolites in the treatment of a variety of health disorders [26]. The immunomodulatory benefits of SCFAs in treating inflammatory bowel disorders (IBD) were investigated by increasing regulatory T cell development and reducing pro-inflammatory cytokine production. Furthermore, researchers demonstrated the importance of bile acid metabolism in controlling glucose homeostasis and insulin sensitivity, implying innovative treatment methods for metabolic diseases. These new advances highlight the significance of understanding the intricate interplay between gut microbiota and host health, paving the path for novel therapeutic approaches that target microbial metabolites [27].

Targeting Metabolites for Disease Management

The gut microbiota is important for human health maintenance and has a role in the pathophysiology of many disorders. The possible therapeutic implications of targeting microbial metabolites for illness management offered thorough insights into the complex interaction between the microbiota and human health. The fermentation of food components by the gut microbiota results in the production of many metabolites, such as trimethylamine N-oxide (TMAO), bile acids, and short-chain fatty acids (SCFAs). These metabolites influence host physiology in a variety of ways, including immune response control, energy metabolism modification, and intestinal barrier maintenance. A potential strategy for the treatment of many illnesses is to target certain bacteria metabolites. For example, SCFAs have been studied for their anti-inflammatory effects and possible significance in the treatment of inflammatory bowel illnesses. Manipulating bile acid metabolism or manipulating the gut microbiota to increase the synthesis of beneficial bile acid metabolites shows promise in the treatment of metabolic illnesses such as obesity and type 2 diabetes. Furthermore, efforts to lower circulating TMAO levels may have therapeutic effects in the prevention and treatment of cardiovascular disorders. Overall, addressing gut microbial metabolites is a unique and promising path for illness treatment, with possible therapeutic approaches that use the microbiota's symbiotic interaction with host physiology [28].

Modulating Gut Microbiota Composition

The billions of bacteria that live in the gastrointestinal system, known as the gut microbiota, are essential to human health and affect many physiological functions. The complex association between the chemical composition of the gut microbiota and the onset of many illnesses, from gastrointestinal problems to systemic ailments like cancer and cardiovascular diseases, has been clarified by recent studies. Promoting health and delaying the onset of disease can be achieved by comprehending and modifying the makeup of the gut microbiota.

The relationship between intestinal immune response and colitis susceptibility and the modification of gut microbiota composition by serotonin signaling was examined. The neurotransmitter serotonin, which is well recognized for its function in mood regulation, has a notable impact on the gastrointestinal system. The results of the study showed that modifications to serotonin signaling pathways might influence the makeup of the gut microbiota, which in turn affects intestinal immune response and colitis susceptibility. This research emphasizes the complex interactions that occur between the nervous system and the gut microbiota and emphasizes how serotonin signaling may be targeted to modify the composition of the gut microbiota and reduce the risk of inflammatory bowel disorders [29].

The use of dietary treatments to modify the makeup of the gut microbiota as a prophylactic against cardiovascular illnesses. The study focused on how foods and herbs, among other dietary components, shape the variety and composition of gut microbiota. It has been discovered that specific dietary patterns high in fiber, polyphenols, and other bioactive chemicals decrease harmful bacteria linked to cardiovascular risk factors including inflammation and dyslipidemia while fostering the growth of advantageous microbial species. These results highlight the possibility of using dietary approaches to change the makeup of the gut microbiota and lower the risk of cardiovascular illnesses [30].

The function of gut microbiota manipulation as a potential approach to colorectal cancer prevention and therapy was examined by Fong *et al.* A growing body of research indicates that colorectal carcinogenesis may be related to dysbiosis of the gut microbiota, which is defined by changes in microbial diversity and composition. The study highlighted a number of methods, such as fecal microbiota transplantation, dietary modifications, probiotics, and prebiotics, for modifying the makeup of the gut microbiota. These therapies may help prevent and cure colorectal cancer by improving host immune responses, re-establishing the balance of gut microbes, and inhibiting carcinogenic processes in the colon [31].

Personalized Approaches

Utilizing individual variations in microbiome composition, metabolism, and host physiology, personalized approaches to the therapeutic implications of gut microbial metabolites aim to customize therapies for better gut health. Researchers mentioned the use of these strategies, which take into account each person's own microbiome profiles and metabolic activity in order to treat gut dysbiosis and enhance general health. Understanding the dynamic interaction between the gut microbiota and its host is essential to tailored therapies. The gut microbiome is made up of several microbial communities that interact with environmental variables, genetics, nutrition, and lifestyle of the host. The synthesis of bile acids, neurotransmitters, short-chain fatty acids (SCFAs), and other bioactive substances is influenced by these interactions. The colon produces SCFAs such as butyrate, propionate, and acetate by microbial fermentation of dietary fiber. They are essential for preserving the integrity of the intestinal barrier, controlling immunological reactions, and controlling the metabolism of energy. Dietary changes to encourage the growth of beneficial bacteria that can produce certain SCFAs unique to a person's microbiome makeup may be part of personalized therapies. Bile acids control immunological signaling, cholesterol metabolism, and fat absorption. They are produced in the liver and broken down by gut microbes. Inflammatory bowel disease (IBD) and colorectal cancer are two gastrointestinal conditions linked to dysregulation of bile acid metabolism. In order to ease gut dysbiosis and restore bile acid balance, personalized treatment techniques may target certain bile acid-metabolizing pathways or change the gut microbiota. Furthermore, the gut-brain axis allows neurotransmitters and neuropeptides produced by gut microorganisms to affect behavior, mood, and thought processes. Psychiatric conditions including anxiety and sadness have been related to imbalances in the synthesis of microbiological neurotransmitters. Probiotic supplements and dietary changes that target gut bacteria's synthesis of neurotransmitter precursors as a means of enhancing mental health outcomes are examples of personalized therapies. Personalized approaches to gut health may include microbiome-based diagnostics and therapies in addition to metabolite-targeted interventions. With the use of cutting-edge sequencing technology, it is possible to characterize each person's microbiome profile and identify the microbial signatures connected to various health or disease states. Then, depending on a person's unique needs, therapeutic treatments, such fecal microbiota transplantation (FMT) or precision probiotics, can be customized to restore microbial balance and support gut health.

Personalized approaches to the therapeutic implications of gut microbiota metabolites have the potential to significantly improve overall health outcomes by treating dysbiosis of the gut. Through the incorporation of insights into the unique composition, metabolism, and interactions between the host and microbiota, tailored therapies can enhance the effectiveness of therapy and advance customized medicine within the realm of gut health [32].

GUT MICROBIAL METABOLITES IN GASTROINTESTINAL DISORDERS

Metabolites produced by gut microbes are essential to the development and pathophysiology of a number of gastrointestinal diseases. Acetate, propionate, and butyrate are examples of short-chain fatty acids (SCFAs), which have been the subject of substantial research in the field of microbial metabolism. These SCFAs have the ability to reduce inflammation and support the integrity of the gut barrier, which may help improve diseases like inflammatory bowel disease (IBD). Colorectal cancer (CRC) and bile acid diarrhea (BAD) are two gastrointestinal disorders that have been linked to changes in bile acid metabolism brought on by dysbiosis [33]. Furthermore, the metabolite trimethylamine-N-oxide (TMAO), which is generated when dietary choline is metabolized by gut microbes, has been connected to the etiology of liver and cardiovascular diseases. Additionally, new data highlights the dual function of indole chemicals produced by gut bacteria, which, depending on their quantity and the particular microbial community involved, can have both positive and negative impacts on gastrointestinal health [34, 35].

Metabolites and Metabolic Diseases

Metabolites serve critical roles in biological functions, and abnormal amounts can contribute to a variety of metabolic disorders. Recent research has focused on understanding the complex interactions between metabolites and metabolic diseases, offering information on new diagnostic indicators and treatment targets. Researchers studied the involvement of amino acid metabolites in the etiology of type 2 diabetes mellitus. They discovered that those with T2DM had lower amounts of many amino acids, particularly branched-chain amino acids (BCAAs), compared to healthy controls. This implies a possible relationship between amino acid metabolism and insulin resistance, emphasizing the significance of tailored therapies in controlling T2DM [36]. The metabolic profiles related to non-alcoholic fatty liver disease (NAFLD). They used metabolomic analysis to identify particular lipid compounds that were highly dysregulated in NAFLD patients, suggesting new biomarkers for disease diagnosis and progression monitoring. Furthermore, their findings highlighted the intricate relationship between lipid metabolism and hepatic steatosis. Furthermore, another study conducted a meta-analysis to explore the relationship between gut microbiota-derived metabolites and obesity. They discovered substantial differences in several metabolites, such as short-chain fatty acids (SCFAs) and bile acids, between obese people and lean controls after analyzing extensive data. This emphasizes the importance of gut microbiota in modifying host metabolism and identifies microbial metabolites as possible targets for anti-obesity treatments [37, 38].

Neurological and Immune System Implications

In recent years, there has been a lot of discussion on the complex relationship between gut microbiota and host health, particularly the implications for brain and immune system function. Therapeutic therapies that target gut microbial metabolites have emerged as viable ways for regulating these complex processes and improving general health. One such technique is to modulate short-chain fatty acids (SCFAs), which are microbial metabolites that have a variety of impacts on human physiology. For example, butyrate, a kind of SCFA, has been found to have anti-inflammatory properties in the gut and elsewhere, potentially improving neuroinflammation and immunological dysregulation. Furthermore, certain dietary treatments, such as high-fiber meals or prebiotic supplementation, can selectively boost SCFA generation by gut bacteria, providing a non-invasive way to regulate host-microbiota interactions. In addition to SCFAs, additional gut microbial metabolites, including tryptophan metabolites and bile acids, have been linked to neuroimmune regulation. For example, some gut bacteria may convert tryptophan into neuroactive chemicals, altering neurotransmitter production and immune cell activity. Similarly, bile acids, which are best known for their role in lipid digestion, have recently been identified as signaling molecules that can regulate immunological responses and neuroinflammation by activating certain receptors. Harnessing the therapeutic potential of gut microbial metabolites is a promising approach to tackling neurological and immune system issues. By targeting these metabolites through dietary treatments, microbial manipulation, or direct supplementation, researchers hope to restore equilibrium to dysregulated host-microbiota interactions and alleviate related health issues [39].

CHALLENGES AND FUTURE DIRECTIONS

The goal of using microorganisms as therapy is to alter the metabolic, nutritional, and physiological pathways to promote host survival and restore dysbiosis [40]. Microbiota-based medicines are being developed more quickly as a result of developments in synthetic biology and our growing understanding of the ecology of host-associated microbial communities [41]. Along with the advantageousness; there are some significant challenges, which need future attention in the promotion of these microbial therapeutics are discussed below.

- The makeup of a microbial community can be changed by immigrant bacteria, antibiotics, illness, and food, as is widely recognized; nevertheless, a set of prediction guidelines explaining the effects of these perturbations has not yet been established.
- Selecting the appropriate microbial chassis for a therapy based on microbiota might be tricky since it is hard to say which microbe will work best in a certain situation. A therapeutic microbe may thus be unable to engraft in the endogenous microbiota or thrive in the intended habitat.
  Distinct cell-based therapeutic applications ought to necessitate distinct assembly organisms. Although some species favor the intestinal lumen, others choose to colonize the mucosal layer [42 - 44].

- Creation of Clinically Significant Sensors: To achieve completely autonomous microbial therapies, biosensors that can identify disease-related biomarkers must be developed. Recombinant bacteria, for instance, can identify biomarkers associated with intestinal inflammation (red diamonds) and facilitate the expression of therapeutic proteins (blue hexagons).
  For cell-based therapeutics, distinct applications should require distinct chassis organisms [42].
- To avoid the loss or malfunction of recombinant genetic material, engineered bacteria need to be resilient both phenotypically and evolutionarily.
- One major obstacle to the practical translation of basic research is the safety and biocontainment of microbiota-based therapeutics.
- Overlapping of metabolic and signaling functions of metabolites [45].
- A significant obstacle linked to the postbiotic methodology is the pleiotropic nature of metabolites [46].
- Research on microbiome therapy was mostly conducted on rodent models, and human trials will need further work. Effective microbiome treatments are dependent on the robustness and stability of the therapeutically relevant microbial strains [46].
- To ensure that clinical trials of microbiome therapies are successful, several safety and regulatory concerns must be investigated. The biosafety of therapies must be addressed by a regulatory framework to lessen side effects and the discharge of modified germs into the environment [40].
- A significant concern is the horizontal transmission of recombinant DNA from the modified microbiome to the natural microbiome [47].
- The discharge of recombinant probiotics into the environment may be detrimental [48].
- Due to the possibility that modified phases could cause them to lose the metabolite function, coordinated research, and regulatory mechanisms are therefore required for both therapeutic maintenance and a safe treatment strategy [49].
- In case of synthetic metabolites, the ability of current in vivo studies to directly anticipate the behaviour of synthetic microbial communities is likewise restricted. Consequently, a combination of artificial gut ecosystems and in vivo animal models should be used to investigate the interactions between intestinal microorganisms, other gut microbiota, and the host [40].

Significant attention towards these subjects is very essential in future research for the development of significantly safe and effective microorganism-based metabolite therapeutics.

Unraveling Complexity in Gut Microbial Metabolite Interactions

The researchers used modern analytical techniques and bioinformatic tools to disentangle the complex network of interactions between various microbial species that live in the gut. They revealed the cooperative and competitive connections between these bacteria through their thorough investigation, emphasizing their tremendous effect on the synthesis and metabolism of gut microbial compounds. The study found that microbial interactions are critical for maintaining gut homeostasis and supporting host health. Certain microbial consortia work together to ferment food substrates and create beneficial metabolites including short-chain fatty acids (SCFAs), which help with gut barrier integrity, immunological modulation, and energy metabolism. Furthermore, the researchers discovered complicated metabolic pathways organized by microbial communities, revealing their function in food utilization and xenobiotic metabolism in the gut environment. However, in addition to these beneficial connections, the study discovered instances of microbial fights in the gut ecosystem. Competition for resources and niche space among microbial taxa can result in dysbiosis and the spread of pathogenic species, which contribute to gut inflammation and disease development. Understanding the dynamics of these microbial fights is critical for determining the causes of a variety of gut-related illnesses, such as inflammatory bowel disease (IBD) and metabolic syndrome. Overall, the study's findings highlight the complexities of gut microbial metabolite interactions and their significant consequences for human health and illness. By uncovering the complexities of microbial partnerships and conflicts within the gut ecosystem, researchers might pave the path for tailored therapies that attempt to modulate gut microbiota composition and activity in order to promote optimum health outcomes [50].

Development of Targeted Therapies

The development of tailored treatment for the gut microbiota is a potential area in precision medicine, with the goal of improving therapeutic efficacy while reducing toxicity. Researchers stressed the importance of knowing the interactions between medications and gut bacteria in developing individualized treatment regimens. Therapeutic treatments can be designed to change the makeup and activity of the gut microbiota by targeting specific microbial communities, improving medication effectiveness, and decreasing side effects [51]. Gebrayel *et al.* (2022) emphasized the importance of microbial medicine in transforming clinical practice. Their comprehensive study highlighted the many ways being developed to modify the gut microbiota for medicinal objectives. Probiotics, prebiotics, postbiotics, and fecal microbiota transplantation (FMT) are among the treatments used to restore microbial balance and enhance patient outcomes.

Targeted therapeutics targeting the gut microbiota need a multidisciplinary approach that incorporates knowledge from microbiology, pharmacology, and systems biology. By understanding the processes underpinning drug-microbiota interactions, researchers can uncover new therapeutic targets and create precision therapies that specifically regulate microbial populations to achieve the desired clinical results. Furthermore, breakthroughs in omics technologies, such as metagenomics and metabolomics, offer useful tools for defining the gut microbiota and monitoring its responsiveness to treatments. These molecular insights enable the discovery of microbial biomarkers that predict medication response, allowing for better patient classification and tailored treatment regimens [32]. Overall, targeted treatment for the gut microbiota has great potential for increasing the effectiveness and safety of pharmaceutical therapies. By using the microbiota's therapeutic potential, doctors may usher in a new age of precision medicine that is personalized to each patient's specific microbial composition [51, 52].

Translational Potential and Implementation

In recent years, there has been an increasing interest in investigating the translational potential and practical use of medicinal treatments targeting gut microbial metabolites. The gut microbiota, which consists of a varied array of bacteria, is critical to human health and illness because it produces a number of compounds that can impact host physiology and immune function. Harnessing the therapeutic potential of these microbial metabolites holds promise for the development of new treatments for a variety of illnesses, including inflammatory bowel disease, metabolic disorders, and even neurological problems. Several recent investigations have given insight into the therapeutic potential of some gut bacteria metabolites.

Researchers investigate a fascinating frontier in cancer treatment: the possible therapeutic effect of gut microbial metabolites, specifically in lymphoma. The complex interplay between the gut microbiota and the immune system has long been recognized, and a new study shows that microbial metabolites might be used as innovative therapeutics. Researchers can unlock the translational potential of these metabolites in lymphoma treatment by better understanding the molecular processes by which they affect immune responses. Furthermore, the study emphasizes the necessity of customized therapy, since gut microbiota composition differs between individuals, demanding specific therapeutic measures to enhance results. Harnessing the therapeutic potential of gut microbial metabolites necessitates a multidimensional strategy that includes preclinical research, clinical trials, and implementation plans. Preclinical research on the mechanisms of action and efficacy of certain microbial metabolites paves the path for clinical trials to assess their safety and efficacy in lymphoma patients. Furthermore, strong translational frameworks are required for the successful integration of microbial metabolite-based therapeutics into clinical practice. This includes creating accurate biomarkers for patient stratification, improving drug delivery systems, and encouraging multidisciplinary partnerships among microbiologists, immunologists, oncologists, and bioinformaticians. Finally, fulfilling the therapeutic promise of gut microbial metabolites requires a concerted effort to bridge the gap between benchtop findings and bedside applications, providing fresh hope for improved cancer treatment results [53].

CONCLUSION

To summarize, the emerging area of therapeutic methods targeting gut microbial metabolites has great potential for transforming disease management and treatment tactics. Researchers have discovered a wide range of metabolites with potential therapeutic uses across several disease domains by unraveling the complicated interplay between the gut microbiota and human health. From immunomodulation to metabolic control and beyond, these microbial-derived metabolites provide new paths for intervention in illnesses ranging from metabolic disorders to inflammatory ailments and even cancer. Furthermore, the development of new delivery methods and tailored therapy modalities is critical to realizing the full therapeutic potential of these microbial metabolites while minimizing possible side effects. As our understanding of the gut-microbiome axis grows, so does the possibility of individualized medication based on specific microbial profiles, ushering in a new age of precision therapies. The translation of these results from bench to bedside, with continued research and collaboration, has the potential to change healthcare, providing fresh hope and improved outcomes for patients worldwide.

CONSENT FOR PUBLICATIONS

We, the undersigned authors, hereby provide our consent for the publication of the book chapter titled **"Therapeutic Approaches Targeting Gut Microbial Metabolites"**. We certify that we made a substantial contribution to the idea, planning, and gathering of the data for the project that is detailed in the book chapter. Furthermore, we declare that the book chapter is entirely original material that has never been published before and is not presently being considered for publication anywhere.

REFERENCES

[1] Smith PM, Howitt MR, Panikov N, *et al.* The microbial metabolites, short-chain fatty acids, regulate colonic Treg cell homeostasis. Science 2013; 341(6145): 569-73. [http://dx.doi.org/10.1126/science.1241165] [PMID: 23828891]

[2] Sun L, Xie C, Wang G, *et al.* Gut microbiota and intestinal FXR mediate the clinical benefits of metformin. Nat Med 2018; 24(12): 1919-29.
[http://dx.doi.org/10.1038/s41591-018-0222-4] [PMID: 30397356]

[3] Parada Venegas D, De la Fuente MK, Landskron G, *et al.* Short Chain Fatty Acids (SCFAs)-Mediated Gut Epithelial and Immune Regulation and Its Relevance for Inflammatory Bowel Diseases. Front Immunol 2019; 10: 277.
[http://dx.doi.org/10.3389/fimmu.2019.00277] [PMID: 30915065]

[4] Vatanen T, Kostic AD, d'Hennezel E, *et al.* Variation in Microbiome LPS Immunogenicity Contributes to Autoimmunity in Humans. Cell 2016; 165(4): 842-53.
[http://dx.doi.org/10.1016/j.cell.2016.04.007] [PMID: 27133167]

[5] Li M, van Esch BCAM, Henricks PAJ, Folkerts G, Garssen J. The Anti-inflammatory Effects of Short Chain Fatty Acids on Lipopolysaccharide- or Tumor Necrosis Factor α-Stimulated Endothelial Cells *via* Activation of GPR41/43 and Inhibition of HDACs. Front Pharmacol 2018; 9: 533.
[http://dx.doi.org/10.3389/fphar.2018.00533] [PMID: 29875665]

[6] Rahman S, O'Connor AL, Becker SL, Patel RK, Martindale RG, Tsikitis VL. Gut microbial metabolites and its impact on human health. Ann Gastroenterol 2023; 36(4): 360-8.
[http://dx.doi.org/10.20524/aog.2023.0809] [PMID: 37396009]

[7] Silva YP, Bernardi A, Frozza RL. The Role of Short-Chain Fatty Acids From Gut Microbiota in Gut-Brain Communication. Front Endocrinol (Lausanne) 2020; 11: 25.
[http://dx.doi.org/10.3389/fendo.2020.00025] [PMID: 32082260]

[8] O'Riordan KJ, Collins MK, Moloney GM, Knox EG, Aburto MR, Fülling C, Morley SJ, Clarke G, Schellekens H, Cryan JF. Short-chain fatty acids: Microbial metabolites for gut-brain axis signaling. Mol Cell Endocrinol. 2022; 546: 111572. ISSN 0303-7207. Available from: https://www.sciencedirect.com/science/article/pii/S0303720722000193
[http://dx.doi.org/10.1016/j.mce.2022.111572]

[9] Blachier F. Amino Acid-Derived Bacterial Metabolites in the Colorectal Luminal Fluid: Effects on Microbial Communication, Metabolism, Physiology, and Growth. Microorganisms 2023; 11(5): 1317.
[http://dx.doi.org/10.3390/microorganisms11051317] [PMID: 37317289]

[10] Portune KJ, Beaumont M, Davila A-M, Tomé D, Blachier F, Sanz Y. Gut microbiota role in dietary protein metabolism and health-related outcomes: The two sides of the coin. Trends Food Sci Technol. 2016; 57(Part B): 213-232. ISSN 0924-2244. Available from: https://www.sciencedirect.com/science/article/pii/S0924224416303612
[http://dx.doi.org/10.1016/j.tifs.2016.08.011]

[11] Larabi AB, Masson HLP, Bäumler AJ. Bile acids as modulators of gut microbiota composition and function. Gut Microbes 2023; 15(1): 2172671.
[http://dx.doi.org/10.1080/19490976.2023.2172671] [PMID: 36740850]

[12] Fogelson KA, Dorrestein PC, Zarrinpar A, Knight R. The Gut Microbial Bile Acid Modulation and Its Relevance to Digestive Health and Diseases. Gastroenterology. 2023; 164(7): 1069-1085. ISSN 0016-5085. Available from: https://www.sciencedirect.com/science/article/pii/S0016508523001610
[http://dx.doi.org/10.1053/j.gastro.2023.02.022]

[13] Staley C, Weingarden AR, Khoruts A, Sadowsky MJ. Interaction of gut microbiota with bile acid metabolism and its influence on disease states. Appl Microbiol Biotechnol 2017; 101(1): 47-64.
[http://dx.doi.org/10.1007/s00253-016-8006-6] [PMID: 27888332]

[14] Schirone M, Esposito L, D'Onofrio F, *et al.* Biogenic Amines in Meat and Meat Products: A Review of the Science and Future Perspectives. Foods 2022; 11(6): 788.
[http://dx.doi.org/10.3390/foods11060788] [PMID: 35327210]

[15] Saha Turna N, Chung R, McIntyre L. A review of biogenic amines in fermented foods: Occurrence and health effects. Heliyon 2024; 10(2): e24501.

[http://dx.doi.org/10.1016/j.heliyon.2024.e24501] [PMID: 38304783]

[16] Özogul Y, Özogul F. Biogenic Amines Formation, Toxicity, Regulations in Food. In: Saad B, Tofalo R, editors. Biogenic Amines in Food: Analysis, Occurrence and Toxicity. The Royal Society of Chemistry. 2019.
[http://dx.doi.org/10.1039/9781788015813-00001]

[17] Ruiz-Capillas C, Herrero A. Impact of Biogenic Amines on Food Quality and Safety. Foods 2019; 8(2): 62.
[http://dx.doi.org/10.3390/foods8020062] [PMID: 30744001]

[18] Donia MS, Fischbach MA. Small molecules from the human microbiota. Science 2015; 349(6246): 1254766.
[http://dx.doi.org/10.1126/science.1254766] [PMID: 26206939]

[19] Collin F, Maxwell A. The Microbial Toxin Microcin B17: Prospects for the Development of New Antibacterial Agents. J Mol Biol 2019; 431(18): 3400-26.
[http://dx.doi.org/10.1016/j.jmb.2019.05.050] [PMID: 31181289]

[20a] Arnison PG, Bibb MJ, Bierbaum G, Bowers AA, *et al.* Ribosomally synthesized and post-translationally modified peptide natural products: overview and recommendations for a universal nomenclature. Nat Prod Rep. 2013; 30(1): 108-60.
[http://dx.doi.org/10.1039/C2NP20085F] [PMID: 23165928] [PMCID: PMC3954855]

[20b] Wang S, Lin S, Fang Q, Gyampoh R, Lu Z, Gao Y, Clarke DJ, Wu K, Trembleau L, Yu Y, Kyeremeh K, Milne BF, Tabudravu J, Deng H. A ribosomally synthesised and post-translationally modified peptide containing a β-enamino acid and a macrocyclic motif. Nat Commun. 2022; 13: 5044.

[21] Jariyasopit N, Khoomrung S. Mass spectrometry-based analysis of gut microbial metabolites of aromatic amino acids. Comput Struct Biotechnol J 2023; 21: 4777-89.
[http://dx.doi.org/10.1016/j.csbj.2023.09.032] [PMID: 37841334]

[22] Chen MX, Wang SY, Kuo CH, Tsai IL. Metabolome analysis for investigating host-gut microbiota interactions. J Formos Med Assoc 2019; 118 (Suppl. 1): S10-22.
[http://dx.doi.org/10.1016/j.jfma.2018.09.007] [PMID: 30269936]

[23] Cuscó A, Catozzi C, Viñes J, Sanchez A, Francino O. Microbiota profiling with long amplicons using Nanopore sequencing: full-length 16S rRNA gene and whole rrn operon. F1000 Res 2018; 7: 1755.
[http://dx.doi.org/10.12688/f1000research.16817.1] [PMID: 30815250]

[24] Vernocchi P, Del Chierico F, Putignani L. Gut Microbiota Profiling: Metabolomics Based Approach to Unravel Compounds Affecting Human Health. Front Microbiol 2016; 7: 1144.
[http://dx.doi.org/10.3389/fmicb.2016.01144] [PMID: 27507964]

[25] Fiorucci S, Biagioli M, Zampella A, Distrutti E. Bile Acids Activated Receptors Regulate Innate Immunity. Front Immunol 2018; 9: 1853.
[http://dx.doi.org/10.3389/fimmu.2018.01853] [PMID: 30150987]

[26] Koh A, De Vadder F, Kovatcheva-Datchary P, Bäckhed F. From Dietary Fiber to Host Physiology: Short-Chain Fatty Acids as Key Bacterial Metabolites. Cell 2016; 165(6): 1332-45.
[http://dx.doi.org/10.1016/j.cell.2016.05.041] [PMID: 27259147]

[27] Gao R, Meng X, Xue Y, *et al.* Bile acids-gut microbiota crosstalk contributes to the improvement of type 2 diabetes mellitus. Front Pharmacol 2022; 13: 1027212.
[http://dx.doi.org/10.3389/fphar.2022.1027212] [PMID: 36386219]

[28] Hou K, Wu ZX, Chen XY, *et al.* Microbiota in health and diseases. Signal Transduct Target Ther 2022; 7(1): 135.
[http://dx.doi.org/10.1038/s41392-022-00974-4] [PMID: 35461318]

[29] Kwon YH, Wang H, Denou E, *et al.* Modulation of Gut Microbiota Composition by Serotonin Signaling Influences Intestinal Immune Response and Susceptibility to Colitis. Cell Mol Gastroenterol Hepatol 2019; 7(4): 709-28.

[http://dx.doi.org/10.1016/j.jcmgh.2019.01.004] [PMID: 30716420]

[30] Panyod S, Wu WK, Chen CC, Wu MS, Ho CT, Sheen LY. Modulation of gut microbiota by foods and herbs to prevent cardiovascular diseases. J Tradit Complement Med 2023; 13(2): 107-18. [http://dx.doi.org/10.1016/j.jtcme.2021.09.006] [PMID: 36970453]

[31] Perillo F, Amoroso C, Strati F, *et al.* Gut microbiota manipulation as a tool for colorectal cancer management: recent advances in its use for therapeutic purposes. Int J Mol Sci 2020; 21(15): 5389. [http://dx.doi.org/10.3390/ijms21155389] [PMID: 32751239]

[32] Matthewman C, Narin A, Huston H, Hopkins CE. Systems to model the personalized aspects of microbiome health and gut dysbiosis. Mol Aspects Med 2023; 91: 101115. [http://dx.doi.org/10.1016/j.mam.2022.101115] [PMID: 36104261]

[33] O'Keefe SJ. The association between dietary fibre deficiency and high-income lifestyle-associated diseases: Burkitt's hypothesis revisited. Lancet Gastroenterol Hepatol 2019; 4(12): 984-96. [http://dx.doi.org/10.1016/S2468-1253(19)30257-2] [PMID: 31696832]

[34] Tang WHW, Wang Z, Levison BS, *et al.* Intestinal microbial metabolism of phosphatidylcholine and cardiovascular risk. N Engl J Med 2013; 368(17): 1575-84. [http://dx.doi.org/10.1056/NEJMoa1109400] [PMID: 23614584]

[35] Berger K, Burleigh S, Lindahl M, *et al.* Xylooligosaccharides Increase *Bifidobacteria* and *Lachnospiraceae* in Mice on a High-Fat Diet, with a Concomitant Increase in Short-Chain Fatty Acids, Especially Butyric Acid. J Agric Food Chem 2021; 69(12): 3617-25. [http://dx.doi.org/10.1021/acs.jafc.0c06279] [PMID: 33724030]

[36] Ding Y, Wang S, Lu J. Unlocking the Potential: Amino Acids' Role in Predicting and Exploring Therapeutic Avenues for Type 2 Diabetes Mellitus. Metabolites 2023; 13(9): 1017. [http://dx.doi.org/10.3390/metabo13091017] [PMID: 37755297]

[37] Ejtahed HS, Angoorani P, Soroush AR, Hasani-Ranjbar S, Siadat SD, Larijani B. Gut microbiota-derived metabolites in obesity: a systematic review. Biosci Microbiota Food Health 2020; 39(3): 65-76. [http://dx.doi.org/10.12938/bmfh.2019-026] [PMID: 32775123]

[38] Pouwels S, Sakran N, Graham Y, *et al.* Non-alcoholic fatty liver disease (NAFLD): a review of pathophysiology, clinical management and effects of weight loss. BMC Endocr Disord 2022; 22(1): 63. [http://dx.doi.org/10.1186/s12902-022-00980-1] [PMID: 35287643]

[39] Sharon G, Sampson TR, Geschwind DH, Mazmanian SK. The Central Nervous System and the Gut Microbiome. Cell 2016; 167(4): 915-32. [http://dx.doi.org/10.1016/j.cell.2016.10.027] [PMID: 27814521]

[40] Yadav M, Chauhan NS. Microbiome therapeutics: exploring the present scenario and challenges. Gastroenterol Rep (Oxf) 2022; 10: goab046. [http://dx.doi.org/10.1093/gastro/goab046] [PMID: 35382166]

[41] Wong AC, Levy M. New Approaches to Microbiome-Based Therapies. mSystems 2019; 4(3): e00122-19. [http://dx.doi.org/10.1128/mSystems.00122-19] [PMID: 31164406]

[42] Li H, Limenitakis JP, Fuhrer T, *et al.* The outer mucus layer hosts a distinct intestinal microbial niche. Nat Commun 2015; 6(1): 8292. [http://dx.doi.org/10.1038/ncomms9292] [PMID: 26392213]

[43] Nava GM, Friedrichsen HJ, Stappenbeck TS. Spatial organization of intestinal microbiota in the mouse ascending colon. ISME J 2011; 5(4): 627-38. [http://dx.doi.org/10.1038/ismej.2010.161] [PMID: 20981114]

[44] Earle KA, Billings G, Sigal M, *et al.* Quantitative imaging of gut microbiota spatial organization. Cell Host Microbe 2015; 18(4): 478-88.

[http://dx.doi.org/10.1016/j.chom.2015.09.002] [PMID: 26439864]

[45] Singh N, Gurav A, Sivaprakasam S, *et al.* Activation of Gpr109a, receptor for niacin and the commensal metabolite butyrate, suppresses colonic inflammation and carcinogenesis. Immunity 2014; 40(1): 128-39.
[http://dx.doi.org/10.1016/j.immuni.2013.12.007] [PMID: 24412617]

[46] Morrison DJ, Preston T. Formation of short chain fatty acids by the gut microbiota and their impact on human metabolism. Gut Microbes 2016; 7(3): 189-200.
[http://dx.doi.org/10.1080/19490976.2015.1134082] [PMID: 26963409]

[47] Steidler L, Neirynck S, Huyghebaert N, *et al.* Biological containment of genetically modified Lactococcus lactis for intestinal delivery of human interleukin 10. Nat Biotechnol 2003; 21(7): 785-9.
[http://dx.doi.org/10.1038/nbt840] [PMID: 12808464]

[48] Ceroni F, Algar R, Stan GB, Ellis T. Quantifying cellular capacity identifies gene expression designs with reduced burden. Nat Methods 2015; 12(5): 415-8.
[http://dx.doi.org/10.1038/nmeth.3339] [PMID: 25849635]

[49] Gladstone EG, Molineux IJ, Bull JJ. Evolutionary principles and synthetic biology: avoiding a molecular tragedy of the commons with an engineered phage. J Biol Eng 2012; 6(1): 13.
[http://dx.doi.org/10.1186/1754-1611-6-13] [PMID: 22947166]

[50] Wang S, Mu L, Yu C, *et al.* Microbial collaborations and conflicts: unraveling interactions in the gut ecosystem. Gut Microbes 2024; 16(1): 2296603.
[http://dx.doi.org/10.1080/19490976.2023.2296603] [PMID: 38149632]

[51] Feng W, Liu J, Ao H, Yue S, Peng C. Targeting gut microbiota for precision medicine: Focusing on the efficacy and toxicity of drugs. Theranostics 2020; 10(24): 11278-301.
[http://dx.doi.org/10.7150/thno.47289] [PMID: 33042283]

[52] Gebrayel P, Nicco C, Al Khodor S, *et al.* Microbiota medicine: towards clinical revolution. J Transl Med 2022; 20(1): 111.
[http://dx.doi.org/10.1186/s12967-022-03296-9] [PMID: 35255932]

[53] Al-Khazaleh AK, Chang D, Münch GW, Bhuyan DJ. The Gut Connection: Exploring the Possibility of Implementing Gut Microbial Metabolites in Lymphoma Treatment. Cancers (Basel) 2024; 16(8): 1464.
[http://dx.doi.org/10.3390/cancers16081464] [PMID: 38672546]

CHAPTER 11

Gut Microbiota and Future Research Directions

Sakuntala Gayen[1], **Soumyadeep Chattopadhyay**[1], **Rudradeep Hazra**[1], **Arijit Mallick**[1] and **Souvik Roy**[1,*]

[1] *Department of Pharmaceutical Technology, NSHM Knowledge Campus, Kolkata-Group of Institutions, 124, B. L. Saha Road, Tara Park, Behala, Kolkata, West Bengal-700053, India*

Abstract: The human intestines anchorage a complex of bacterial communities called gut microbiota. Gut microbiota is a prime regulator that preserves homeostasis in the intestine and the extra-intestine host-microbial interface. By contrast, the dysregulation of gut microbiota is accompanied by the assembling of various toxic substances and oncogenic proteins, which encourage several inflammatory responses and tumorigenesis. Moreover, gut microbiota correlates with the pathogenesis and progression of many disease conditions, including diabetes, obesity, inflammatory bowel diseases, cardiovascular disease, and neurological disorders. Besides that, different approaches have been intimated for the modulation of gut microbiome characteristics including treatment with antibiotics, prebiotic and probiotic supplements, nutritional interventions, and fecal microbiota transplantation (FMT) to control normal homeostasis of gut microbiota. Recently, it has been shown that gut microbiota has a significant connection to the regulation of the immune system in pathogenic conditions, and it has been identified as a potent therapeutic biomarker in the context of immunotherapy. This review emphasized the potential role of gut microbiome in the regulation of disease pathogenesis and therapeutic approaches. In connection with this, the recent study has elucidated emerging technologies for gut microbiome research, immunotherapeutic strategies, and the effects of nanomedicines on gut microbiota as a future perspective.

Keywords: Culturomics, Fecal microbiota transplantation, Gut microbiota, Homeostasis, Host-microbial interface, Immunotherapy, Immunomodulation, *In-vitro* holobiont system, Metagenomics, Nanomedicines.

INTRODUCTION

Human gut microbiota is considered a complex bacterial community in the gastrointestinal arena. The intestinal community mainly consists of 10^{13} microbes, primarily obtained from the phyla *Bacteroidetes* and *Firmicutes* [1, 2]. Microorganisms in the gut microbiota interact with various host cells, which can significantly regulate physiological function in response to nutrient metabolisms and gut barrier regulation. The diversity of gut microbiota mainly depends upon several factors such as age, diet, environmental factors, and human lifestyle [3]. In addition, the gut microbiome is in charge of controlling how the host and microbiome interact and how they talk to immune, hormonal, neural, endocrine,

[*] **Corresponding author Souvik Roy:** Department of Pharmaceutical Technology, NSHM Knowledge Campus, Kolkata-Group of Institutions, 124, B. L. Saha Road, Tara Park, Behala, Kolkata, West Bengal-700053; E-mail: souvikroy35@gmail.com

Sandipan Dasgupta & Moitreyee Chattopadhyay (Eds.)

and metabolic pathways. The gut microbiota can help improve the interactions between the host and microbiome, which could boost the host's immune system to fight off pathogens. Dysbiosis of the gut microbiome is significantly correlated with the manifestation and progression of many disease conditions, like cardiovascular disease, diabetes, anxiety, depression, obesity, inflammatory bowel syndrome, and cancer [4, 5].

Intriguingly, the gut microbiota contributes to the relationship to maintain immune homeostatic conditions, demonstrated in germ-free animals resulting in the impairment of regulatory T-cells (Tregs) development as well as the downregulation of gut-associated lymphoid tissues (GALT) proliferation. Besides that, host-immune responses are substantially accompanied by the control of the gut microbiome environment [6]. For instance, IgA (Immunoglobulin A) is secreted by gut plasma cells and shows reactivity to a wide spectrum of microbes, whereas this immunoglobulin A may increase the translocation of specific commensals into the lymphoid tissue to promote the antigenic appearance and uphold the gut microbiome diversity [7, 8]. The alteration of the gut microbiota environment causes the downregulation of good bacterial survival and function with upsurges of bad bacterial activities. Therefore, fecal microbial transplantation and prebiotic management significantly increase the magnitude of beneficial bacterial restoration in the intestine, changing this dysregulation and combating disease prevalence [9].

The immune surveillance theory identifies the evasion of tumor immuneresponses as a fundamental mechanism within the tumor microenvironment. This is because gut microbiota interacts directly with human immune systems, stopping tumor immune escape through their structures and byproducts. These factors play a pivotal role in facilitating disease progression and poor prognosis. Additionally, the microbiota in the gut can effectively change the immune system by producing metabolites [6, 10]. This recent article has reviewed the potential mechanistic understanding of gut microbiota in response to disease progression as well as the correlation with recent therapeutic strategies. Furthermore, this study also described the emerging technologies associated with gut microbiome research, as well as the potential role of immunotherapy and the effect of nanomedicines on gut microbiota.

Microbiota in Health

The intestinal-gut microbial balance is directly associated with human health and disease progression. The human digestive tract is home to a large community of microbes that play a big role in breaking down nutrients, extracting them, and immune system regulation [11]. Extensive studies have suggested that microbiota can significantly interact with several biological processes *via* several mechanistic pathways. Furthermore, the biosynthesis of bioactive molecules like amino acids, vitamins, and lipids also depends upon gut microbial regulation [12].

In healthy conditions, the gut microbiome elicits resilience, stability, and symbiotic interactions with the hosts. The gut microbial community consists of bacteria, yeasts, and viruses. The healthy microbial community often exhibits higher taxonomical diversity, stable core microbiota, and high microbial gene prosperity [13]. Moreover, it has been reported that the relative distribution of microbiomes is different between individuals, which may be associated with age and environmental factors like pH and medicine usage. Additionally, the presence of gut microbiota may also vary in different anatomical parts of the gastrointestinal tract. For instance, *Proteobacteria* like *Enterobacteriaceae* are found in the small intestine and *Bacteriodetes* like *Bacteroidaceae*, *Prevotellaceae* and *Rikenellaceae* are present in the colonic environment [14]. These changes depend on the environment. For example, the small intestines have a short transit time and a high concentration of bile, while the colon has slower flow rates, a lighter pH, and large communities of anaerobic microbes [15]. Moreover, gut microbiota could differ by age. Normally, we observe a significant microbiota diversity between childhood and adulthood, which decreases at an older age [13]. Children's gut microbiota diversity increases due to the presence of *Akkermansia muciniphila*, *Bacteroides*, *Veillonella*, *Clostridium coccoides spp*., and *Clostridium botulinum spp* [16]. An adult's gut microbial community consists of three dominant microbial phyla, such as *Firmicutes*, *Bacteroidetes* and *Actinobacteria*. The dietary and immune systems remarkably change in older age people, which can affect the healthy gut microbial composition. Especially, elder people have been shown to have increased *Clostridium* and *Proteobacteria* and decreased *Bifidobacterium* microbiota [17]. In the last two decades, extemporaneous efforts in biomedicine have been undertaken to develop the interplay of commensal bacteria living in and on the human body with their own human physiology. Also, Laudes and his colleagues reported some examples of future clinical applications in several entities, which suggest the microbiome-based molecules as potential targets for intervention studies, either as a standalone therapy or in addition to disease-specific drugs to make them work better [18].

Microbiota in the Development of Diseases

The gut microbiota communities encompass trillions of microorganisms, utilizing advanced sequencing technologies and bioinformatics [5]. These microorganisms have a significant impact on our physiology, both healthy and diseased. They facilitate multiple functions, some of which include modulating metabolic activities, defending against potential infections, bolstering the immune system, and so on. As a result, they promote either direct or indirect effects on our physiology [19]. Furthermore, research on the microbiome focuses on the connection between microbial compositional deviations in various disease conditions. Interaction with external stimuli can alter the gut microbial ecosystem, leading to dysregulation of the body's immune responses and manifestation of disease conditions [20, 21]. Several pieces of evidence show that changing the environment of the gut microbiota can lead to lung diseases, heart disease, diabetes, brain disorders, inflammatory bowel disease (IBD), cancer, long-term kidney diseases, and liver diseases (Fig. **1**) [1].

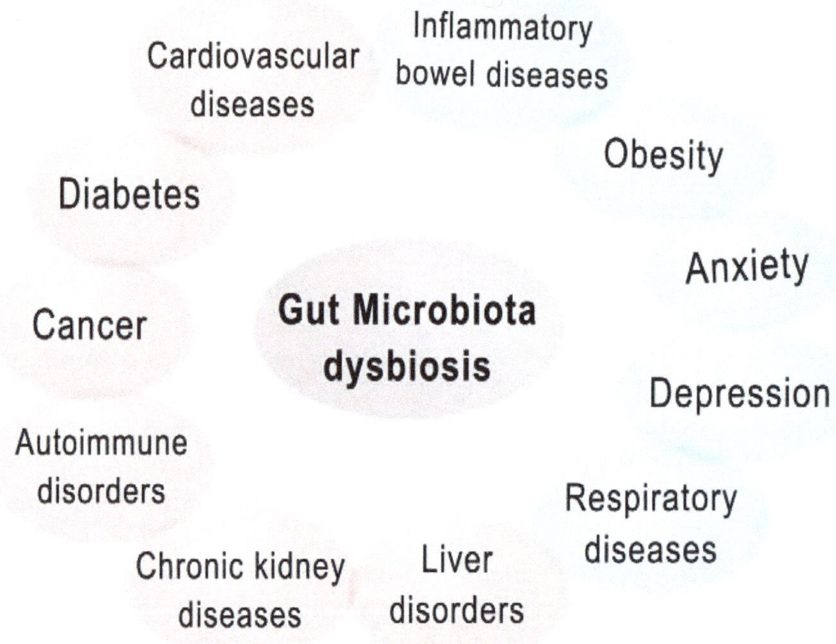

Fig. (1). Dysbiosis of the gut microbial ecosystem causes the manifestation of several disease conditions.

While commensal microbes are aberrantly permeable into the gut ecosystem and enhance the production of microbial-derived metabolites, virulence factors, and other luminal compounds that significantly disrupt the gut microbial function, facilitate immune-related inflammatory diseases like allergy, inflammation, and autoimmune diseases facilitated by molecular mimicry and deactivation of T-cell responses [22]. The interaction between gut microbiota and host cross-regulates the physiological and immunological functional barriers. T-cells play an important role in systemic and mucosal immunity [23]. *Bacteroides fragilis*, *Bifidobacterium infantis*, and *Firmicutes* are some of the good bacteria that can make more regulatory T-cells (Tregs). . These Tregs include FOXP3-expressing Tregs and anti-inflammatory IL-10-producing Tregs, which help to stop pathological inflammation caused by abnormal effector T-cell responses and make the gut barrier stronger [19, 24]. Moreover, various microbial-derived metabolites, like neuromodulators and neurotransmitters, such as short-chain fatty acids (SCFAs) formed by *Bacillus*, *Saccharomyces*, *Lactobacillus*, *Escherichia*, *Bifidobacterium,* and biogenic amines (like dopamine, histamine, and serotonin) as well as other amino acid-derived metabolites such as GABA and tryptophan, act as a safeguard of the gut barrier integrity from the destructive responses of pro-inflammatory cytokines by abnormal immune-related inflammatory responses. Whereas, butyrate is capable of activating antigen-specific CD8+ T-cells, improving the intestinal defense mechanism against pathogens. Additionally, other metabolites of the gut microbiome affect effector T-cell function in various pathways, such as ascorbate encouraging apoptotic activation of T-cells, repression of CD8+ T-cell proliferation, and downstream of IFN-γ production by mevalonate, and upstream of Treg cells activity by glutamate [23 - 25].

Microbiota in theDevelopment of Immune Responses

The microbial communities in different organs exhibit distinctive characteristics and compositions that interact with multiple biological processes in the host. The immune system consists of innate and adaptive immune responses, which extensively interact with the microbiota. Naturally occurring immune responses help keep the environment stable by lowering the number of harmful bacteria that live there and ensuring that adaptive immune responses to microbiota stay strong [26]. Toll-like receptor 5 (TLR5), secretory IgA (sIgA), inflammasomes, and autophagy are some of the mediators that control these immune responses [27].

As a paradigm, secretory IgA (sIgA) can bind strongly with commensal bacteria, creating complexes with bacterial parts and tolerogenic dendritic cells. Moreover, sIgA can represent an anti-inflammatory molecule, that significantly decreases the inflammatory responses caused by immense bacterial loads in the organ. Furthermore, the dysbiosis of the microbiota can modify sIgA responses, closely correlated with bacterial growth [28]. The research by Hapfelmeier and his colleague showed that the reversible microbial colonization technique in GF mice led to sIgA immune responses that were specific to the microbiota [29]. Furthermore, the adaptive immune system is an alternative to controlling healthy microbiota and immune balance. An important part of adaptive immunity is the development and differentiation of T and B cells, which makes the immune system less sensitive to microbiota. Depending on the bacterial species, the CD4+ T-cells can differentiate into distinct subsets and subsequently release pro-inflammatory cytokines such as interferon (IFN) and interleukin 17A (IL-17A) [30].

The gastrointestinal tract contains a significant number of immune cells that have the potential to interact with the gut microbiota. The maturation of the immune system leads to the development of a commensal microbial community. The gut microbiota can substantially trigger the immune system, which is facilitated through neutrophil migration and subsequently influences T-cell differentiation into regulatory T-cells and various helper T-cells (Th1, Th2, and Th17) [31]. The disorder of microbiota development can substantially impede the maturation of immune cells, which may cause the development of immunological tolerance and autoimmune disorders. Furthermore, the gut microbiota could produce heterogeneous molecules that may stimulate immune responses and activate inflammation or chronic tissue damage [32]. Additionally, the gut microbiota can explain immune-related adverse events, and help us to understand the complex interactions between the microbiome, systemic immune system, and immunotherapy in the context of cancer. More functional studies and prospective clinical studies are essential to translate preclinical interventions targeting the gut microbiota into clinical studies in humans. However, researchers cannot always use experimental treatments in clinics because people and rodents have different immune systems and gut microbiomes [33].

EMERGING TECHNOLOGIES ON GUT MICROBIOME RESEARCH

Recently, researchers in the field of microbial ecology have turned their attention to studying commensal microbiomes that interact positively with human hosts [34, 35]. Holobionts are groups of microbes that live together in complex communities. These communities are important for keeping the balance between host and microbes because they are where interactions between microbes and hosts happen [36, 37]. The imbalance occurs in these mechanisms due to either the introduction of pathogens or extreme environmental changes, which could contribute to an alteration of the microbial community's composition that has been imitated through the loss of microbial diversity to induce dysbiosis, leading to facilitate negative regulation of human physiology, thereby propagating diseases [38, 39].

Recent advancements in genomic sequencing, facilitated by computational biology pipelines, have led to exponential growth in gut microbiome research. Moreover, the mechanisms of microbial pathways altering the host biology remain to be completely accomplished [40]. Interestingly, the high-throughput sequencing technologies deliver critical information regarding both the composition and function of the gut microbiota and their impact on the host immune system. The different methodologies of high-throughput sequencing technologies in gut microbiome research include culturomics, metagenomics, multi-omics, and *in-vitro* holobiont systems, which aim to accomplish a better understanding of the host-microbiome interactions in both healthy and diseased conditions (Fig. **2**) [41, 42].

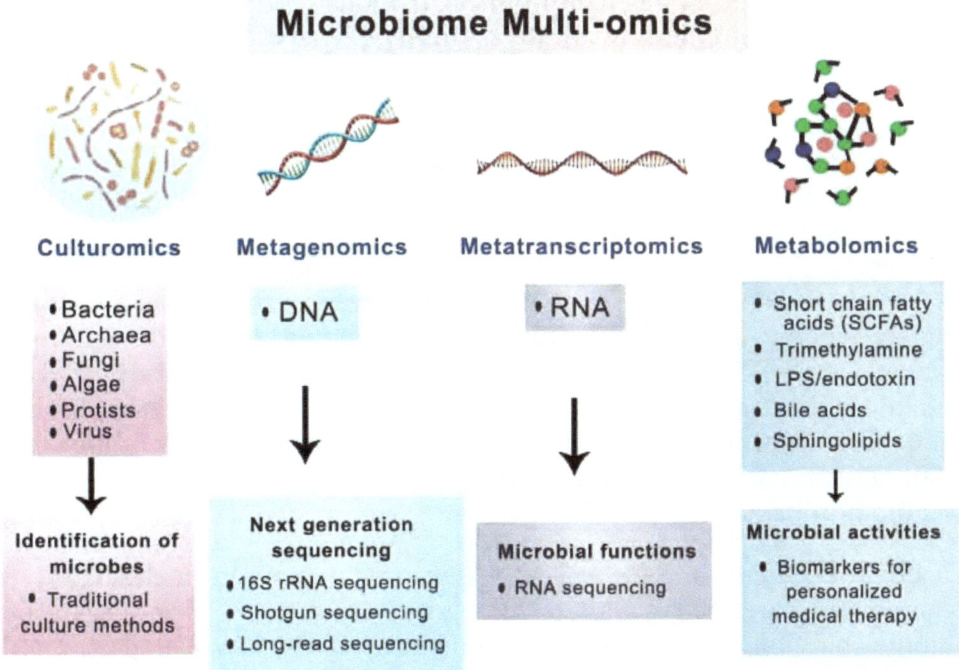

Fig. (2). Emerging technologies in gut microbiome research.

Culturomics

Culturomics comprises a traditional culture method that can facilitate the accurate identification of previously challenging microbes. Prior to the advancements in sequencing technologies, researchers estimated that approximately 80% of bacteria in the human gut remained uncultured [43]. Moreover, recent high-throughput computerized innovation has identified hundreds of novel bacterial species in the last few ages [44]. This technique allows for the aliquotation of a single fecal sample into several microchambers, each with unique culture settings, and then incubation. Scientists have developed a culturomics technique to culture the bacterium in a high-throughput setting [45]. In the beginning, researchers tried 212 different culture conditions in culturomics and obtained more than 30,000 colonies from 341 different bacterial species. More than half of these species knew they had first been found in the human gut. The culturomics technique has continuously grown, including ethanol addition to fecal samples for developing the sporulated bacteria, as a result of the isolation of 69 newer bacterial species [46]. High-throughput techniques successfully acknowledge the expanded knowledge of gut microbiota; however, this study is relatively labor-intensive compared to other microbiome methods. Therefore, researchers have evaluated several groups for optimizing culturomics, demonstrating a methodologically limited number of conditions with substantially preserved bacterial diversities [47].

Metagenomics

Recently, most studies on microbiome research have primarily utilized next-generation sequencing metagenomics to develop community-wide ecological maps that provide information on the microbial determinants of health and disease [48 - 50]. This high-throughput, culture-free technology showcases two specific genome sequencing approaches: amplicon sequencing involved with unique variable areas of the bacterial 16S rRNA / internal transcribed spacer (ITS) as a phylogenetic marker. Shotgun sequencing, on the other hand, imprisons the entire breadth of DNA within a sample and breaks all genomes present in the sample into small DNA fragments, which are then independently sequenced and analyzed by using bioinformatic tools [51, 52].

It has been proven that using the 16S rRNA genome as a phylogenetic marker is a better and more cost-effective way to study gut microbiota [53] The breakthrough microbiome study on inflammatory bowel diseases (IBD) has been performed to characterize fecal samples, ileum, as well as rectal mucosal microbiomes of pediatric Crohn's disease patients [54, 55]. Gevers *et al.* reported that IBD disease activity was detected by utilizing a simple microbiome dysbiosis index from 16S sequencing. This investigation also demonstrated the aptitude of 16S rRNA sequencing to recognize the microbial low-biomass samples, including rectal and ileum biopsies [56]. Moreover, some technical considerations with amplicon sequencing could produce various outcomes. The microbial 16S rRNA genome consists of nine hypervariable regions (V1-V9), and thus it may be essential for recognizing the common primers that aid other researchers in comparing the outcomes [57]. The human microbiome project characterized 300 healthy individuals across the various sites of the human body (skin, nasal passage, gastrointestinal tract, oral cavity, and urinary tract) using both V1-3 and V3-5 primers. In the gut microbial study, V3-4 and V4 primers were most widely utilized, as they have the advantage of recognizing both several bacterial species and archaea [58]. While the amplicon sequencing procedure is capable of providing only a partial genome architecture. Despite its limitations, amplicon sequencing cannot provide a detailed explanation of every amplicon at the bacterial species level. Recently, the advancement of amplicon sequencing, united with long read sequencing methods, is associated with providing the full-length sequencing of the complete V1-V9 genes and subsequently highlighting the all-amplified sequencing for all species. Furthermore, it was discovered that other target areas, such as 23S and ITS, could be linked with long-read sequencing methods, suggesting that the amplicon sequencing techniques could achieve the strain-level resolution that would be needed in future clinical settings [59, 60].

The limitations of amplicon sequencing suggest that several scientists are substantially dependent on shotgun sequencing. In this advanced technology, read all the genomic DNA in a sample preparation from one particular area of DNA. This analysis also represented the resolution at the sub-species strain level and provided functional intuitions. The pan-genome analysis by the shotgun sequencing method was conducted by Hall et al., utilizing 266 fecal samples obtained from 20 IBD patients, 16 control samples, and no subspecies strains of *Ruminococcus gnavus*. This study reported that *R gnavus* strains specifically identified 199 IBD-specific microbial genes linked to oxidative stress, iron acquisition, adhesions, and mucous utilization [61]. Moreover, the shotgun technique can identify the pathognomic bacterial species in IBD, but*R gnavus* strains are still required for a better understanding of host-microbial interactions at strain-level resolution [62].

Additionally, shotgun technologies can also enable profiling of fungi, viruses, and several types of micro-organisms [63, 64]. Both amplicon and shotgun sequencing methods are short-read sequencing methods. The emergent information represents the long-read sequencing, which facilitates the identification of a wide variety of species and explicitly distinguishes between the strains within a species [65]. The utilization of long-read sequencing was exclusively feasible for the identification of small bacterial genomes [66]. Metagenomic analysis of fecal samples from patients with or without cancer showed unique virome sequencing as compared with cancer-free controls [67, 68]. Hence, the research on gut microbiome is predicted to grow significantly on these more sophisticated methodologies with evaluating the host-microbiome interactions in healthy and diseased conditions.

Multi-omics Microbiome Integrated Analysis

Internal validations of microbial records are frequently conducted in microbiome investigations, particularly in those that demonstrate the characterization of patients' samples with low biomass using experimental validation techniques and microbiome multi-omics such as culturomics, meta-transcriptomics, and metabolomics [69, 70]. Mishra *et al.* represented the profile of microbiome communities in human fetal tissue of the second trimester of gestation by applying 16S rRNA sequencing. This study demonstrated the additional microbial information for identifying the presence of these microbes and electron microscopy, culturomics, and *in-vitro* investigational validation methods confirming the function of these microbial strains. Researchers have discovered that early exposure to microbe plays a crucial role in priming the immune system. For example, gut microbiota during the second trimester of pregnancy makes memory T-cells work [71].

Multi-omics also covers the function of microbiota in the gut microbial ecosystem, verifying through the metagenomic readouts, that genes are expressed and translated into proteins [72, 73]. Schirmer and his research team conducted a study on IBD meta-transcriptomics, which represented the meta-transcriptional profiles of RNA isolated from fecal samples, transcribed into cDNA, and then sequenced. This study provides information on gut microbiota community dynamics, such as IBD-specific transcriptional activities [74]. Furthermore, it has been shown that microbial-specific transcriptional analysis is extensively correlated with environmental signals like altered oxygen levels, and inflammation may not affect the DNA level. Moreover, the limitations of the interpretation of fecal meta-transcriptomics readouts include the variation that occurs when the subject-specific transit times differ, as fecal samples only capture extractable, non-degradable RNA restricted to the presence of micro-organisms in fecal samples [74, 75].

Furthermore, one of the important groups of metabolites obtained as short-chain fatty acids (SCFAs) include butyrate, acetate, and propionate, which are obtained after fermentation of carbohydrates by the gut microbiota in the colon [76, 77]. SCFAs play a crucial role in the gut microbiota to diversify the immunomodulation by the regulation of histone acetylation and alteration of T-cell function in the gut [78, 79]. Notably, SCFAs have extensively emerged as a promising treatment approach for IBD because they modulate the intestinal gut microbiome ecosystem [80].

IgA-Seq uses sequencing of the 16S rRNA gene to find and separate the groups of bacteria that are covered in endogenous host IgA [81]. IgA-Seq can directly pair with 16S amplicon sequencing and microbial fluorescence-stimulated cell sorting, exploiting IgA-coated microbial taxa that can most precisely identify the pathogenic gut microbiome-associated inflammatory responses in IBD [82]. Recently, this strategy could ingeniously focus on microbial research that has shown interactions with the host-mucosal immune responses. Therefore, IgA-Seq demonstrates an innovative strategy to integrate microbial sequencing with other investigational biological approaches, which additionally accomplishes a better understanding of host-microbial interactions in healthy and disease conditions [83, 84].

In-vitro Holobiont System

Another strategy to represent host-microbial interactions is the high-throughput *in-vitro* holobiont systems. Three well-known methods are used in a microbial study, including a simulator of the human intestinal microbial ecosystem (SHIME), human microbial X (cross) talk (HuMix), and rapid assay of the individual microbiome (RapidAIM) [37, 85]. SHIME is an *in-vitro* gut model that summarizes the physiological state of the human gut. This model encompasses five dynamic simulating sections namely, small intestine, stomach, ascending colon, transverse colon, and descending colon. The high-throughput methods SHIME has emerged as a promising technique for the study of prebiotics, probiotics and oral therapeutic metabolisms [86]. Through their research, Abbeele and his team have shown that different probiotics can colonize the gut when mixed with mucin to make a more dynamic system. This scheme aids in the investigation of micro-organisms that benefit from mucosal adhesion, as well as the study of microbial stability over a longer period [87].

HuMix is a three-dimensional organotypic model of human colonic epithelium utilizing microfluidics-dependent principles. It comprises three microchambers: microbiota, epithelial cells, and perfusion, wherein the microbes and intestinal cells are co-cultured and detached with a nanoporous membrane. This study's results significantly simplify the monitoring of oxygen levels in real time, a crucial step in understanding the changes in oxygen levels in various parts of the gastrointestinal (GI) tract and in inflammatory diseases such as IBD [88]. Shah and his colleagues reported using HuMix to determine host-microbiome interactions by co-culturing *Lactobacillus rhamnosus* GG and Caco-2 cells for transcriptomics, metabolomics, and immunological readouts [89]. The HuMix *in-vitro* holobiont study promises to accomplish the systematic evaluation of host-microbial interactions that promote transcriptional microbiomes in novel therapeutic discovery [90].

Furthermore, RapidAIM is a rapid and scalable assay method that extemporaneously evaluates the response of the gut microbiome to drugs. Using the RapidAIM technique, the development of a pipeline to co-culture individual fecal samples in uniform non-selective media and a variety of therapeutic drugs could subsequently enter into high-throughput meta-proteomics analysis to estimate the drug concentrations as well as microbial biomass levels. This analysis could provide better insights on microbial–drug responses. Lately, this analysis conveys a promise for personalized medicine in the near future, as depending on the microbial pharmacogenomics, the drugs can be prescribed based on the microbial profiles [69, 91].

GUT MICROBIOTA INFLUENCES IMMUNOTHERAPEUTIC RESPONSES

Immunotherapy has emerged as an effective treatment for several cancer types. Ample studies have demonstrated a significant correlation between gut microbiota and patient's response to immunotherapy. The gut microbiome's taxonomical compositions, community structures, and molecular functions have all been found to be important biomarkers for predicting immunotherapeutic response and immune-related adverse effects. Unlike other omics, the gut microbiota not only serves as a biomarker but also presents a potential target for enhancing the effectiveness of immunotherapy [92, 93]. Indeed, the gut microbiota synthesizes a myriad of small molecules and metabolites, and plays an important role in several human physiological procedures like metabolism, immunity, inflammation, and neurology [94 - 96]. The gut microbiota and its metabolites have a direct correlation with regulating local and systemic immunity that significantly led to the investigation of cancer immunotherapy and immune checkpoint blockade (ICB) therapy [97 - 99]. The extensive variations in the gut microbiome among adult individuals are an alternative approach as a potential source to contribute to the phenotypic variations in gut microbiome that encourage tumorigenesis and drug resistance [100]. Ample reviews have shown that the gut microbiota can significantly modulate immune responses by interacting with immune checkpoint blockade (ICB) therapy in preclinical as well as clinical investigations [101 - 103]. ICB therapy can improvise the traditional cancer therapeutic strategies which is a breakthrough in the treatment of different types of cancer [104 - 106]. ICB can unleash the body's own immune responses to efficiently obstruct the tumoral immune escape by targeting programmed cell death 1 (PD-1) and its ligand (programmed death ligand 1/2, PD-L1/2), cytotoxic T-lymphocyte antigen-4 (CTLA-4) and B7-1/2 interactions, and others lymphocyte activating gene-3 (LAG-3), T-cell immunoglobulin and mucin domain containing 3 (TIM-3) immune checkpoint molecules. The modulation of gut microbiome ecology promotes the newer emergent targets for developing anti-tumor immune responses and increases ICB effectiveness to facilitate immunomodulatory actions (Fig.**3**) [107, 108].

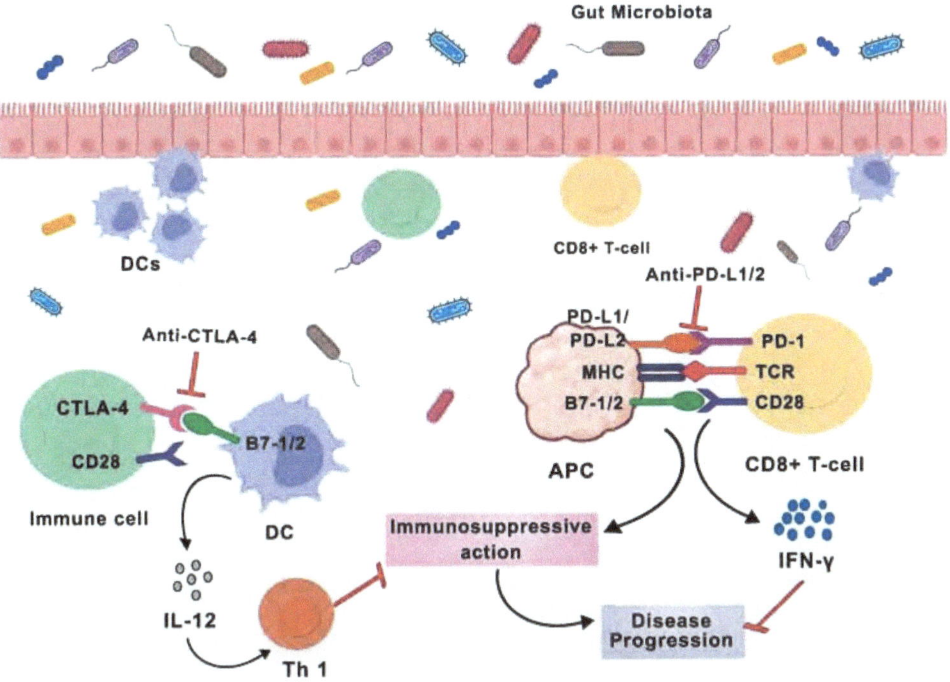

Fig. (3). Potential role of Immunotherapy in gut microbiome research. DCs – Dendritic cells, APC – Antigen-presenting cells, PD-1 – Programmed cell death 1, PD-L1/2 – Programmed death ligand 1 / 2, CTLA-4 – Cytotoxic T-lymphocyte antigen 4, IFN-γ – Interferon γ, IL-12 – Interleukin 12, Th 1 – Helper T-cells.

Over the past few decades, many studies have shown that the gut microbiome can change CD8+ T lymphocytes, helper T cells 1 (Th1), and immune responses that are linked to tumors, which makes the immune system better at fighting them [109]. The composition of gut microbiome ecology influences anti-PD-L1 treatment. The oral administration of *Bifidobacterium* promotes anticancer immune responses by blocking PD-1 / PD-L1 interactions *via* increasing dendritic cell maturation and enhancing CD8+ T-cell priming as well as expanding in the tumor microenvironment [110]. Another study demonstrated that anti-CTLA-4 therapy could significantly attenuate the antitumoral efficacy of ICB therapy, and subsequently, supplementation of *Bacteroides fragilis* in germ-free or treatment with antibiotics in melanoma mice may improve anti-CTLA-4 activity. The microbiota-dependent anti-tumoral action relies on helper T-cell stimulation in the tumor drainage lymph node, which leads to the maturation of intra-tumoral dendritic cells [111]. Early studies demonstrated that the composition and diversity of the gut microbiota ecosystem have been explorative of responses to

ICB immunotherapy. Intriguingly, the fecal microbiota transplantation (FMT) with ICB-treated patients to germ-free and antibiotic-treated mouse models might enhance antitumoral immune responses as well as alleviate the effectiveness of ICB therapy, whereby patients are non-responsive to FMT. Patients with renal cell cancer (RCC) and non-small cell lung cancer (NSCLC) had a wide range of microbiota that responded better to anti-PD-1 therapy . A similar study has depicted that oral administration of *Akkermansia muciniphila* followed by FMT to non-responding ICB patients reinvigorated the efficacy of anti-PD-1 [112]. The composition and diversity of microbial ecology can affirmatively be associated with the anti-PD-1 treatment responses in melanoma cancer patients. The significant abundance of *Faecalibacterium* and *Ruminococcaceae* bacteria in the gut demonstrated a higher number of CD4+ and CD8+ T-cells in the periphery of ICB-responding patients [113]. In metastatic melanoma patients, *Collinsella aerofaciens, Enterococcus faecium,* and *Bifidobacterium longum* have been more abundant than the baseline feces of responders [114].

Prospective investigations suggested a substantial correlation between the gut microbiota and ICB therapy in hepatocellular cancer (HCC), renal cell cancer (RCC), melanoma, and non-small cell lung cancer (NSCLC) patients from 2019 to 2020 [115 - 117]. At that time, retrospective revision indicated that antibiotics remarkably attenuated the survival and decreased the efficacy of ICB therapy in patients with advanced solid tumor by encouraging the promotion of antibiotic-dependent dysbiosis and poor therapeutic efficiency of ICB. Moreover, two clinical investigations significantly reported that FMT with ICB therapy plus anti-PD-1 therapy astonishingly deactivated the resistance to PD-1 inhibitors in melanoma [118 - 121].

Additionally, the gut microbiota can significantly enhance adoptive T-cell transfer (ACT) immunotherapy, immune-cell-dependent immunotherapy, and CpG-oligodeoxynucleotide (CpG-ODN) immunotherapy [122]. In contrast, antibiotics may make ACT therapy less effective in mice. However, adding bacterial LPS improves the effectiveness of the therapy by changing the signaling through toll-like receptor 4 (TLR4). Furthermore, the gut microbiota upheld ACT therapy *via* upregulating the abundance of CD8α+dendritic cells, thus increasing interleukin 1 (IL-1) production [123]. Another study demonstrated that the gut microbiome can stimulate TLR4, which directly or indirectly promotes TLR9-dependent immune responses of tumor-associated myeloid cells in CpG-ODN immunotherapy. The activity of CpG-ODN is dampened by antibiotic exposure through attenuating tumor necrosis factor (TNF) and interleukin 12 (IL-12) activation [124]. Moreover, gut microbiome-dependent metabolism of bile acids enhanced the stimulation of CXCR6+ natural killer cells to augment anti-tumoral effects in HCC [125].

Several studies suggested that gut microbiota can change ICB responses by altering innate as well as adaptive immune responses and enhancing anticancer immune responses in the tumor microenvironment. The immune cells, including CD8+ and CD4+ T-lymphocytes, dendritic cells, natural killer cells, and macrophages, play a pivotal role in modulating immune responses in association with gut microbiota [126, 127]. Multiple investigations have reported that CD8+ T-lymphocytes are produced by the gut microbiota in the tumor microenvironment. As a paradigm, in melanoma patients, the higher abundance of favorable microbiota such as *Ruminococcaceae, Faecalibacterium,* or *Clostridiales,* superior antigen presentation with improvising effector CD4+ and CD8+ T-lymphocyte activity in peripheral blood and tumor microenvironments to enhance antitumoral activity of ICB [113]. The clinical trials report has suggested that *phyla Firmicutes* and *Actinobacteria* have been supplemented with FMT in combination with PD-1 blockade therapy. The combination therapy of FMT and PD-1 blockade can substantially increase mucosal-associated invariant T-lymphocytes (MAITs) and CD56+CD8+ T-lymphocytes in peripheral blood mononuclear cells (PBMCs) and upstream of the expression of human leukocyte antigen (HLA) class-II genes CD74 and GZMK on CD8+ T-lymphocyte at tumoral regions [128]. Moreover, *Bifidobacterium* and their eleven strains may also boost the effector CD8+ T-lymphocyte activation on dendritic cells to modulate ICB therapeutic responses [129]. *One of the byproducts of B. pseudolongum microbes, inosine, made ICB work better and activated Th1 transcriptional differentiation, which improved the body's ability to fight cancer* [130]. Additionally, *Bacteroides fragilis* can improve IL-12-mediated Th1 immune response by augmenting the mobilization of dendritic cells that activate the immune system to ICB therapy [111]. Furthermore, the oral administration of *A. muciniphila* in FMT non-responding mice restored anti-PD-1 efficacy by encouraging CCR9+CXCR3+CD4+ T-cell recruitment into cancer cells [112]. *Faecalibacterium* encouraged the proportion of CD4+ T-cells and serum CD25 while decreasing Treg cell proportion at peripheral sites that promoted the long-term clinical benefits of ipilimumab [131].

Furthermore, Microbiota-derived IFN-1 signaling facilitates the transition from innate to adaptive immune responses. Microbiota-derived stimulator of interferon genes (STING) agonists can initiate IFN-1 signaling through intra-tumoral monocytes that raise mononuclear phagocyte-mediated anticancer macrophages (Macs) and increase the crosstalk between the monocyte IFN-1 natural killer cells and dendritic cells [132, 133]. Interestingly, feeding a high-fiber diet causes the mono-colonization with cdAMP-produced *A. muciniphila* or transferred fecal microbiota from ICB respondents with enhanced antitumor immunity to ICB therapy [132]. Notably, *Bifidobacterium* extensively colonizes the tumoral sites and encourages CD47-dependent immunotherapy *via* the activation of STING signaling and IFN-1 production [134]. *Bacteroides fragilis* helped macrophages change into the M1 phenotype and increased the expression of CD80 and CD86 in cells, which helped the body's natural defenses [110]. Moreover, gut microbiota metabolites or antigens with immunomodulators have been utilized to mobilize and stimulate dendritic cells (DCs) to convert immature DCs to mediate immune tolerance [135]. For example, oral supplementation of *Bifidobacterium* enhanced DC stimulation that facilitated the activation of tumor-specific CD8+ T-cell immunity and increased the therapeutic efficacy of anti-PD-L1 therapy in mice with an "unfavorable" gut microbiota [110]. Additionally, *Bacteroides fragilis* improved anticancer immunity of CTLA-4 inhibitors *via* enhancing DCs maturation and stimulation of IL-12-dependent Th1 cells immunity (Fig. **3**) [136].

GUT MICROBIOTA AND NANOMEDICINES

Nanomedicines can enter into micro-organisms by distinct routes of administration and demonstrate varying magnitudes of effect on organelles, cells, tissues, and organs. Nanomedicines eventually come into contact with the gut microbiota once they reach the gut lumen [137]. Considerable evidence has confirmed that gut microbiota plays an important intermediate role in developing the positive effects of nanomedicines. Modulating the gut microbiome in a beneficial way could make nanomedicines more effective in treating cancer [138]. Ample studies reported that the gut microbiota interferes with the nanomedicines to bolster the immune responses in cancer. For instance, the treatment with cyclophosphamide in mice causes translocation of specific gram-positive bacteria into lymphoid tissues, thus encouraging to generate T helper 17 (pTH17), whereas germ-free mice pretreated with antibiotics lead to promote resistance to cyclophosphamide. The study's results showed that the gut microbiota is very important for cancer treatment because it changes how the immune system reacts to cyclophosphamide [139]. Another study showed that the microbiota in the gut can effectively control the myeloid-derived cells that invade tumors. However, when the gut microbiota is interrupted after antibiotic treatment, it makes it harder for the body's immune system to respond to CpG-oligonucleotide-dependent immunotherapy in subcutaneous tumors [140]. *Bifidobacterium* could activate T-cells in PD-1-based anticancer immunity through the maturation of dendritic cells and cytokine production. Researchers have also demonstrated the tumor-suppressive action of *Lactobacillus johnsonii, Bifidobacterium pseudolongum,* and *Olsnella* species in immunotherapy. *Bifidobacterium* can improve immunotherapeutic responses through the systemic transportation of *B. pseudolongum*-derived inosine to activate T-lymphocyte-specific immune responses [130]. Taking all considerations into account, gut microbiota can significantly enhance anti-tumor immune responses through several mechanistic pathways and develop gut microbiota-specific treatment strategies for cancer.

Interfering with gut microbiota allows nanomedicines to develop anti-tumor immunity. Thus, nanomedicines could modify the specific gut microbial species and immune cells that would be a potential avenue for future cancer therapy.

Gut microbiota dysbiosis, on the other hand, lowers the number of good bacteria and the variety of bacteria that help with inflammatory responses [141]. The overall interactions between the gut microbiota and nanomedicines are mutual. Some nanomedicines can alter the gut microbiota ecosystem, which facilitates several intestinal disorders like colorectal cancer and enteritis [142]. Nanomedicines have the potential to upset the microbe balance in the gut, leading to the activation of inflammatory signaling pathways [143]. For example, tungsten oxide nanoparticles (WO_3NPs) have demonstrated therapeutic efficiency in DSS (dextran sulfate sodium)-induced IBD in C57BL/6J mice through altering gut microbial homeostasis and decreasing intestinal inflammation [144]. An earlier investigation revealed that tungstate treatment downregulates the explosive proliferation of facultative anaerobes *Enterobacteriaceae* in a colitis-induced mice model by preventing molybdenum cofactor-dependent microbial respiratory pathways [145]. Moreover, the exposure of nanomedicines could persuade inflammatory actions through either decreasing *Firmicutes*-induced anti-inflammatory effects or increasing proinflammatory *Bacteroidetes* effects on the gut [146 - 148]. The study conducted by Li and his colleague on the effects of nanomedicines in gut microbiota involved different concentrations of intravenous cadmium telluride quantum dots (CdTe QDs) administered in Balb/c mice. The finding of the study suggested that variations of gut microbial ecosystems due to the effects of CdTe QDs may alter the gut and liver immune system and lipid metabolisms [149]. Based on all relevant evidence, nanomedicines have a significant impact on gut microbiota. They either work with gut microbiota to boost the immune system or upset the balance of gut microbiota to cause disease.

CONCLUSION AND FUTURE PERSPECTIVES

In recent years, there has been a gradual increase in the investigation of gut microbiota, which has accomplished the emergence of novel strategies, including high-throughput sequencing methods (16S rRNA and shotgun sequencing methods), gut microbiota influences immune cell activation, and the interactions of nanomedicines and gut microbiota. The cohort investigations by metagenomic methods have to continue for translating microbiota in healthy and disease states. The multi-omics studies like meta-transcriptomics, metabolomics, culturomics, and synthetic biology have uncovered the "microbial dark matter" in microbiomes and provided a comprehensive explanation of microbes, genes, proteins, and metabolites of human gut microbiota and also demonstrated the complete interpretations of host-microbial interactions. Furthermore, the crosstalk between the gut microbiota and innate and adaptive immune systems increases intermediatory activities of innate immunity, augmenting anticancer effects of adaptive immunity and enhancing tumor cells' immunogenicity by reprogramming tumor-specific immune responses and improving ICB responses. Additionally, microbiota-derived circulating metabolites can alter several human physiological activities and disseminate from their original site in the gut to display local and systemic anticancer immune responses and significantly enhance ICB efficacy. Therapeutic approaches that combine gut microbiota with ICB, like probiotic usage, FMT, bacterial genetic engineering, and appropriate antibiotic selection, may emerge as new avenues for the gut microbiota and its metabolites to be used as excellent ICB adjuvants. The mechanisms underlying the synergy of gut microbiota and ICB with accurate determination of immunosuppressive and immunostimulant strains are predicted to develop more effective combination treatment approaches for ICB and the advancement of personalized medicine therapy. Additionally, targeting gut microbiota is a novel strategy for cancer nanomedicines, wherein microbiota serves as an important aspect that significantly affects its therapeutic activities. Hence, there are still some obstacles in the way of using nanomedicines for gut microbiota interventions in cancer treatment.

CONSENT FOR PUBLICATION

All authors have consented to publish the book chapter "Gut Microbiota And Future Research Directions" in this book.

REFERENCES

[1] Afzaal M, Saeed F, Shah YA, *et al.* Human gut microbiota in health and disease: Unveiling the relationship. Front Microbiol 2022; 13: 999001. [http://dx.doi.org/10.3389/fmicb.2022.999001] [PMID: 36225386]

[2] Thursby E, Juge N. Introduction to the human gut microbiota. Biochem J 2017; 474(11): 1823-36. [http://dx.doi.org/10.1042/BCJ20160510] [PMID: 28512250]

[3] Hasan N, Yang H. Factors affecting the composition of the gut microbiota, and its modulation. PeerJ 2019; 7: e7502. [http://dx.doi.org/10.7717/peerj.7502] [PMID: 31440436]

[4] Fujisaka S, Watanabe Y, Tobe K. The gut microbiome: a core regulator of metabolism. J Endocrinol 2023; 256(3): e220111. [http://dx.doi.org/10.1530/JOE-22-0111] [PMID: 36458804]

[5] Hou K, Wu ZX, Chen XY, *et al.* Microbiota in health and diseases. Signal Transduct Target Ther 2022; 7(1): 135. [http://dx.doi.org/10.1038/s41392-022-00974-4] [PMID: 35461318]

[6] Lin L, Zhang J. Role of intestinal microbiota and metabolites on gut homeostasis and human diseases. BMC Immunol 2017; 18(1): 2. [http://dx.doi.org/10.1186/s12865-016-0187-3] [PMID: 28061847]

[7] León ED, Francino MP. Roles of Secretory Immunoglobulin A in Host-Microbiota Interactions in the

Gut Ecosystem. Front Microbiol 2022; 13: 880484.
[http://dx.doi.org/10.3389/fmicb.2022.880484] [PMID: 35722300]

[8] Yang Y, Palm NW. Immunoglobulin A and the microbiome. Curr Opin Microbiol 2020; 56: 89-96.
[http://dx.doi.org/10.1016/j.mib.2020.08.003] [PMID: 32889295]

[9] Yu D, Meng X, de Vos WM, Wu H, Fang X, Maiti AK. Implications of Gut Microbiota in Complex Human Diseases. Int J Mol Sci 2021; 22(23): 12661.
[http://dx.doi.org/10.3390/ijms222312661] [PMID: 34884466]

[10] Rooks MG, Garrett WS. Gut microbiota, metabolites and host immunity. Nat Rev Immunol 2016; 16(6): 341-52.
[http://dx.doi.org/10.1038/nri.2016.42] [PMID: 27231050]

[11] Zhang YJ, Li S, Gan RY, Zhou T, Xu DP, Li HB. Impacts of gut bacteria on human health and diseases. Int J Mol Sci 2015; 16(4): 7493-519.
[http://dx.doi.org/10.3390/ijms16047493] [PMID: 25849657]

[12] Rowland I, Gibson G, Heinken A, *et al.* Gut microbiota functions: metabolism of nutrients and other food components. Eur J Nutr 2018; 57(1): 1-24.
[http://dx.doi.org/10.1007/s00394-017-1445-8] [PMID: 28393285]

[13] Rinninella E, Raoul P, Cintoni M, *et al.* What is the Healthy Gut Microbiota Composition? A Changing Ecosystem across Age, Environment, Diet, and Diseases. Microorganisms 2019; 7(1): 14.
[http://dx.doi.org/10.3390/microorganisms7010014] [PMID: 30634578]

[14] Wang B, Yao M, Lv L, Ling Z, Li L. The human microbiota in Health and Disease. Engineering (Beijing) 2017; 3(1): 71-82.
[http://dx.doi.org/10.1016/J.ENG.2017.01.008]

[15] Milani C, Duranti S, Bottacini F, *et al.* The First Microbial Colonizers of the Human Gut: Composition, Activities, and Health Implications of the Infant Gut Microbiota. Microbiol Mol Biol Rev 2017; 81(4): e00036-17.
[http://dx.doi.org/10.1128/MMBR.00036-17] [PMID: 29118049]

[16] Amabebe E, Robert FO, Agbalalah T, Orubu ESF. Microbial dysbiosis-induced obesity: role of gut microbiota in homoeostasis of energy metabolism. Br J Nutr 2020; 123(10): 1127-37.
[http://dx.doi.org/10.1017/S0007114520000380] [PMID: 32008579]

[17] Nagpal R, Mainali R, Ahmadi S, *et al.* Gut microbiome and aging: Physiological and mechanistic insights. Nutr Healthy Aging 2018; 4(4): 267-85.
[http://dx.doi.org/10.3233/NHA-170030] [PMID: 29951588]

[18] Laudes M, Geisler C, Rohmann N, Bouwman J, Pischon T, Schlicht K. Microbiota in Health and Disease—Potential Clinical Applications. Nutrients 2021; 13(11): 3866.
[http://dx.doi.org/10.3390/nu13113866] [PMID: 34836121]

[19] Shreiner AB, Kao JY, Young VB. The gut microbiome in health and in disease. Curr Opin Gastroenterol 2015; 31(1): 69-75.
[http://dx.doi.org/10.1097/MOG.0000000000000139] [PMID: 25394236]

[20] Lau K, Srivatsav V, Rizwan A, *et al.* Bridging the Gap between Gut Microbial Dysbiosis and Cardiovascular Diseases. Nutrients 2017; 9(8): 859.
[http://dx.doi.org/10.3390/nu9080859] [PMID: 28796176]

[21] Durack J, Lynch SV. The gut microbiome: Relationships with disease and opportunities for therapy. J Exp Med 2019; 216(1): 20-40.
[http://dx.doi.org/10.1084/jem.20180448] [PMID: 30322864]

[22] Kho ZY, Lal SK. The Human Gut Microbiome – A Potential Controller of Wellness and Disease. Front Microbiol 2018; 9: 1835.
[http://dx.doi.org/10.3389/fmicb.2018.01835] [PMID: 30154767]

[23] Zheng D, Liwinski T, Elinav E. Interaction between microbiota and immunity in health and disease. Cell Res 2020; 30(6): 492-506.
[http://dx.doi.org/10.1038/s41422-020-0332-7] [PMID: 32433595]

[24] Yang W, Cong Y. Gut microbiota-derived metabolites in the regulation of host immune responses and immune-related inflammatory diseases. Cell Mol Immunol 2021; 18(4): 866-77.
[http://dx.doi.org/10.1038/s41423-021-00661-4] [PMID: 33707689]

[25] Wang J, Zhu N, Su X, Gao Y, Yang R. Gut-Microbiota-Derived Metabolites Maintain Gut and Systemic Immune Homeostasis. Cells 2023; 12(5): 793.
[http://dx.doi.org/10.3390/cells12050793] [PMID: 36899929]

[26] Yoo J, Groer M, Dutra S, Sarkar A, McSkimming D. Gut Microbiota and Immune System Interactions. Microorganisms 2020; 8(10): 1587.
[http://dx.doi.org/10.3390/microorganisms8101587] [PMID: 33076307]

[27] Alexander KL, Targan SR, Elson CO III. Microbiota activation and regulation of innate and adaptive immunity. Immunol Rev 2014; 260(1): 206-20.
[http://dx.doi.org/10.1111/imr.12180] [PMID: 24942691]

[28] Pietrzak B, Tomela K, Olejnik-Schmidt A, Mackiewicz A, Schmidt M. Secretory IgA in Intestinal Mucosal Secretions as an Adaptive Barrier against Microbial Cells. Int J Mol Sci 2020; 21(23): 9254.
[http://dx.doi.org/10.3390/ijms21239254] [PMID: 33291586]

[29] Hapfelmeier S, Lawson MAE, Slack E, *et al.* Reversible microbial colonization of germ-free mice reveals the dynamics of IgA immune responses. Science 2010; 328(5986): 1705-9.
[http://dx.doi.org/10.1126/science.1188454] [PMID: 20576892]

[30] Zhao Q, Elson CO. Adaptive immune education by gut microbiota antigens. Immunology 2018; 154(1): 28-37.
[http://dx.doi.org/10.1111/imm.12896] [PMID: 29338074]

[31] Lazar V, Ditu LM, Pircalabioru GG, *et al.* Aspects of Gut Microbiota and Immune System Interactions in Infectious Diseases, Immunopathology, and Cancer. Front Immunol 2018; 9: 1830.
[http://dx.doi.org/10.3389/fimmu.2018.01830] [PMID: 30158926]

[32] Jiao Y, Wu L, Huntington ND, Zhang X. Crosstalk Between Gut Microbiota and Innate Immunity and Its Implication in Autoimmune Diseases. Front Immunol 2020; 11: 282.
[http://dx.doi.org/10.3389/fimmu.2020.00282] [PMID: 32153586]

[33] Li Z, Xiong W, Liang Z, *et al.* Critical role of the gut microbiota in immune responses and cancer immunotherapy. J Hematol Oncol 2024; 17(1): 33.
[http://dx.doi.org/10.1186/s13045-024-01541-w] [PMID: 38745196]

[34] Aggarwal N, Kitano S, Puah GRY, Kittelmann S, Hwang IY, Chang MW. Microbiome and Human Health: Current Understanding, Engineering, and Enabling Technologies. Chem Rev 2023; 123(1): 31-72.
[http://dx.doi.org/10.1021/acs.chemrev.2c00431] [PMID: 36317983]

[35] Berg G, Rybakova D, Fischer D, *et al.* Microbiome definition re-visited: old concepts and new challenges. Microbiome 2020; 8(1): 103.
[http://dx.doi.org/10.1186/s40168-020-00875-0] [PMID: 32605663]

[36] Schneider T. The holobiont self: understanding immunity in context. Hist Philos Life Sci 2021; 43(3): 99.
[http://dx.doi.org/10.1007/s40656-021-00454-y] [PMID: 34370107]

[37] Simon JC, Marchesi JR, Mougel C, Selosse MA. Host-microbiota interactions: from holobiont theory to analysis. Microbiome 2019; 7(1): 5.
[http://dx.doi.org/10.1186/s40168-019-0619-4] [PMID: 30635058]

[38] Vijay A, Valdes AM. RETRACTED ARTICLE: Role of the gut microbiome in chronic diseases: a

narrative review. Eur J Clin Nutr 2022; 76(4): 489-501.
[http://dx.doi.org/10.1038/s41430-021-00991-6] [PMID: 34584224]

[39] Chen Y, Zhou J, Wang L. Role and Mechanism of Gut Microbiota in Human Disease. Front Cell Infect Microbiol 2021; 11: 625913.
[http://dx.doi.org/10.3389/fcimb.2021.625913] [PMID: 33816335]

[40] Mabwi HA, Kim E, Song DG, *et al.* Synthetic gut microbiome: Advances and challenges. Comput Struct Biotechnol J 2021; 19: 363-71.
[http://dx.doi.org/10.1016/j.csbj.2020.12.029] [PMID: 33489006]

[41] Huang Y, Sheth RU, Zhao S, *et al.* High-throughput microbial culturomics using automation and machine learning. Nat Biotechnol 2023; 41(10): 1424-33.
[http://dx.doi.org/10.1038/s41587-023-01674-2] [PMID: 36805559]

[42] Szóstak N, Szymanek A, Havránek J, *et al.* The standardisation of the approach to metagenomic human gut analysis: from sample collection to microbiome profiling. Sci Rep 2022; 12(1): 8470.
[http://dx.doi.org/10.1038/s41598-022-12037-3] [PMID: 35589762]

[43] Lagier JC, Dubourg G, Million M, *et al.* Culturing the human microbiota and culturomics. Nat Rev Microbiol 2018; 16(9): 540-50.
[http://dx.doi.org/10.1038/s41579-018-0041-0] [PMID: 29937540]

[44] Alkatheri AH, Yap PSX, Abushelaibi A, Lai KS, Cheng WH, Erin Lim SH. Microbial Genomics: Innovative Targets and Mechanisms. Antibiotics (Basel) 2023; 12(2): 190.
[http://dx.doi.org/10.3390/antibiotics12020190] [PMID: 36830101]

[45] Lagier JC, Armougom F, Million M, *et al.* Microbial culturomics: paradigm shift in the human gut microbiome study. Clin Microbiol Infect 2012; 18(12): 1185-93.
[http://dx.doi.org/10.1111/1469-0691.12023] [PMID: 23033984]

[46] Browne HP, Forster SC, Anonye BO, *et al.* Culturing of 'unculturable' human microbiota reveals novel taxa and extensive sporulation. Nature 2016; 533(7604): 543-6.
[http://dx.doi.org/10.1038/nature17645] [PMID: 27144353]

[47] Diakite A, Dubourg G, Dione N, *et al.* Optimization and standardization of the culturomics technique for human microbiome exploration. Sci Rep 2020; 10(1): 9674.
[http://dx.doi.org/10.1038/s41598-020-66738-8] [PMID: 32541790]

[48] Yen S, Johnson JS. Metagenomics: a path to understanding the gut microbiome. Mamm Genome 2021; 32(4): 282-96.
[http://dx.doi.org/10.1007/s00335-021-09889-x] [PMID: 34259891]

[49] Ko KKK, Chng KR, Nagarajan N. Metagenomics-enabled microbial surveillance. Nat Microbiol 2022; 7(4): 486-96.
[http://dx.doi.org/10.1038/s41564-022-01089-w] [PMID: 35365786]

[50] Srinivas M, O'Sullivan O, Cotter PD. SinderenDv, Kenny JG. The Application of Metagenomics to Study Microbial Communities and Develop Desirable Traits in Fermented Foods. Foods 2022; 11(20): 3297.
[http://dx.doi.org/10.3390/foods11203297] [PMID: 37431045]

[51] Sergeant MJ, Constantinidou C, Cogan T, Penn CW, Pallen MJ. High-throughput sequencing of 16S rRNA gene amplicons: effects of extraction procedure, primer length and annealing temperature. PLoS One 2012; 7(5): e38094.
[http://dx.doi.org/10.1371/journal.pone.0038094] [PMID: 22666455]

[52] Callahan BJ, Wong J, Heiner C, *et al.* High-throughput amplicon sequencing of the full-length 16S rRNA gene with single-nucleotide resolution. Nucleic Acids Res 2019; 47(18): e103.
[http://dx.doi.org/10.1093/nar/gkz569] [PMID: 31269198]

[53] Osman MA, Neoh H, Ab Mutalib NS, Chin SF, Jamal R. 16S rRNA Gene Sequencing for Deciphering the Colorectal Cancer Gut Microbiome: Current Protocols and Workflows. Front Microbiol 2018; 9:

767.
[http://dx.doi.org/10.3389/fmicb.2018.00767] [PMID: 29755427]

[54] Conrad MA, Bittinger K, Ren Y, *et al.* The intestinal microbiome of inflammatory bowel disease across the pediatric age range. Gut Microbes 2024; 16(1): 2317932.
[http://dx.doi.org/10.1080/19490976.2024.2317932] [PMID: 38404111]

[55] Lane ER, Zisman T, Suskind D. The microbiota in inflammatory bowel disease: current and therapeutic insights. J Inflamm Res 2017; 10: 63-73.
[http://dx.doi.org/10.2147/JIR.S116088] [PMID: 28652796]

[56] Gevers D, Kugathasan S, Denson LA, *et al.* The treatment-naive microbiome in new-onset Crohn's disease. Cell Host Microbe 2014; 15(3): 382-92.
[http://dx.doi.org/10.1016/j.chom.2014.02.005] [PMID: 24629344]

[57] López-Aladid R, Fernández-Barat L, Alcaraz-Serrano V, *et al.* Determining the most accurate 16S rRNA hypervariable region for taxonomic identification from respiratory samples. Sci Rep 2023; 13(1): 3974.
[http://dx.doi.org/10.1038/s41598-023-30764-z] [PMID: 36894603]

[58] Zeevi D, Korem T, Godneva A, *et al.* Structural variation in the gut microbiome associates with host health. Nature 2019; 568(7750): 43-8.
[http://dx.doi.org/10.1038/s41586-019-1065-y] [PMID: 30918406]

[59] Hård J, Mold JE, Eisfeldt J, *et al.* Long-read whole-genome analysis of human single cells. Nat Commun 2023; 14(1): 5164.
[http://dx.doi.org/10.1038/s41467-023-40898-3] [PMID: 37620373]

[60] Singer E, Bushnell B, Coleman-Derr D, *et al.* High-resolution phylogenetic microbial community profiling. ISME J 2016; 10(8): 2020-32.
[http://dx.doi.org/10.1038/ismej.2015.249] [PMID: 26859772]

[61] Hall AB, Yassour M, Sauk J, *et al.* A novel Ruminococcus gnavus clade enriched in inflammatory bowel disease patients. Genome Med 2017; 9(1): 103.
[http://dx.doi.org/10.1186/s13073-017-0490-5] [PMID: 29183332]

[62] Lloyd-Price J, Arze C, Ananthakrishnan AN, *et al.* Multi-omics of the gut microbial ecosystem in inflammatory bowel diseases. Nature 2019; 569(7758): 655-62.
[http://dx.doi.org/10.1038/s41586-019-1237-9] [PMID: 31142855]

[63] Coker OO, Nakatsu G, Dai RZ, *et al.* Enteric fungal microbiota dysbiosis and ecological alterations in colorectal cancer. Gut 2019; 68(4): 654-62.
[http://dx.doi.org/10.1136/gutjnl-2018-317178] [PMID: 30472682]

[64] Nakatsu G, Zhou H, Wu WKK, *et al.* Alterations in Enteric Virome Are Associated With Colorectal Cancer and Survival Outcomes. Gastroenterology 2018; 155(2): 529-541.e5.
[http://dx.doi.org/10.1053/j.gastro.2018.04.018] [PMID: 29689266]

[65] Allaband C, McDonald D, Vázquez-Baeza Y, *et al.* Microbiome 101: Studying, Analyzing, and Interpreting Gut Microbiome Data for Clinicians. Clin Gastroenterol Hepatol 2019; 17(2): 218-30.
[http://dx.doi.org/10.1016/j.cgh.2018.09.017] [PMID: 30240894]

[66] Bertrand D, Shaw J, Kalathiyappan M, *et al.* Hybrid metagenomic assembly enables high-resolution analysis of resistance determinants and mobile elements in human microbiomes. Nat Biotechnol 2019; 37(8): 937-44.
[http://dx.doi.org/10.1038/s41587-019-0191-2] [PMID: 31359005]

[67] Chen F, Li S, Guo R, *et al.* Meta-analysis of fecal viromes demonstrates high diagnostic potential of the gut viral signatures for colorectal cancer and adenoma risk assessment. J Adv Res 2023; 49: 103-14.
[http://dx.doi.org/10.1016/j.jare.2022.09.012] [PMID: 36198381]

[68] Ezzatpour S, Mondragon Portocarrero AC, Cardelle-Cobas A, *et al.* The Human Gut Virome and Its

Relationship with Nontransmissible Chronic Diseases. Nutrients 2023; 15(4): 977.
[http://dx.doi.org/10.3390/nu15040977] [PMID: 36839335]

[69] Kwa WT, Sundarajoo S, Toh KY, Lee J. Application of emerging technologies for gut microbiome research. Singapore Med J 2023; 64(1): 45-52.
[http://dx.doi.org/10.4103/singaporemedj.SMJ-2021-432] [PMID: 36722516]

[70] Ferrocino I, Rantsiou K, McClure R, *et al.* The need for an integrated multi□OMICs approach in microbiome science in the food system. Compr Rev Food Sci Food Saf 2023; 22(2): 1082-103.
[http://dx.doi.org/10.1111/1541-4337.13103] [PMID: 36636774]

[71] Mishra A, Lai GC, Yao LJ, *et al.* Microbial exposure during early human development primes fetal immune cells. Cell 2021; 184(13): 3394-3409.e20.
[http://dx.doi.org/10.1016/j.cell.2021.04.039] [PMID: 34077752]

[72] Gao X, Sun R, Jiao N, *et al.* Integrative multi-omics deciphers the spatial characteristics of host-gut microbiota interactions in Crohn's disease. Cell Rep Med 2023; 4(6): 101050.
[http://dx.doi.org/10.1016/j.xcrm.2023.101050] [PMID: 37172588]

[73] Muñoz-Benavent M, Hartkopf F, Van Den Bossche T, *et al.* gNOMO: a multi-omics pipeline for integrated host and microbiome analysis of non-model organisms. NAR Genom Bioinform 2020; 2(3): lqaa058.
[http://dx.doi.org/10.1093/nargab/lqaa058] [PMID: 33575609]

[74] Schirmer M, Franzosa EA, Lloyd-Price J, *et al.* Dynamics of metatranscription in the inflammatory bowel disease gut microbiome. Nat Microbiol 2018; 3(3): 337-46.
[http://dx.doi.org/10.1038/s41564-017-0089-z] [PMID: 29311644]

[75] Abu-Ali GS, Mehta RS, Lloyd-Price J, *et al.* Metatranscriptome of human faecal microbial communities in a cohort of adult men. Nat Microbiol 2018; 3(3): 356-66.
[http://dx.doi.org/10.1038/s41564-017-0084-4] [PMID: 29335555]

[76] Lange O, Proczko-Stepaniak M, Mika A. Short-Chain Fatty Acids—A Product of the Microbiome and Its Participation in Two-Way Communication on the Microbiome-Host Mammal Line. Curr Obes Rep 2023; 12(2): 108-26.
[http://dx.doi.org/10.1007/s13679-023-00503-6] [PMID: 37208544]

[77] Portincasa P, Bonfrate L, Vacca M, *et al.* Gut Microbiota and Short Chain Fatty Acids: Implications in Glucose Homeostasis. Int J Mol Sci 2022; 23(3): 1105.
[http://dx.doi.org/10.3390/ijms23031105] [PMID: 35163038]

[78] Liu X, Shao J, Liao YT, *et al.* Regulation of short-chain fatty acids in the immune system. Front Immunol 2023; 14: 1186892.
[http://dx.doi.org/10.3389/fimmu.2023.1186892] [PMID: 37215145]

[79] Akhtar M, Chen Y, Ma Z, *et al.* Gut microbiota-derived short chain fatty acids are potential mediators in gut inflammation. Anim Nutr 2022; 8: 350-60.
[http://dx.doi.org/10.1016/j.aninu.2021.11.005] [PMID: 35510031]

[80] Shin Y, Han S, Kwon J, *et al.* Roles of Short-Chain Fatty Acids in Inflammatory Bowel Disease. Nutrients 2023; 15(20): 4466.
[http://dx.doi.org/10.3390/nu15204466] [PMID: 37892541]

[81] Jackson MA, Pearson C, Ilott NE, *et al.* Accurate identification and quantification of commensal microbiota bound by host immunoglobulins. Microbiome 2021; 9(1): 33.
[http://dx.doi.org/10.1186/s40168-020-00992-w] [PMID: 33516266]

[82] Shapiro JM, de Zoete MR, Palm NW, *et al.* Immunoglobin A targets a unique subset of the microbiota in inflammatory bowel disease. Cell Host Microbe 2021; 29(1): 83-93.e3.
[http://dx.doi.org/10.1016/j.chom.2020.12.003] [PMID: 33385335]

[83] Gupta S, Gupta SL, Singh A, *et al.* IgA Determines Bacterial Composition in the Gut, Crohn's & Colitis 360. 2023; 5(3): otad030.

[84] Pröbstel AK, Zhou X, Baumann R, *et al.* Gut microbiota–specific IgA $^+$ B cells traffic to the CNS in active multiple sclerosis. Sci Immunol 2020; 5(53): eabc7191. [http://dx.doi.org/10.1126/sciimmunol.abc7191] [PMID: 33219152]

[85] Robinson JM, Cameron R. The Holobiont Blindspot: Relating Host-Microbiome Interactions to Cognitive Biases and the Concept of the "Umwelt". Front Psychol 2020; 11: 591071. [http://dx.doi.org/10.3389/fpsyg.2020.591071] [PMID: 33281689]

[86] Reygner J, Joly Condette C, Bruneau A, *et al.* Changes in Composition and Function of Human Intestinal Microbiota Exposed to Chlorpyrifos in Oil as Assessed by the SHIME® Model. Int J Environ Res Public Health 2016; 13(11): 1088. [http://dx.doi.org/10.3390/ijerph13111088] [PMID: 27827942]

[87] Van den Abbeele P, Roos S, Eeckhaut V, *et al.* Incorporating a mucosal environment in a dynamic gut model results in a more representative colonization by lactobacilli. Microb Biotechnol 2012; 5(1): 106-15. [http://dx.doi.org/10.1111/j.1751-7915.2011.00308.x] [PMID: 21989255]

[88] Steinway SN, Saleh J, Koo BK, Delacour D, Kim DH. Human Microphysiological Models of Intestinal Tissue and Gut Microbiome. Front Bioeng Biotechnol 2020; 8: 725. [http://dx.doi.org/10.3389/fbioe.2020.00725] [PMID: 32850690]

[89] Shah P, Fritz JV, Glaab E, *et al.* A microfluidics-based in vitro model of the gastrointestinal human–microbe interface. Nat Commun 2016; 7(1): 11535. [http://dx.doi.org/10.1038/ncomms11535] [PMID: 27168102]

[90] Carper DL, Appidi MR, Mudbhari S, Shrestha HK, Hettich RL, Abraham PE. The Promises, Challenges, and Opportunities of Omics for Studying the Plant Holobiont. Microorganisms 2022; 10(10): 2013. [http://dx.doi.org/10.3390/microorganisms10102013] [PMID: 36296289]

[91] Li L, Ning Z, Zhang X, *et al.* RapidAIM: a culture- and metaproteomics-based Rapid Assay of Individual Microbiome responses to drugs. Microbiome 2020; 8(1): 33. [http://dx.doi.org/10.1186/s40168-020-00806-z] [PMID: 32160905]

[92] Zhang M, Liu J, Xia Q. Role of gut microbiome in cancer immunotherapy: from predictive biomarker to therapeutic target. Exp Hematol Oncol 2023; 12(1): 84. [http://dx.doi.org/10.1186/s40164-023-00442-x] [PMID: 37770953]

[93] Xie Y, Liu F. The role of the gut microbiota in tumor, immunity, and immunotherapy. Front Immunol 2024; 15: 1410928. [http://dx.doi.org/10.3389/fimmu.2024.1410928] [PMID: 38903520]

[94] Jugder BE, Kamareddine L, Watnick PI. Microbiota-derived acetate activates intestinal innate immunity *via* the Tip60 histone acetyltransferase complex. Immunity 2021; 54(8): 1683-1697.e3. [http://dx.doi.org/10.1016/j.immuni.2021.05.017] [PMID: 34107298]

[95] Erny D, Dokalis N, Mezö C, *et al.* Microbiota-derived acetate enables the metabolic fitness of the brain innate immune system during health and disease. Cell Metab 2021; 33(11): 2260-2276.e7. [http://dx.doi.org/10.1016/j.cmet.2021.10.010] [PMID: 34731656]

[96] Morais LH, Schreiber HL IV, Mazmanian SK. The gut microbiota–brain axis in behaviour and brain disorders. Nat Rev Microbiol 2021; 19(4): 241-55. [http://dx.doi.org/10.1038/s41579-020-00460-0] [PMID: 33093662]

[97] He Y, Fu L, Li Y, *et al.* Gut microbial metabolites facilitate anticancer therapy efficacy by modulating cytotoxic CD8$^+$ T cell immunity. Cell Metab 2021; 33(5): 988-1000.e7. [http://dx.doi.org/10.1016/j.cmet.2021.03.002] [PMID: 33761313]

[98] Stower H. Microbiome transplant-induced response to immunotherapy. Nat Med 2021; 27(1): 21. [PMID: 33442010]

[99] Fehervari Z. Microbiota shape tumor immunity. Nat Immunol 2021; 22(12): 1469. [http://dx.doi.org/10.1038/s41590-021-01082-1] [PMID: 34811539]

[100] Mallott EK, Amato KR. Host specificity of the gut microbiome. Nat Rev Microbiol 2021; 19(10): 639-53. [http://dx.doi.org/10.1038/s41579-021-00562-3] [PMID: 34045709]

[101] Allen-Vercoe E, Coburn B. A Microbiota-Derived Metabolite Augments Cancer Immunotherapy Responses in Mice. Cancer Cell 2020; 38(4): 452-3. [http://dx.doi.org/10.1016/j.ccell.2020.09.005] [PMID: 32976777]

[102] Xu X, Lv J, Guo F, *et al.* Gut Microbiome Influences the Efficacy of PD-1 Antibody Immunotherapy on MSS-Type Colorectal Cancer *via* Metabolic Pathway. Front Microbiol 2020; 11: 814. [http://dx.doi.org/10.3389/fmicb.2020.00814] [PMID: 32425919]

[103] Baruch EN, Youngster I, Ben-Betzalel G, *et al.* Fecal microbiota transplant promotes response in immunotherapy-refractory melanoma patients. Science 2021; 371(6529): 602-9. [http://dx.doi.org/10.1126/science.abb5920] [PMID: 33303685]

[104] He X, Xu C. Immune checkpoint signaling and cancer immunotherapy. Cell Res 2020; 30(8): 660-9. [http://dx.doi.org/10.1038/s41422-020-0343-4] [PMID: 32467592]

[105] Xin Yu J, Hubbard-Lucey VM, Tang J. Immuno-oncology drug development goes global. Nat Rev Drug Discov 2019; 18(12): 899-900. [http://dx.doi.org/10.1038/d41573-019-00167-9] [PMID: 31780841]

[106] Nathan P, Hassel JC, Rutkowski P, *et al.* Overall Survival Benefit with Tebentafusp in Metastatic Uveal Melanoma. N Engl J Med 2021; 385(13): 1196-206. [http://dx.doi.org/10.1056/NEJMoa2103485] [PMID: 34551229]

[107] Wei SC, Duffy CR, Allison JP. Fundamental Mechanisms of Immune Checkpoint Blockade Therapy. Cancer Discov 2018; 8(9): 1069-86. [http://dx.doi.org/10.1158/2159-8290.CD-18-0367] [PMID: 30115704]

[108] Wang M, Du Q, Jin J, Wei Y, Lu Y, Li Q. LAG3 and its emerging role in cancer immunotherapy. Clin Transl Med 2021; 11(3): e365. [http://dx.doi.org/10.1002/ctm2.365] [PMID: 33784013]

[109] Aghamajidi A, Maleki Vareki S. The Effect of the Gut Microbiota on Systemic and Anti-Tumor Immunity and Response to Systemic Therapy against Cancer. Cancers (Basel) 2022; 14(15): 3563. [http://dx.doi.org/10.3390/cancers14153563] [PMID: 35892821]

[110] Sivan A, Corrales L, Hubert N, *et al.* Commensal *Bifidobacterium* promotes antitumor immunity and facilitates anti–PD-L1 efficacy. Science 2015; 350(6264): 1084-9. [http://dx.doi.org/10.1126/science.aac4255] [PMID: 26541606]

[111] Zhou Y, Liu X, Gao W, *et al.* The role of intestinal flora on tumor immunotherapy: recent progress and treatment implications. Heliyon 2024; 10(1): e23919. [http://dx.doi.org/10.1016/j.heliyon.2023.e23919]

[112] Vétizou M, Pitt JM, Daillère R, *et al.* Anticancer immunotherapy by CTLA-4 blockade relies on the gut microbiota. Science 2015; 350(6264): 1079-84. [http://dx.doi.org/10.1126/science.aad1329] [PMID: 26541610]

[113] Routy B, Le Chatelier E, Derosa L, *et al.* Gut microbiome influences efficacy of PD-1–based immunotherapy against epithelial tumors. Science 2018; 359(6371): 91-7. [http://dx.doi.org/10.1126/science.aan3706] [PMID: 29097494]

[114] Gopalakrishnan V, Spencer CN, Nezi L, *et al.* Gut microbiome modulates response to anti–PD-1 immunotherapy in melanoma patients. Science 2018; 359(6371): 97-103. [http://dx.doi.org/10.1126/science.aan4236] [PMID: 29097493]

[115] Matson V, Fessler J, Bao R, *et al.* The commensal microbiome is associated with anti–PD-1 efficacy

in metastatic melanoma patients. Science 2018; 359(6371): 104-8.
[http://dx.doi.org/10.1126/science.aao3290] [PMID: 29302014]

[116] Jin Y, Dong H, Xia L, *et al.* The Diversity of Gut Microbiome is Associated With Favorable Responses to Anti–Programmed Death 1 Immunotherapy in Chinese Patients With NSCLC. J Thorac Oncol 2019; 14(8): 1378-89.
[http://dx.doi.org/10.1016/j.jtho.2019.04.007] [PMID: 31026576]

[117] Song P, Yang D, Wang H, *et al.* Relationship between intestinal flora structure and metabolite analysis and immunotherapy efficacy in Chinese NSCLC patients. Thorac Cancer 2020; 11(6): 1621-32.
[http://dx.doi.org/10.1111/1759-7714.13442] [PMID: 32329229]

[118] Derosa L, Routy B, Fidelle M, *et al.* Gut Bacteria Composition Drives Primary Resistance to Cancer Immunotherapy in Renal Cell Carcinoma Patients. Eur Urol 2020; 78(2): 195-206.
[http://dx.doi.org/10.1016/j.eururo.2020.04.044] [PMID: 32376136]

[119] Lalani AKA, Xie W, Braun DA, *et al.* Effect of Antibiotic Use on Outcomes with Systemic Therapies in Metastatic Renal Cell Carcinoma. Eur Urol Oncol 2020; 3(3): 372-81.
[http://dx.doi.org/10.1016/j.euo.2019.09.001] [PMID: 31562048]

[120] Pinato DJ, Howlett S, Ottaviani D, *et al.* Association of Prior Antibiotic Treatment With Survival and Response to Immune Checkpoint Inhibitor Therapy in Patients With Cancer. JAMA Oncol 2019; 5(12): 1774-8.
[http://dx.doi.org/10.1001/jamaoncol.2019.2785] [PMID: 31513236]

[121] Tinsley N, Zhou C, Tan G, *et al.* Cumulative Antibiotic Use Significantly Decreases Efficacy of Checkpoint Inhibitors in Patients with Advanced Cancer. Oncologist 2020; 25(1): 55-63.
[http://dx.doi.org/10.1634/theoncologist.2019-0160] [PMID: 31292268]

[122] Zhao S, Gao G, Li W, *et al.* Antibiotics are associated with attenuated efficacy of anti-PD-1/PD-L1 therapies in Chinese patients with advanced non-small cell lung cancer. Lung Cancer 2019; 130: 10-7.
[http://dx.doi.org/10.1016/j.lungcan.2019.01.017] [PMID: 30885328]

[123] Kuczma MP, Ding ZC, Li T, *et al.* The impact of antibiotic usage on the efficacy of chemoimmunotherapy is contingent on the source of tumor-reactive T cells. Oncotarget 2017; 8(67): 111931-42.
[http://dx.doi.org/10.18632/oncotarget.22953] [PMID: 29340102]

[124] Uribe-Herranz M, Bittinger K, Rafail S, *et al.* Gut microbiota modulates adoptive cell therapy *via* CD8α dendritic cells and IL-12. JCI Insight 2018; 3(4): e94952.
[http://dx.doi.org/10.1172/jci.insight.94952] [PMID: 29467322]

[125] Lu Y, Yuan X, Wang M, *et al.* Gut microbiota influence immunotherapy responses: mechanisms and therapeutic strategies. J Hematol Oncol 2022; 15(1): 47.
[http://dx.doi.org/10.1186/s13045-022-01273-9] [PMID: 35488243]

[126] Ma C, Han M, Heinrich B, *et al.* Gut microbiome–mediated bile acid metabolism regulates liver cancer *via* NKT cells. Science 2018; 360(6391): eaan5931.
[http://dx.doi.org/10.1126/science.aan5931] [PMID: 29798856]

[127] Fenton TM, Jørgensen PB, Niss K, *et al.* Immune Profiling of Human Gut-Associated Lymphoid Tissue Identifies a Role for Isolated Lymphoid Follicles in Priming of Region-Specific Immunity. Immunity 2020; 52(3): 557-570.e6.
[http://dx.doi.org/10.1016/j.immuni.2020.02.001] [PMID: 32160523]

[128] Zheng D, Liwinski T, Elinav E. Interaction between microbiota and immunity in health and disease. Cell Res 2020; 30(6): 492-506.
[http://dx.doi.org/10.1038/s41422-020-0332-7] [PMID: 32433595]

[129] Davar D, Dzutsev AK, McCulloch JA, *et al.* Fecal microbiota transplant overcomes resistance to anti–PD-1 therapy in melanoma patients. Science 2021; 371(6529): 595-602.
[http://dx.doi.org/10.1126/science.abf3363] [PMID: 33542131]

[130] Tanoue T, Morita S, Plichta DR, *et al.* A defined commensal consortium elicits CD8 T cells and anti-cancer immunity. Nature 2019; 565(7741): 600-5. [http://dx.doi.org/10.1038/s41586-019-0878-z] [PMID: 30675064]

[131] Mager LF, Burkhard R, Pett N, *et al.* Microbiome-derived inosine modulates response to checkpoint inhibitor immunotherapy. Science 2020; 369(6510): 1481-9. [http://dx.doi.org/10.1126/science.abc3421] [PMID: 32792462]

[132] Chaput N, Lepage P, Coutzac C, *et al.* Baseline gut microbiota predicts clinical response and colitis in metastatic melanoma patients treated with ipilimumab. Ann Oncol 2017; 28(6): 1368-79. [http://dx.doi.org/10.1093/annonc/mdx108] [PMID: 28368458]

[133] Lam KC, Araya RE, Huang A, *et al.* Microbiota triggers STING-type I IFN-dependent monocyte reprogramming of the tumor microenvironment. Cell 2021; 184(21): 5338-5356.e21. [http://dx.doi.org/10.1016/j.cell.2021.09.019] [PMID: 34624222]

[134] Di Domizio J, Belkhodja C, Chenuet P, *et al.* The commensal skin microbiota triggers type I IFN–dependent innate repair responses in injured skin. Nat Immunol 2020; 21(9): 1034-45. [http://dx.doi.org/10.1038/s41590-020-0721-6] [PMID: 32661363]

[135] Shi Y, Zheng W, Yang K, *et al.* Intratumoral accumulation of gut microbiota facilitates CD47-based immunotherapy *via* STING signaling. J Exp Med 2020; 217(5): e20192282. [http://dx.doi.org/10.1084/jem.20192282] [PMID: 32142585]

[136] Schaupp L, Muth S, Rogell L, *et al.* Microbiota-Induced Type I Interferons Instruct a Poised Basal State of Dendritic Cells. Cell 2020; 181(5): 1080-1096.e19. [http://dx.doi.org/10.1016/j.cell.2020.04.022] [PMID: 32380006]

[137] Pitt JM, Vétizou M, Gomperts Boneca I, Lepage P, Chamaillard M, Zitvogel L. Enhancing the clinical coverage and anticancer efficacy of immune checkpoint blockade through manipulation of the gut microbiota. OncoImmunology 2017; 6(1): e1132137. [http://dx.doi.org/10.1080/2162402X.2015.1132137] [PMID: 28197360]

[138] Feng X, Zhang Y, Zhang C, *et al.* Nanomaterial-mediated autophagy: coexisting hazard and health benefits in biomedicine. Part Fibre Toxicol 2020; 17(1): 53. [http://dx.doi.org/10.1186/s12989-020-00372-0] [PMID: 33066795]

[139] McQuade JL, Daniel CR, Helmink BA, Wargo JA. Modulating the microbiome to improve therapeutic response in cancer. Lancet Oncol 2019; 20(2): e77-91. [http://dx.doi.org/10.1016/S1470-2045(18)30952-5] [PMID: 30712808]

[140] Viaud S, Saccheri F, Mignot G, *et al.* The intestinal microbiota modulates the anticancer immune effects of cyclophosphamide. Science 2013; 342(6161): 971-6. [http://dx.doi.org/10.1126/science.1240537] [PMID: 24264990]

[141] Iida N, Dzutsev A, Stewart CA, *et al.* Commensal bacteria control cancer response to therapy by modulating the tumor microenvironment. Science 2013; 342(6161): 967-70. [http://dx.doi.org/10.1126/science.1240527] [PMID: 24264989]

[142] Helmink BA, Khan MAW, Hermann A, Gopalakrishnan V, Wargo JA. The microbiome, cancer, and cancer therapy. Nat Med 2019; 25(3): 377-88. [http://dx.doi.org/10.1038/s41591-019-0377-7] [PMID: 30842679]

[143] Liu S, Cao S, Guo J, *et al.* Graphene oxide–silver nanocomposites modulate biofilm formation and extracellular polymeric substance (EPS) production. Nanoscale 2018; 10(41): 19603-11. [http://dx.doi.org/10.1039/C8NR04064H] [PMID: 30325394]

[144] Shin NR, Whon TW, Bae JW. Proteobacteria: microbial signature of dysbiosis in gut microbiota. Trends Biotechnol 2015; 33(9): 496-503. [http://dx.doi.org/10.1016/j.tibtech.2015.06.011] [PMID: 26210164]

[145] Qin Y, Zhao R, Qin H, *et al.* Colonic mucus-accumulating tungsten oxide nanoparticles improve the

colitis therapy by targeting Enterobacteriaceae. Nano Today 2021; 39: 101234. [http://dx.doi.org/10.1016/j.nantod.2021.101234]

[146] Zhu W, Winter MG, Byndloss MX, *et al.* Precision editing of the gut microbiota ameliorates colitis. Nature 2018; 553(7687): 208-11. [http://dx.doi.org/10.1038/nature25172] [PMID: 29323293]

[147] Ma Y, Zhang J, Yu N, *et al.* Effect of Nanomaterials on Gut Microbiota. Toxics 2023; 11(4): 384. [http://dx.doi.org/10.3390/toxics11040384] [PMID: 37112611]

[148] Mukherjee S, Joardar N, Sengupta S, Sinha Babu SP. Gut microbes as future therapeutics in treating inflammatory and infectious diseases: Lessons from recent findings. J Nutr Biochem 2018; 61: 111-28. [http://dx.doi.org/10.1016/j.jnutbio.2018.07.010] [PMID: 30196243]

[149] Li X, Wei H, Hu Y, *et al.* Dysbiosis of gut microbiota and intestinal damage in mice induced by a single intravenous exposure to CdTe quantum dots at low concentration. J Appl Toxicol 2022; 42(11): 1757-65. [http://dx.doi.org/10.1002/jat.4352] [PMID: 35618442]

SUBJECT INDEX

A

B

E

F

G

H

I

L

M

N

O

P

www.ingramcontent.com/pod-product-compliance
Lightning Source LLC
Chambersburg PA
CBHW050809220326
41598CB00006B/161
* 9 7 8 9 8 1 5 3 2 4 5 6 3 *